AF342684

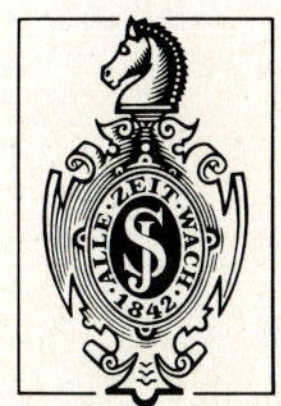
ALLE ZEIT WACH
1842

Cancer Diagnosis

Early Detection

Edited by Peter Bannasch

With 49 Figures

Springer-Verlag
Berlin Heidelberg New York
London Paris Tokyo
Hong Kong Barcelona
Budapest

Prof. Dr. Peter Bannasch
Abteilung für Cytopathologie
Deutsches Krebsforschungszentrum
Im Neuenheimer Feld 280
W-6900 Heidelberg, FRG

The publication of this book was supported by the Arbeitsgemeinschaft der Großforschungseinrichtungen (AGF).

Institutions participating in the AGF-Koordinierungsausschuß Krebsforschung

DKFZ Deutsches Krebsforschungszentrum Heidelberg
GBF   Gesellschaft für Biotechnologische Forschung Braunschweig
GSF   Gesellschaft für Strahlen- und Umweltforschung Neuherberg
KFA   Kernforschungsanlage Jülich
KfK   Kernforschungszentrum Karlsruhe

ISBN 3-540-54503-4 Springer-Verlag Berlin Heidelberg New York
ISBN 0-387-54503-4 Springer-Verlag New York Berlin Heidelberg

Library of Congress Cataloging-in-Publication Data. Cancer diagnosis:early detection/edited by Peter Bannasch. p. cm. Includes bibliographical references and index. ISBN 3-540-54503-4 — ISBN 0-387-54503-4 1. Cancer–Diagnosis–Congresses. 2. Cancer–Prevention–Congresses. 3. Medical screening–Congresses. I. Bannasch, Peter. [DNLM: 1. Neoplasms–diagnosis–congresses. QZ 241 C2138] RC270.C33 1992 616.99′4075-dc20 DNLM/DLC for Library of Congress 92-2201 CIP

Typesetting: Best-set Typesetter Ltd., Hong Kong
21/3130-5 4 3 ·2 1 0 – Printed on acid-free paper

Preface

Early detection of cancer has been recognized as an important area of preventive medicine for quite some time. In a few sites, such as the cervix, the breast, and the skin, it has been shown beyond doubt that early detection and secondary prevention of cancer are realistic goals. However, the general success of this approach is limited and requires substantial additional effort in research and public health education.

The present volume is based on an International Symposium on Cancer Diagnosis – Early Detection, which was organized by the Committee Coordinating Cancer Research in Großforschungseinrichtungen of the Federal Republic of Germany. The meeting was held at the German Cancer Research Center in Heidelberg, June 3–15, 1991. I am grateful to all members of the Scientific Committee who gave valuable advice in preparing the program of the conference: Gunther Bastert (Heidelberg), John Collins (Braunschweig), Heinz Höfler (Munich/Neuherberg), Ernst Jung (Mannheim), Gerhard van Kaick (Heidelberg), Stefan Meuer (Heidelberg), Michael Wannenmacher (Heidelberg), and Wolfgang Wilmanns (Munich/Neuherberg). I am obliged to Volker Diehl (Cologne), Gunther Bastert (Heidelberg), Hans K. Müller-Hermelink (Würzburg), Manfred Schwab (Heidelberg), and Georg Dhom (Homburg/Saar) for serving as chairmen of the sessions. I am also grateful to Horst Metzler and the administration of the German Cancer Research Center for all their efforts to guarantee a smooth running of the Conference. My special thanks go to the speakers, the rapporteurs of the discussions, and to all the participants who contributed to the success of the meeting and provided the basis for this book. Finally, I am indebted to Heide Zerban for careful editorial help, and to Adelheid Duhm of Springer-Verlag for excellent cooperation and much support in achieving rapid publication of the proceedings.

Heidelberg, February 1992   PETER BANNASCH

Contents

Session 7
Epidemiology
Chairman: J. Wahrendorf

List of Contributors

ACKERMANN, R., Department of Urology, Heinrich-Heine-University, Medical School, Moorenstr. 5, W-4000 Düsseldorf, FRG

ANTON, H.-W., Universitäts-Frauenklinik, Voßstr. 9, W-6900 Heidelberg, FRG

BANNASCH, P., Deutsches Krebsforschungszentrum, Abteilung für Cytopathologie, Im Neuenheimer Feld 280, W-6900 Heidelberg, FRG

BASTERT, G., Universitäts-Frauenklinik, Voßstr. 9, W-6900 Heidelberg, FRG

BAUMANN, R., Institute of Pathology, University Clinics, University of Mainz, W-6500 Mainz, FRG

BHONSLE, R.B., Tata Institute of Fundamental Research, National Centre of the Government of India for Nuclear Science and Mathematics, Homi Bhabha Road, Bombay 400 005, India

BISCHOF DELALOYE, A., Division Autonome de Médicine Nucléaire, Centre Hospitalier Universitaire Vaudois, CH-1011 Lausanne, Switzerland

BLEUL, C., Deutsches Krebsforschungszentrum, Institut für Virusforschung, Im Neuenheimer Feld 280, W-6900 Heidelberg, FRG

BONGARTZ, G., Westfälische Wilhelms-Universität, Institut für Klinische Radiologie, Albert-Schweitzer-Str. 33, W-4400 Münster, FRG

BRAUCH, H., Deutsches Krebsforschungszentrum, Institut für Experimentelle Pathologie, Im Neuenheimer Feld 280, W-6900 Heidelberg, FRG

CARTER, R.L., Institute of Cancer Research and Royal Marsden Hospital, Sutton, Surrey, U.K.

CHANG-CLAUDE, J., Deutsches Krebsforschungszentrum, Institut für Epidemiologie und Biometrie, Im Neuenheimer Feld 280, W-6900 Heidelberg, FRG

CLEMM, C., Medizinische Klinik III, Klinikum Großhadern, Universität München, Marchioninistr. 15, W-8000 München 70, FRG

DAFTARY, D.K., Tata Institute of Fundamental Research, National Centre of the Government of India for Nuclear Science and Mathematics, Homi Bhabha Road, Bombay 400 005, India

DELALOYE, B., Division Autonome de Médicine Nucléaire, Centre Hospitalier Universitaire Vaudois, CH-1011 Lausanne, Switzerland

DESAI, P.B., Tata Memorial Centre, Tata Memorial Hospital and Cancer Research Institute, Dr. Ernest Borges Road, Parel, Bombay 400 012, India

DHOM, G., Am Webersberg 20, W-6650 Homburg/Saar, FRG

DÖRKEN, B., Abteilung Innere Medizin V, Medizinische Universitäts-Klinik, Hospitalstr. 3, W-6900 Heidelberg, FRG

EBERT, T., Department of Urology, Heinrich-Heine-University, Medical School, Moorenstr. 5, W-4000 Düsseldorf, FRG

FOURNIER, D. VON, Universitäts-Frauenklinik, Voßstr. 9, W-6900 Heidelberg, FRG

GADEMANN, G., Radiologische Universitätsklinik, Abteilung Klinische Radiologie, Im Neuenheimer Feld 400, W-6900 Heidelberg, FRG

GERHARTZ, H.H., Institut für Klinische Hämatologie, GSF-Forschungszentrum für Umwelt und Gesundheit, Marchioninistr. 25, W-8000 München 70, FRG

GISSMANN, L., Deutsches Krebsforschungszentrum, Institut für Virusforschung, Im Neuenheimer Feld 280, W-6900 Heidelberg, FRG

HAGE, C., Institute of Pathology, University Clinics, University of Mainz, W-6500 Mainz, FRG

HÖFLER, H., GSF Institut für Pathologie, Pathologisches Institut der TU, Klinikum rechts der Isar, Ismaninger Str. 22, W-8000 München 80, FRG

HUK, W.J., Department of Neuroradiology, Neurosurgical Hospital, University of Erlangen-Nürnberg, Schwabachanlage 6, W-8520 Erlangen, FRG

JAHN, U.R., Deutsches Krebsforschungszentrum, Abteilung für Cytopathologie, Im Neuenheimer Feld 280, W-6900 Heidelberg, FRG

JOCHMUS, I., Department of Pathology, Georgetown University, Washington DC, USA

JUNG, E.G., Department of Dermatology, University of Heidelberg, Mannheim Medical School, W-6800 Mannheim, FRG

JUNIEN, C., INSERM U 73 Génétique et Pathologie Foetale, Chateau de Longchamp, Bois de Boulogne, F-75016 Paris, France

JUNKERMANN, H., Universitäts-Frauenklinik, Voßstr. 9, W-6900-Heidelberg, FRG

KAICK, G. VAN, Deutsches Krebsforschungszentrum, Institut für Radiologie und Pathophysiologie, Im Neuenheimer Feld 280, W-6900 Heidelberg, FRG

KATO, H., Department of Medicine, National Cancer Center Hospital, 1-1 Tsukiji 5 chome, Chuo-ku, Tokyo, 104, Japan

KAUFMANN, M., Universitäts-Frauenklinik, Voßstr. 9, W-6900-Heidelberg, FRG

KINDERMANN, G., I. Universitäts-Frauenklinik München, Klinikum Innenstadt, Maistr. 11, W-8000 München 20, FRG

KOSS, L.G., Department of Pathology, Montefiore Medical Center and the Albert Einstein College of Medicine, 111 East 210 Street, Bronx, NY 10467, USA

LAMERZ, R., Medizinische Klinik II, Klinikum Großhadern, Universität München, Marchioninistr. 15, W-8000 München 70, FRG

LICHTER, P., Institut für Virusforschung, Deutsches Krebsforschungszentrum, Im Neuenheimer Feld 280, W-6900 Heidelberg, FRG

LOHMANN, D., GSF-Institut für Pathologie, Pathologisches Institut der TU, Klinikum rechts der Isar, Ismaninger Str. 22, W-8000 München 80, FRG

LUZ, A., GSF-Institut für Pathologie, W-8042 Neuherberg, FRG

MANDAHL, N., Department of Clinical Genetics, University Hospital, S-22185 Lund, Sweden

MEHTA, F.S., Tata Institute of Fundamental Research, National Centre of the Government of India for Nuclear Science and Mathematics, Homi Bhabha Road, Bombay 400 005, India

MEUER, S., Deutsches Krebsforschungszentrum, Institut für Radiologie und Pathophysiologie, Im Neuenheimer Feld 280, W-6900 Heidelberg, FRG

MILLER, A.B., Department of Preventive Medicine and Biostatistics, University of Toronto, Toronto, Ontario M5S 1AB, Canada

MÖLLER, P., Pathologisches Institut, Abteilung für Allgemeine und Pathologische Anatomie, Im Neuenheimer Feld 220/221, W-6900 Heidelberg, FRG

MOLL, R., Institute of Pathology, University Clinics, University of Mainz, W-6500 Mainz, FRG

MORIYA, N., Department of Medicine, National Cancer Center Hospital, 1-1 Tsukiji 5 chome, Chuo-ku, Tokyo, 104, Japan

MÜLLER, M., Deutsches Krebsforschungszentrum, Institut für Virusforschung, Im Neuenheimer Feld 280, W-6900 Heidelberg, FRG

MURTI, P.R., Tata Institute of Fundamental Research, National Centre of the Government of India for Nuclear Science and Mathematics, Homi Bhabha Road, Bombay 400 005, India

NÜSSLER, V., Medizinische Klinik III, Klinikum Großhadern, Universität München, Marchioninistr. 15, W-8000 München 70, FRG

PETERS, P.E., Institut für Klinische Radiologie, Westfälische Wilhelms-Universität, Albert-Schweitzer-Str. 33, W-4400 Münster, FRG

RUMMENY, E., Institut für Klinische Radiologie, Westfälische Wilhelms-Universität, Albert-Schweitzer-Str. 33, W-4400 Münster, FRG

RUSTIN, G.J.S., Department of Medical Oncology, Charing Cross Hospital, Fulham Palace Road, London W6 8RF, U.K.

SASAKO, M., Department of Surgery, National Cancer Center Hospital, 1-1 Tsukiji 5 chome, Chuo-ku, Tokyo, 104, Japan

SAUER, H., Institut für Klinische Hämatologie, GSF-Forschungszentrum für Umwelt und Gesundheit, Marchioninistr. 25, W-8000 München 70, FRG

SCHMETZER, H., Medizinische Klinik III, Klinikum Großhadern, Universität München, Marchioninistr. 15, W-8000 München 70, FRG

SCHMITZ-DRÄGER, B.J., Department of Urology, Heinrich-Heine-University, Medical School, Moorenstr. 5, W-4000 Düsseldorf, FRG

SCHWAB, M., Deutsches Krebsforschungszentrum, Institut für Experimentelle Pathologie, Im Neuenheimer Feld 280, W-6900 Heidelberg, FRG

SHAH, K.V., Johns Hopkins Medical Institutions, Baltimore, MD, USA

STRAUSS, L.G., Deutsches Krebsforschungszentrum, Institut für Radiologie und Pathophysiologie, Im Neuenheimer Feld 280, W-6900 Heidelberg, FRG

VISCIDI, R.K., Johns Hopkins Medical Institutions, Baltimore, MD, USA

WERNECKE, K., Institut für Klinische Radiologie, Westfälische Wilhelms-Universität, Albert-Schweitzer-Str. 33, W-4400 Münster, FRG

WIESMANN, W., Institut für Klinische Radiologie, Westfälische Wilhelms-Universität, Albert-Schweitzer-Str. 33, W-4400 Münster, FRG

WILMANNS, W., Medizinische Klinik III, Klinikum Großhadern, Universität München, Marchioninistr. 15, W-8000 München 70, FRG

YOSHIDA, S., Department of Medicine, National Cancer Center Hospital, 1-1 Tsukiji 5 chome, Chuo-ku, Tokyo, 104, Japan

ZERBAN, H., Deutsches Krebsforschungszentrum, Abteilung für Cytopathologie, Im Neuenheimer Feld 280, W-6900 Heidelberg, FRG

What does "Early" Stand for in Cancer Diagnosis?

P. BANNASCH and G. VAN KAICK

Cancer is a chronic disease the development of which passes through different stages and may take several decades. One of the main shortcomings in the clinical management of cancer is that the disease usually does not lead to early symptoms or complaints which would stimulate the patient to ask for medical care. Thus, cancer is often only diagnosed in advanced stages for which curative therapy is not available. Since most cancers emerge slowly their diagnosis at early stages should in principle be possible and provide the basis for more effective therapy. Consequently, early detection has been recognized as a major challenge in the fight against cancer and has been introduced in the health care programs of many countries.

What does "early" mean in the context of cancer diagnosis? From a theoretical point of view, the demonstration of the primary molecular and cellular changes leading to a specific type of cancer would be ideal. Some recent results which may eventually lead to this ambitious aim will be considered at this symposium. In present practice, however, "early" indicates an ill-defined time point relative to the later clinical manifestation of cancer. Hence, early detection may have at least three different meanings:

- The detection of precancerous changes, permitting intervention before the endstage of the disease becomes manifest
- The diagnosis of small, localized cancers without metastatic spread, which are accessible to curative therapy
- The early detection of recurrent cancers

The detection of precancerous changes is certainly the most desirable approach to early diagnosis, resulting in secondary prevention of the disease when appropriate therapeutic measures are taken. Mass screening for cervical cancer by cytological examination of smears is the most convincing example for this approach. It has been calculated that the incidence of cervical cancer may be reduced dramatically, by about 93%, if women are screened annually over the age range 20–64 years (Miller 1991). Unfortunately, however, for no other type of cancer have potential approaches to the detection of precancerous changes been comparably successful.

The early diagnosis of small localized cancers of certain sites, such as the breast or prostate, has also been included in screening programs in many countries. In a recent evaluation of screening for cancer, Miller and colleagues (1990) stated that physical examination and mammography every 1–3 years can reduce breast cancer mortality substantially in women aged 50–70. In women under 50 there is little evidence for benefit, at least in the first 10 years after screening is initiated. This has called into question the cost effectiveness of screening for breast cancer under the age of 50.

In the case of cancer of the prostate, which accounts for about 8% of the cancer mortality in males in the Federal Republic of Germany, evaluation of the success of the digital rectal examination is precluded by the poor motivation of men to participate in the screening programs offered (Isele 1990). The value of transrectal ultrasonography for early diagnosis of prostate cancer is controversial, but the method is certainly more expensive than digital rectal examination. Whereas some authors feel that increasing utilization of screening programs might reduce mortality from prostate cancer, Miller argues that because of the frequency of latent prostate cancer in elderly men mortality from treatment of these conditions might offset any benefit from screening.

The examples of breast and prostate cancer show some major problems which have to be considered in all efforts to improve early detection of cancer, namely possible adverse effects of the medical intervention, the cost-benefit ratio, and the acceptance of the procedures proposed on the part of the population. A number of other problems (Miller 1991), such as adequacy of facilities, organization of quality control and availability of appropriate treatment, all have a considerable impact on the success of secondary prevention of cancer.

The early detection of recurrent cancers is essential when additional therapy can be offered. Finally, the identification and follow-up of high-risk groups, including patients who have been cured of one type of cancer by radiation and/or chemotherapy but are at significantly greater risk of developing second neoplasms, is another important aspect of secondary prevention.

In spite of the existence of some useful approaches to early detection of cancer, there is little doubt that the general success is limited, calling for much more research and careful epidemiological evaluation of the results in this important area of preventive medicine.

References

Isele H (ed) (1990) Onkologie für den Hausarzt. Themen der Vor-, Nach- und Mitsorge. Zuckschwerdt, Munich

Miller AB (1991) Epidemiological approaches to primary and secondary prevention of cancer. J Cancer Res Clin Oncol 117:177–185

Miller AB, Chamberlain J, Day NE, Hakama M, Prorok PC (1990) Report on a workshop of the UICC project on evaluation of screening for cancer. Int J Cancer 66:761–769

SESSION 1

Clinical Aspects I

Chairman: V. DIEHL

Skin Cancer and Melanoma

E.G. Jung

Introduction

The starting points and the end products of skin carcinogenesis are well known. In between, there is a cascade of events that are not known at all and which are not experimentally reproducible. The results of carcinogenesis are the keratinocyte-borne actinic keratoses, precancerous states, the basal cell carcinomas (BCC), the squamous cell carcinomas (SCC), the very rare Merkel-cell tumors and the melanocyte-borne lentigo maligna (LMM) as well as the various forms of malignant melanomas (nodular, NM; superficial spreading, SSM).

For tumor prevention and early detection of the precursors, it is necessary to explore the pathogenesis of these tumors. Three pathogenetic paradigms can be distinguished and described as risks of skin tumors. In two, the nature and degree of *UV exposure* play a major role. This must be reduced. The third risk is characterized by specific *melanoma precursors*. These must be detected early and precisely. They can then be excised before manifestation of an invasive tumor.

Evidence for Photocarcinogenesis

Apart from the location of most skin tumors in previously overirradiated skin areas, there is substantial epidemiological evidence for a strong correlation between solar irradiation of the skin and carcinogenesis, although with a lag phase of years or decades. The data on skin tumors collected from all continents and over several decades can be summarized as follows (Fitzpatrick 1988, Glass and Hoover 1989, Jung 1986, Sober 1987, Weinstock 1989):

- Mostly located in skin areas exposed to light
- More frequent among outdoor workers than indoor workers
- Far more frequent among white people than among blacks and orientals
- Dramatically higher incidence in whites at more equatorial latitudes
- White sun-sensitive phenotypes are at higher risk (skin types I and II)
- Increasing incidence in whites with exaggerated sunning habits since childhood
- High risk in patients with Xeroderma pigmentosum (2000 fold)
- Action spectrum in the UVB (and UVC)

Armed with these data and evidence, skin photocarcinogenesis can be described in model terms on the basis of two fundamentally different risk patterns.

1. Cumulative Total Lifetime Exposure to Sunlight

Photo-induced damage occurs by repeated exposures to UV distributed throughout life and acting cumulatively. The damage spreads extensively on the areas exposed to light and becomes manifest relatively late in life with multiple foci. Besides actinic elastosis (heliosis), actinic keratoses, BCC, and SCC are manifested as precanceroses and carcinomas of the keratinocyte system. Of the melanomas, only the LMM are located here. In view of their age of manifestation, morphodynamics, multilocular disposition, and strictly light-related location, the LMM correspond to the photo-induced damage mentioned here, and they account for 5%–10% of cutaneous melanomas (Jung 1988, 1989, Sober 1987).

Experimental data on keratinocytes and fibroblasts show that the effectiveness of the cellular repair systems and their overtaxing play a major role (Thielmann et al. 1987). The excision repair, measured as unscheduled DNA synthesis (UDS), can repair a light-induced DNA damage during the first hours after irradiation without errors. This enzymatic repair system of cell nuclei is limited to between 1/2 and 1 MED (minimal erythema dose) and is exhausted by repeated irradiation at short intervals (Hönigsmann et al. 1987). It can no longer repair all the DNA damage caused by UV, and thus the damage persists, and other error-prone repair systems are induced or activated. In this way, oncogenic point mutations and the development of a malignant clonus in the epidermis as well as in the melanocytes may occur.

Xeroderma Pigmentosum. The autosomal-recessive disease Xeroderma pigmentosum (XP) is the genetic model of this risk group (Jung 1986). This condition is rare but very characteristic. With increased sensitivity to light, these patients suffer from chronic photo-induced damage to the skin after a single or after very few UV exposures. Besides the pigment incontinence, epidermal atrophy, and actinic elastosis, multiple benign and malignant tumors of the skin develop regularly and in large numbers. Half of the XP patients develop one or several lentigo malignas (LM) and melanomas, exclusively of the LMM type. It is calculated that the light-dependent risk of melanoma is raised by a factor of 2000 in patients with XP and by far exceeds the differences in risk due to racial pigmentation (Jung 1986).

The other striking difference of photocarcinogenesis between XP patients and normal white subjects is the shortened lag phase in XP between irradiation and appearance of skin malignancies in childhood and adolescence. This can be demonstrated and even differentiated regarding the complementation groups of XP.

Events in the Lag Phase Between Photodamage and Malignancy. Immediately after the UV exposure (time measured in seconds and minutes), photochemical damage in the DNA but also in the RNA, proteins and membranes, are covalently fixed and start to elicit biological reactions on the cellular level.

The best known and the most destructive damage is the formation of cyclobutane dimers on the DNA, followed by the initiation of excision repair processes.

During the first hours, about 50% of the dimers are removed and replaced error-free, whereas the final dimer-removing efficacy of 90% is achieved after 24 h. This process, enabling the cells to resume their functions, may be optimized after an UVB irradiation corresponding to 0.5–1 MED. If the irradiation dose is higher, the excision repair mechanism is overtaxed, and more and more dimers persist, either inducing cell death or the induction of error-prone repair mechanisms (Hönigsmann et al. 1987, Thielmann et al. 1987). These errors might lead to somatic point mutations, initiating oncogenic clones of keratinocytes as well as of melanocytes.

In the keratinocyte compartment, such point mutations are of special interest only in the basal cell layer; in the upper layers, the cells, damaged or not, are removed by the natural processes of differentiation and desquamation, at least during the next 3–4 weeks.

Keratinocytes are, in vivo and in culture, relatively UV resistant, whereas the melanocytes, themselves not sufficiently protected by melanosomes, are more sensitive to UV irradiation. UVB irradiation acts on melanocytes as a promotor and stimulates melanin production as well as mitosis and even migration. This is the basis of suntanning and is used in vitiligo treatment. Epidermal melanocytes are therefore UV sensitive and have not enough time to repair DNA damage before they are promoted. The efficacy of UV-induced malignant clones must therefore be high.

The situation in keratinocytes is completely different. They are less UV sensitive and additionally enjoy the protection of transferred melanosomes. UVB does not act as a promotor of keratinocyte growth, differentiation, and function. In contrast, the keratinocytes undergo an arrest of their cell cycle of at least 24 h (used in psoriasis therapy), enabling optimal repair processes before they are reintegrated into the mitotic cycle. Keratinocytes are less UV sensitive than melanocytes and have enough time for an optimal recovery from UV damage. The efficacy of UV-induced malignant clones should therefore be low. However, these clones nevertheless evidently occur and lead to keratinocyte-derived skin malignancies. They must be found in a special keratinocyte compartment with higher UV susceptibility and less melanosome protection. Candidates for such a population are the basal keratinocytes in their most sensitive phase of mitosis or immediately after the M-phase. These cells are highly UV sensitive, and their melanosome content is only half that in the mother cell.

Another and very important control mechanism of eliminating oncogenic cells and clones, before they reach an invasive stage, is immune surveillance. Animal experiments show that the cell-mediated immune reaction is of special importance. This can be clinically documented by considering the sun damage in immunosuppressed patients after renal transplantation. There is evidence

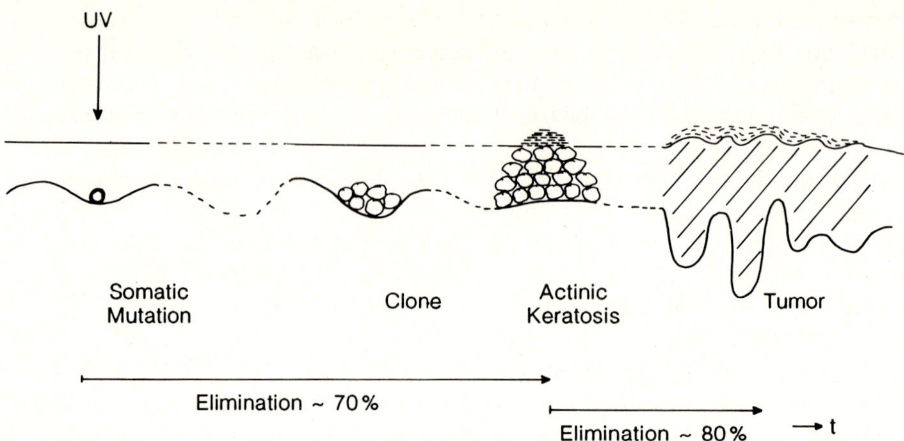

Fig. 1. Events in the lag phase between primary photodamage and malignancy

that the lag phase between UV irradiation and the appearance of skin tumors is remarkably shortened, and the number of lesions is increased.

Sun-induced oncogenic cells and clones are nevertheless produced in a tremendous excess, as can be learned by studying XP. Most of this damage is repaired, or the cells are removed from the epidermal compartment during the next steps, either by inflammation, immune surveillance, or mechanically by excoriation. Calculations suggest that no more than 6% of the incipient oncogenic foci survive to realize a skin cancer (Fig. 1). Let me express that only the fittest clone may give rise to a clinically manifest lesion. And then thousands of well-trained and very professional dermatologists are waiting to remove these lesions definitively and cure the patients.

2. Particularly Intense Exposure in Early Life

As indicated by epidemiological observations, case control studies, and investigations on patients who have undergone "migration" (Jung 1989, Sober 1987), one or several (as a rule only a few) excessive exposures to UV in childhood and in youth (Mackie et al. 1989) leading to severe sunburns (which can be remembered by the patients and which mostly received medical treatment), appear to characterize a further risk of melanoma. In locations which do not have to be typical for usual light exposure, nodular (NM) and superficially spreading melanomas (SSM) occur solitarily between the 20th and the 50th year of life. This is earlier than LMM (Fig. 2). However, excessive exposure to sunlight may also activate or provoke melanomas in dysplastic nevi (Kopf et al. 1985). This appears to be correlated with a reduction of the age of melanoma manifestation. Without being able to present exact figures on the risk of excessive UV exposure in youth, it is suspected that most NM and SSM of the skin arise from this risk type.

DNSy ▪ Melanoma in DNS
NM ▪ Nodular Melanoma
LMM ▪ Lentigo maligna Melanoma
SSM ▪ Superficial spreading Melanoma

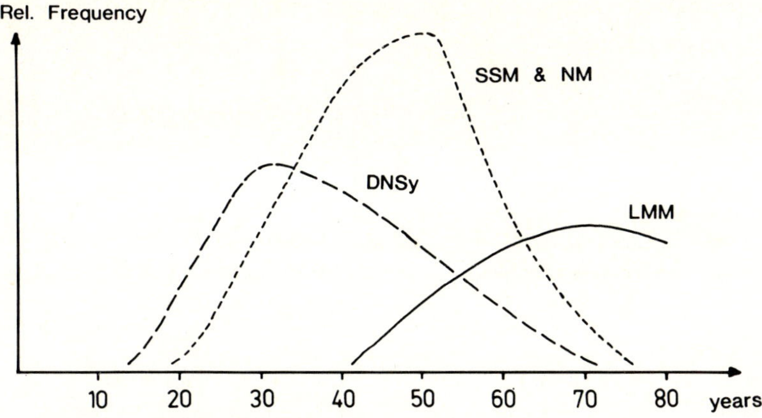

Fig. 2. Age of manifestation of the different melanoma types

Dysplastic Nevus Syndrome (DNS)

Dysplastic Nevi

- multiple (10 to >100)
- buttocks, trunk, head
- increase in number and size (in adults)

Genetic

- autosomal
- dominant or polygenetic
- associated with fair complexion

Melanoma in DN

- early appearance (20-40 y)
- often multiple
- up to 100% (>70 y)

Fig. 3. Synopsis of the dysplastic nevus syndrome (DNS)

In this context, it is helpful to examine the congenital dysplastic nevus syndrome (DNS). This is an autosomal and polygenic syndrome with multiple dysplastic nevi which spread and proliferate in a bizarre, irregular way wich changes of shape and color even after adolescence (Figs. 3, 4). Carriers of this syndrome develop solitary or multiple melanomas from dysplastic nevi with an age of manifestation between the 25th and 40th year of life (Jung 1988, 1989). On extrapolation, at least one melanoma will be manifest in each carrier of DNS at the age of 70 years (Kraemer et al. 1983). The clinical and histological activity and the number of dysplastic nevi are substantially raised at skin sites with exposure to sunburn compared with covered skin areas (Kopf et al. 1985). Melanomas based on DNS probably account for 20% or more of NM and SSM.

<u>Dysplastic Nevi (DN)</u>

Polycyclic, irregular borders (>5 mm)
Polychromasia (black, brown, rose)
Regression and satellites
Surface flat and lichenoid

Fig. 4. Synopsis of dysplastic nevi (DN)

Relative Risk (RR)	Multicenter Study (1079 Cases, 778 Controls)	Mannheim Study (204 Cases, 200 Controls)
Sun exposure		
recreational	1.2	1.8
professional	2.7	2.1
Skin type I versus IV	2.0	4.9
Red hair	4.7	2.9
NZN		
<10	1.0	1.0
10 - 50	2.3	4.3
>50	4.8	14.9

Fig. 5. Predictive values of risk factors for melanoma. *NZN*, nevocytic nevi. German Melanoma Register: Case Control Studies 1989–91

In the "particularly intense exposure" type of photocarcinogenesis, the main and almost the unique risk is from melanoma. On the other hand, more than 90% of the melanomas (excluding LMM) is probably partially or completely initiated and promoted by such a periodic burst of extensive sun exposure leading to severe sunburn. In the case of DNS, the precursor lesions, the dysplastic nevi, are genetically preformed, and it is possible that the excessive sun exposure acts as a promotor. Further insights may be found on the cytogenetic level as well as with molecular biology.

The excision repair (UDS) and the colony forming ability (CFA) are in the normal range in solitary melanomas, familial melanoma, and DNS, whereas increased chromsomal anomalies (translocations involving chromosomes 1, 6, and 7) are found in melanocytes as well as in fibroblasts in patients with DNS. Moreover, cytogenetic indications of hypermutability are regularly found under experimental UV exposure (UVB, UVC, but not UVA) of cultivated cells and cell lines, which enable an approach to cytogenetic detection and description of the endogenous risk. The hypermutability is the same in DNS patients with and without manifest melanoma, indicating that it is due to the syndrome and does not arise in the course of the disease or during tumor progression (Bohnert and Weiss 1990, Bröcker et al. 1989, Jung et al. 1986, Perera et al. 1986). In DNS, an excessive UV exposure in youth very probably leads to the manifestation or to a decisive promotion of the pre-existent, endogenous risk.

In DNS, a first or a leading mutation can be assumed in the genome. This shows autosomal inheritance, might be located on the short arm of chromosome 1 (1p) (Bale et al. 1989), and might be an UV-labile molecular repressor (anti-oncogene). The spectrum of secondary induced oncogene activations (N-*ras*; C-*myc*), the chromosomal instability, and the UV-inducible hypermutability may result from further, UV-driven promotion and acceleration (Bohnert and Weiss 1990, Bröcker et al. 1989, Schrier et al. 1990, Steijlen et al. 1989, Yamamura and Mishima 1990). The first mutation leads to chromosomal instability and to hypermutability. One or several excessive UV exposures early in life are to be considered as a second exogenously induced somatic mutation with consecutive growth promotion. This may explain the reduced age of manifestation, the familial occurrence, and the multiplicity of melanomas in DNS.

An analogous situation is found in the "two-hit model" in *Xiphophorus* and other pigment-tumor-prone fishes as well as in selected human tumors such as neuroblastoma and retinoblastoma (Jung 1988).

Nevocytic Nevus as Risk Indicator for Melanoma

Apart from the UV-induced melanoma risk, there is a more unusual melanoma risk based on the number and the atypia of benign nevocytic nevi. The relative melanoma risk for patients with DNS with at least 3 atypical and dysplastic nevi is increased 500-fold (Mackie et al. 1989), and the melanoma will manifest during adult life (Kraemer et al. 1983). The melanomas occurring in large congenital nevi, in 10%–20% of the patients with bathing-trunk nevi, will manifest during the first 10 years of life (Jung 1988, 1989). Beside these special conditions, there is strong evidence that the number of benign nevi is the best risk indicator for developing melanoma (Mackie et al. 1989, Weiss et al. 1990, 1991). This is clearly shown in recent studies based on the data of the German Melanoma Register (organized and conducted by C. Garbe and C. Orfanos, Berlin) (Fig. 5).

The Mannheim case control study with 204 melanoma patients and 200 control persons assessed the significance of melanoma risk factors for an ethnically homogeneous population from a geographically small region. In a multivariate analysis of the data, the total number of benign nevi proved to be the most predictive parameter with a relative risk (RR) of 14.9 (total number of nevi greater than 50). The constitutional factors red hair color and skin type I were less predictive with a relative risk of 2.9 and 4.9, respectively. Occupational and recreational sun exposure were of ancillary importance (RR 1.8 and 2.1). The assessment of the risk for the various subtypes of melanoma, however, showed a clear difference in the predictive value of the mentioned risk factors. The risk of developing SSM is nearly exclusively defined by the number of benign nevi (RR 24.8); red hair color was of subordinate importance (RR 4.2); whereas the risk for LMM is dependent on skin type I (RR 12.9) and sun exposure (RR 3.4).

Therefore, patients with large congenital nevi, patients with a familial history and the personal criteria of DNS, as well as all persons with more than 50 nevi have to be regularly examined. Atypical pigment lesions have to be surgically removed and histologically certified.

Summary

Keratinocyte-derived skin tumors, basal cell carcinomas (BCC), squamous cell carcinomas (SCC), Merkel-cell tumors, as well as malignant melanomas have dramatically increased in number in recent decades. There is substantial experimental and epidemiological evidence for the influence of UV irradiation as the major cause of this trend. For tumor prevention and early detection of their precursors, it is necessary to explore their pathogenesis. Three paradigms can be distinguished and described as risks of skin tumors. In two, the nature and degree of UV exposure play a major role. This must be reduced. The third is characterized by specific melanoma precursors, which should be detected early. They can then be excised before manifestation of an invasive tumor. The *cumulative total lifetime exposure* is correlated with the appearance of keratinocyte-derived tumors and lentigo maligna melanomas (LMM). The rare autosomal-recessive disease Xeroderma pigmentosum (XP) is the genetic model for this risk group.

Particularly intense exposure in early life may be responsible for most of the melanomas of the skin. In this context, it is helpful to examine the congenital dysplastic nevus syndrome (DNS). Carriers of this syndrome have a very high risk of developing melanomas during life.

The number of benign nevocytic nevi is the strongest risk indicator for developing melanoma. The relative risk is 14.9 when the total number of nevi is higher than 50. Apart from these cases, to be regularly examined, melanoma occurs in 10%–20% of patients with large congenital nevi during childhood.

References

Bale SJ, Dracopoli NC, Tucker MA, Clark WA, Fraser MC, Stanger BZ, Green P, Donis-Keller H, Housman DE, Greene MH (1989) Mapping the gene for hereditary cutaneous malignant melanoma-dysplastic nevus to chromosome 1q. N Engl J Med 320:1367–1372

Bohnert E, Weiss J (1990) Zytogenetische Befunde beim Syndrom der dysplastischen Nävi (DNS). In: Orfanos CE, Garbe C (eds) Das maligne Melanom der Haut. Zuckschwerdt, Munich, pp 153–157

Bröcker EB, Ruiter DJ, Johnson JP, Suter L, Sorg C (1989) Marker der Melanom-progression (Abstr). Hautarzt 40:381

Fitzpatrick TB (1988) The validity and practicality of sun-reactive skin types I through VI. Arch Dermatol 124:869–874

Glass AG, Hoover RN (1989) The emerging epidemic of melanoma and squamous cell skin cancer. JAMA 262:2097–2100

Hönigsmann H, Brenner W, Tanew A, Ortel B (1987) UV-induced unscheduled DNA synthesis in human skin. Dose response, correlation with erythema, time course and split dose exposure in vivo. J Photochem Photobiol [B] 1:33–39

Jung EG (1986) Xeroderma pigmentosum. Int J Dermatol 25:629–634

Jung EG (1988) Ist das Melanom-Risiko kalkulierbar? Z Haut Geschlechtskr 63:559–562

Jung EG (1989) Wie kann man Melanome verhindern? Dtsch Med Wochenschr 114:393–397

Jung EG, Bohnert E, Boonen H (1986) Dysplastic nevus syndrome. Ultraviolet hypermutability confirmed in vitro by elevated sister chromatid exchanges. Dermatologica 173:297–300

Kopf AW, Lindsay AC, Rogers GS, Friedman RJ, Rigel DS, Levenstein M (1985) Relationship of nevocytic nevi to sun exposure in dysplastic nevus syndrome. J Am Acad Dermatol 12:656–663

Kraemer KH, Greene MH, Tarone R, Edler DE, Clark WH Jr, Guerry D (1983) Dysplastic nevi and cutaneous melanoma risk. Lancet 2:1076–1077

MacKie RM, Freudenberger T, Aitchison TC (1989) Personal risk-factor chart for cutaneous melanoma. Lancet:487–490

Perera MI, Um KI, Greene MH, Waters HL, Bredberg A, Kraemer KH (1986) Hereditary dysplastic nevus syndrome. Lymphoid cell ultraviolet hypermutability in association with increased melanoma susceptibility. Cancer Res 46:1005–1009

Schrier PI, Versteeg R, Peltenburg LTC, Plomp AC, van't Veer LJ, Krüse-Wolters KM (1990) Empfindlichkeit von Melanomzellinien gegenüber natürlichen Killerzellen und der mögliche Einfluß von Onkogenaktivierungen. In: Orfanos CE, Garbe C (eds) Das maligne Melanom der Haut. Zuckschwerdt, Munich, pp 176–188

Sober AJ (1987) Solar exposure in the etiology of cutaneous melanoma. Photodermatology 4:23–27

Steijlen PM, Hamm H, van Erp PEJ, Johnson JP, Ruiter DJ, Bröcker EB (1989) Immunohistologic evidence for the malignant potential of congenital melanocytic nevi. J Invest Dermatol 92:366–370

Thielmann HW, Edler L, Burkhardt MR, Jung EG (1987) DNA repair synthesis in fibroblast strains from patients with actinic keratosis, squamous cell carcinoma, basal cell carcinoma, or malignant melanoma after treatment with ultraviolet light, N-acetoxy-2-acetyl-aminofluorene; methyl methanesulfonate, and N-methyl-N-nitrosourea. J Cancer Res Clin Oncol 113:171–186

Weinstock MA (1989) The epidemic of squamous cell carcinoma. JAMA 262:2138–2140

Weiss J et al. (1990) Risikofaktoren für die Entwicklung maligner Melanome in der Bundesrepublik Deutschland. Hautarzt 41:309–313

Weiss J, Bertz J, Jung EG (1991) Malignant melanoma in southern Germany: different predictive value of risk factors for melanoma subtypes. Dermatologica (in press)

Yamamura K, Mishima Y (1990) Antigen dynamics in melanocytic and nevocytic melanoma oncogenesis: anti-ganglioside and anti-ras p21 antibodies as markers of tumor progression. J Invest Dermatol 94:174–182

Cancer of the Oral Cavity*

D.K. Daftary, P.R. Murti, R.B. Bhonsle, and F.S. Mehta

Introduction

The term oral cancer refers to all malignancies that arise in the oral cavity. Squamous cell carcinoma, however, is the most common, accounting for well over 90%. In this paper the term oral cancer is used to describe squamous cell carcinoma comprising ICD (9th revision) site groups 140, 141, 143–145. Oral cancer is one of the ten most common cancers globally (WHO 1984). Its distribution, however, varies from one geographic area to another. It ranks 6th and 9th among men and women in North America while it ranks 1st and 3rd in middle to south Asia (Parkin et al. 1984).

In several Southeast Asian countries, oral cancer is the most frequent cancer. According to WHO estimates, about 100000 oral cancers occur each year in India, Pakistan, Bangladesh, Nepal, Sri Lanka, Thailand, Singapore, Vietnam, Kampuchea, and other countries in this region (WHO 1984). This paper gives an overview of this disease with special focus on the role of oral precancer in the pathogenesis and its prevention.

Epidemiology

The occurrence of oral cancer exhibits notable geographic variations. Utilizing data from *Cancer Incidence in Five Continents*, vol. 4 (Waterhouse et al. 1982) (latest edition 1988), *National Cancer Registries of India* (Indian Council of Medical Research 1989, 1990), and other sources, a brief account of its morbidity is given below. For the sake of brevity, the incidence rates are presented for only select population groups; furthermore, as the incidence rates among women are generally lower than among men in non-Asian regions, women were excluded from the analysis for these areas.

In the European region, the incidence rates of oral cancer among men ranged from 10.4 per 100000 to 17.2 per 100000 (Table 1) and in the Americas, from 12.4 to 25 per 100000 (Table 2). In the Asian region the incidence rate among men varied from 7.4 to 18 per 100000 (Table 3), while among women, it was 6.7 to 10.5 per 100000 (Table 4). In this region the incidence rates were

*This study was supported in whole by funds from the National Institutes of Health, USA, under Indo-US Fund Research Agreement no. 01-022N.

Table 1. Incidence rates of oral cancer (ICD 140, 141, 143–145) among men in some select populations in Europe (Waterhouse et al. 1982)

Population	Incidence per 100 000
France, Bas-Rhin	17.2
Romania, Cluj	13.2
France, Doubs	11.6
Italy, Varese	10.8
The Netherlands	10.7
Yugoslavia, Slovenia	10.6
Hungary, Szabolcs-Szatmár	10.4

Range: 10.4 to 17.2

Table 2. Incidence rates of oral cancer (ICD 140, 141, 143–145) among men in some select populations in the Americas (Waterhouse et al. 1982)

Population	Incidence per 100 000
Canada, Newfoundland	25.0
Brazil, São Paulo	17.3
Canada, Saskatchewan	15.8
USA, Utah	13.6
Puerto Rico	13.4
Canada, Manitoba	12.4

Range: 12.4 to 25.0

Table 3. Incidence rates of oral cancer (ICD 140, 141, 143–145) among men in some select populations in the Asian region

Population	Incidence per 100 000
India	
Poona	18.0
Bombay (1976–1980)	16.3
Singapore, Indians (Waterhouse et al. 1982)	13.2
India (Indian Council of Medical Research 1990)	
Bombay (1987)	12.8
Madras (1987)	11.3
Bangalore (1987)	7.4

Range: 7.4 to 18.0

Table 4. Incidence rates of oral cancer (ICD 140, 141, 143–145) among women in some select populations in the Asian region

Population	Incidence per 100 000
India	
Bangalore (1987) [Indian Council of Medical Research 1990]	10.5
Bombay (1976–1980) [Waterhouse et al. 1982]	10.3
Madras (1987) [Indian Council of Medical Research 1990]	9.6
Singapore, Indians [Waterhouse et al. 1982]	8.6
Bombay (1987) [Indian Council of Medical Research 1990]	6.7

Range: 6.7 to 10.5

Table 5. Leading cancers in five hospital-based Cancer Registries in India (Indian Council of Medical Research 1989)

Registry	Men		Women	
	Percentage	Site	Percentage	Site
Bangalore	19.0	Pharynx	42.0	Cervix uteri
	10.3	Esophagus	13.7	Oral cavity
	9.1	Lung	10.3	Breast
	7.4	Oral cavity	6.3	Esophagus
	4.9	Larynx	9.8	Ovary
Bombay	19.8	Pharynx	29.7	Cervix uteri
	12.4	Oral cavity	21.9	Breast
	8.1	Esophagus	7.3	Oral cavity
	6.5	Larynx	5.5	Esophagus
	6.1	Lung	3.8	Pharynx
Madras	19.9	Pharynx	46.8	Cervix uteri
	15.5	Oral cavity	13.3	Breast
	9.9	Esophagus	10.7	Oral cavity
	7.0	Stomach	3.3	Pharynx
	6.0	Lung	3.3	Esophagus
Dibrugarh	37.6	Pharynx	22.9	Cervix uteri
	17.0	Esophagus	12.9	Esophagus
	6.9	Primary (?)	12.5	Breast
	6.4	Oral cavity	11.4	Pharynx
	5.1	Stomach	6.0	Oral cavity
Trivandrum	18.1	Oral cavity	24.2	Cervix uteri
	11.4	Lung	18.2	Breast
	8.4	Pharynx	14.2	Oral cavity
	5.6	Stomach	5.1	Ovary
	5.5	Esophagus	3.7	Thyroid

higher in India or for people of Indian origin in Singapore. The problem of oral cancer in India can be better appreciated from the ranking of cancers. In five *Cancer Registry* areas, among all cancers oral cancer ranked 1st to 5th among men and women, respectively (Table 5). In Australia and the Oceania region the incidence among men varied from 9.1 to 13.3 per 100 000 (Table 6). It must be noted, however, that involvement of specific intraoral locations exhibited notable differences in these populations.

Oral cancer is also common in other countries in the Asian region. This disease represented 48.2% of all cancers in Sri Lanka (Balendra 1949), 18.4% in Bangladesh (Huq 1965), 18.2% in Pakistan (Zaidi et al. 1974), 14% in Thailand (Piyaratn 1959), and 11% in Malaysia (Ahluwalia and Dugid 1966).

Etiology

Several factors such as alcohol consumption, syphilis, orodental factors, dietary deficiency states, tobacco, candidiasis, viruses, sunlight, immunologic and genetic factors have been mentioned as playing an etiologic or contributory role in the pathogenesis of oral cancer; the evidence, however, is overwhelming with regard to the etiologic role of tobacco. There are voluminous epidemiologic data demonstrating a strong association between certain forms

Table 6. Incidence rates of oral cancer (ICD 140, 141, 143–145) among men in two populations in Australia (Waterhouse et al. 1982)

Population	Incidence per 100 000
South Australia	13.3
New South Wales	9.1

Range: 9.1 to 13.3

Table 7. Relative and attributable risks for oral cancer (WHO 1984)

Habits	Relative risk	Attributable risk (%)
None	1	–
Betel quid without tobacco	1–4	1
Smoking only	3–6	8
Betel quid + tobacco	8–15	30
Betel quid + smoking	4–25	2
Betel quid + tobacco + smoking	20	50
Total	–	91

of tobacco use and oral cancer, comprising ecological observations and cross-sectional, descriptive, case control, prospective, dose-response, and intervention studies. Several independent evaluations reviewed these data (International Agency for Research on Cancer 1985, 1986, US Department of Health and Human Services 1986, 1989, US Public Health Services 1986) and confirmed unequivocally that there exists a causal relationship between certain forms of tobacco use and oral cancer. The attributable risk estimates for oral cancer from tobacco for some countries in the South-East region was 91%; it was highest (50%) for the combined habit of chewing betel-quid with tobacco and tobacco smoking (Table 7).

It is also possible that nutritional status, viruses (especially HSV, HPV, and HIV) might play an important contributory role in the causation of oral cancer, but their exact role needs to be clarified fully.

Clinical Aspects

As with incidence, there are marked geographic variations in regard to sex, age, and site distribution.

Sex Distribution. Oral cancer predominantly affects men, as borne out by higher incidence rates (Indian Council of Medical Research 1989, 1990, Waterhouse et al. 1982). In some countries, notably in India, the incidence rates among women are higher compared with those among women in the non-Asian regions. The gender differences in some population groups could be a direct consequence of the sex distribution of tobacco habits. For instance, in an Indian study the male:female ratio of oral cancer patients was proportional to

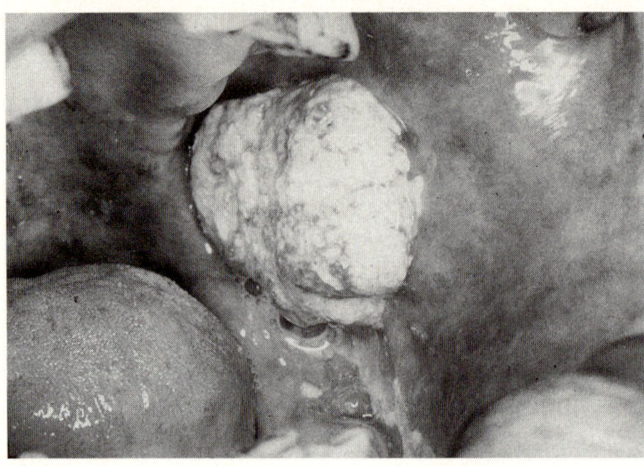

Fig. 1. Exophytic cancer in the buccal mucosa of a betel-quid chewer

the prevalence of tobacco habits in the general population (Mehta et al. 1971). A similar view was expressed by Fleming et al. (1982) on the basis of their observations in South Africa.

Age Distribution. Oral cancer generally occurs in individuals over the age of 40 years. In Western countries, it occurs more often in those aged over 75 years (Krolls and Hoffman 1976, Langdon et al. 1977), while in Asia it generally arises earlier. Currently, there is an upsurge in the use of smokeless tobacco products in America and Europe, especially among the young. This habit starts among teenagers, and correspondingly cases began to appear in 3rd and 4th decades (Davis and Severson 1987, Hakulinen et al. 1986, MacFarlane et al. 1987, Moller 1989).

Site Distribution. Cancer of the vermilion border of the lip is most common in certain population groups in the USA, Canada, and Australia, usually light-skinned people engaged in outdoor work. It is believed that exposure to sunlight (actinic radiation) and tobacco smoking are responsible for this site involvement. An inverse relationship between vermilion border cancer and intraoral cancer has been observed (Pindborg 1980). In Western countries, intraoral cancer most commonly affects the tongue and the floor of the mouth, followed by the buccal mucosa and the mandibular alveolus. The site distribution in Southeast Asia generally depends on the type of tobacco habits practiced by the individuals. Hirayama (1966) demonstrated that among Indians who chew betel quid, buccal mucosa (a location that affords intimate contact with betel quid) was involved in well over 80% of cases. Other forms of tobacco use also showed a similar site versus habit relationship. We observed that the hard palate was most commonly affected among those who smoked reverse, i.e., with the lighted end inside the mouth; involvement of the hard palate is otherwise uncommon.

Clinically, a majority of oral cancers tend to be exophytic (Fig. 1) and ulcerative-infiltrative lesions; some of them are verrucous carcinoma, which is a

Table 8. Extent of oral cancer (including lip) among men (M) and women (F) observed in hospital-based Cancer Registries in India in 1986 (Indian Council of Medical Research 1989)

Registry	Patient evaluated for extent of disease		Localized		Regional spread		Disseminated (advanced)	
	M (n)	F (n)	M (%)	F (%)	M (%)	F (%)	M (%)	F (%)
Chandigarh	39	25	28	32	72	64	0	4
Dibrugarh	53	21	40	43	57	57	4	0
Trivandrum	405	268	21	22	78	77	1	1
Bangalore	202	427	9	8	65	60	26	32
Bombay	640	312	26	26	70	71	5	3
Madras	283	226	10	6	87	92	3	2
Total	1622	1279	20	16	74	72	6	12

variant of squamous cell carcinoma. Ulcerative-infiltrative lesions are known to metastasize more frequently than exophytic lesions. Verrucous carcinoma is slow-growing and rarely metastasizes. Sometimes, oral precancerous lesions may coexist with oral cancer. Indian data from long-term studies showed that in most instances oral cancer originates from oral precancer (see below).

Metastasis and Survival. The extent of lymph node involvement determines the prognosis. More often than not, a high percentage (60%–71%) of lymph node involvement is observed at first diagnosis (Fahmy et al. 1983, Spiro et al. 1974, Wahi et al. 1965), involving mostly the cervical chain of lymph nodes. In a study of 500 oral cancer patients (Paymaster 1962), 12% had involvement of the submental lymph nodes, 32% of the submaxillary nodes, 10% of the superior group of deep cervical chain, and 30% of the jugular group of lymph nodes. In the remainder, other nodes in the cervical and supraclavicular region were affected.

The crude 5-year survival rates for intraoral cancer range from 30% to 40%; it is higher (80%) for lip cancer (Johnson 1990). The survival rate depends on the size of the lesion, the degree of its histologic differentiation, and the staging. Data from 2921 oral cancers in both genders in India shows that 18% of the oral cancers were localized, 73% exhibited regional spread, and 9% were disseminated at diagnosis (Table 8). Evans et al. (1982) demonstrated a decrease in the 5-year survival rates from 78% in stage I lesions to 20% for stage IV lesions.

Role of Oral Precancer

The term oral precancer encompasses a group of lesions or conditions which are precursors to oral cancer. They share the same etiologic factors as well as the same site versus habit relationship. For example, among betel-quid chewers in India, oral cancer and leukoplakia (see below) occur in the buccal mucosa,

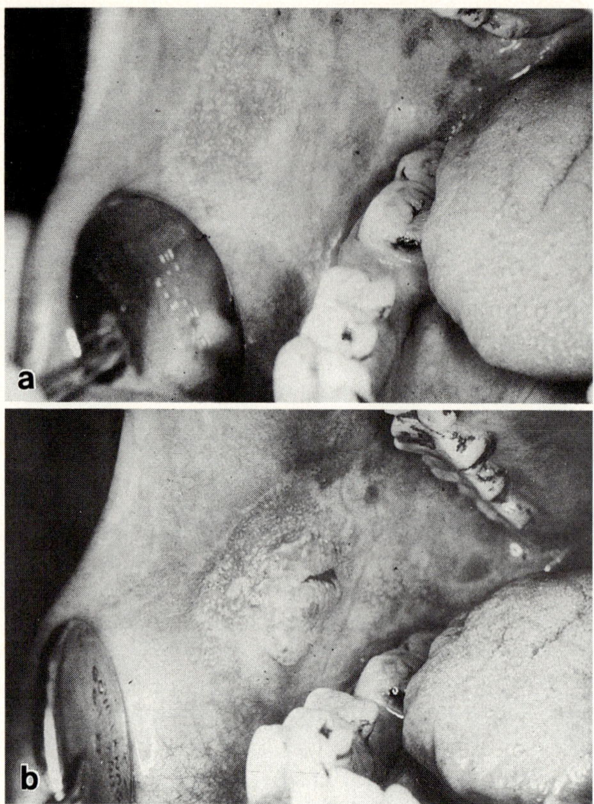

Fig. 2. **a** Nodular leukoplakia characterized by white nodules on an erythematous base in the buccal mucosa. **b** Three years later, cancer developed in this lesion

a location that has intimate contact with betel quid. During the past 25 years, extensive cross-sectional (Mehta et al. 1971) and prospective studies on precancer were conducted (Gupta et al. 1980, 1989). In a 10-year follow-up study of two population groups, each consisting of 10000 individuals, 24 oral cancers were observed, and all of them originated from a pre-existing precancerous lesion or condition (Gupta et al. 1980). Mallaowalla et al. (1976) reported that 68% of the 22 oral cancers in their study developed from precancer, namely, leukoplakia. In another 8-year follow-up study of 12000 tobacco users, we found that the relative risk for developing oral cancer from precancer or other tobacco-related lesions as compared to tobacco users was 69.2 (Gupta et al. 1989). Thus, oral precancer plays a vital role in the pathogenesis of oral cancer.

Oral precancer is divided into (i) precancerous lesions and (ii) precancerous conditions (Pindborg 1980). A precancerous lesion is defined as morphologically altered tissue in which cancer is more likely to occur compared with its apparently normal counterpart. Erythroplakia and leukoplakia are examples of precancerous lesions. A precancerous condition is defined as a generalized state associated with a significantly increased risk of cancer. Submucous fibriosis syphilis and sideropenic dysphagia fall into this category. Oral lichen planus is regarded as a possible precancerous condition.

Table 9. Relative risk estimates in various precancerous lesions and conditions (Gupta et al. 1989)

Precursor lesion/condition	Total no.	Average follow-up period (years)	Oral cancers	MT rate per 100 000 per year	Relative risk
Nodular leukoplakia	13	2.8	6	16 216.2	3243.2
Submucous fibrosis	25	6.0	3	1 986.7	397.3
Others[a]	26	2.6	1[b]	1 515.2	303.0
Ulcerated leukoplakia	105	4.4	1	218.8	43.8
Homogeneous leukoplakia	489	4.8	3	128.1	25.6
Lichen planus	344	3.7	1	78.9	15.8
None of the above	10 145	7.8	4	5.0	1.0

MT, malignant transformation.
[a] Includes nonspecific diagnosis, such as red area, ulcers, and benign growth.
[b] Preceding lesion, red area.

Erythroplakia consists of a bright red, velvety plaque which cannot be characterized clinically or pathologically as being due to any other condition (WHO 1978). Histologically, most of these lesions tend to show squamous cell carcinomas or severe dysplasias (Shafer and Waldron 1975).

Leukoplakia is defined as a raised white patch of oral mucosa measuring 5 mm or more in diameter, which cannot be scraped off and which cannot be attributed to any other diagnosable disease. This definition does not carry any histologic connotation (WHO 1978). Leukoplakias are distinguished into several clinical types (Axell et al. 1984, Mehta et al. 1971). Such a distinction is essential as the malignant transformation varies among the different clinical types. About 3%–6% of the leukoplakias progress to cancer (WHO 1978). Nodular leukoplakias (Fig. 2) or leukoplakias exhibiting erosive or erythroplastic components and idiopathic leukoplakia are more prone to cancer development. Nodular leukoplakias exhibited a highest relative risk of 3243.2 as compared with 43.8 for ulcerated leukoplakia and 25.6 for homogeneous leukoplakia (Table 9).

Submucous fibrosis is a chronic oral mucosal condition marked by mucosal rigidity of varying intensity due to the fibroelastic transformation of the juxta-epithelial tissue. This condition predominantly occurs among Indians and other Asians. Areca nut (*Areca catechu*) chewing in any form is regarded as an etiologic agent for this condition; tobacco use by the affected individuals may lead to the development of oral cancer. This is a high-risk precancerous condition with a malignant transformation rate of 7.6% (median observation of 10 years) (Murti et al. 1985). The relative risk for cancer development in this condition was 397.3 (Table 9).

Syphilis exhibits a variety of oral manifestations in its different stages. They are characterized by epithelial atrophy due to syphilitic endarteritis; such an epithelium is more prone to the action of carcinogens. However, with the advancement of treatment methods for syphilis, it is rare now to find progression of syphilis to the extent that oral cancer would develop.

Sideropenic dysphagia is primarily due to iron deficiency. It is almost exclusively found in middle-aged women of Scandinavian and European stock. There is epithelial atrophy in this condition or in iron deficiency without sideropenic dysphagia, which presumably leads to the development of oral cancer.

Oral lichen planus lesions are suspected of possessing some cancer potential. Interestingly, oral lichen planus is strongly associated with tobacco use (Bhonsle et al. 1979, Gupta et al. 1980); however, malignant transformation rates (Murti et al. 1986) and the relative risk (Table 9) were not significant enough to confirm its malignant potential.

Prevention of Oral Cancer

By virtue of its location in an easily accessible part of the body, oral cancer lends itself to early detection. Unfortunately, patients with this disease report for treatment when in the later stages, especially in the developing world, leading to poor survival rates. Fortunately, identification of tobacco as a causal factor and the observation that oral cancer in most instances originates from precancer place this disease in the preventable category. A large-scale intervention study among 12 000 tobacco users in each of three selected areas was conducted (Mehta et al. 1982). They were motivated to give up their tobacco habits utilizing a variety communication inputs. In the Ernakulam district, which is an area of high oral cancer incidence (Gupta et al. 1980), 2% discontinued the habit at the end of 2 years of intervention (Mehta et al. 1982), 9.4% at the end of 5 years (Gupta et al. 1986), 12.3% at the end of 8 years (Gupta et al. 1990), and about 14.3% at the end of 10 years. Correspondingly, the incidence of leukoplakia dropped significantly, implying a reduction in the risk for oral cancer. In recent times, the role of chemopreventive agents like β-carotene and vitamin A derivatives is being tested by other investigators.

The early detection and management of precancerous lesions and conditions constitute the secondary prevention of this disease. Early detection involves routine and periodic examination of people at risk, namely, individuals over the age of 35 years who are tobacco users. In that context, it is strongly desirable for all health professionals to incorporate routine examination of the mouth; the problem, however, lies in its limited reach, especially in the developing world where a vast majority of people in rural areas do not seek medical attention for various reasons. To overcome this problem, the feasibility of incorporating early detection of oral cancer by the paramedical workers (basic health workers) of the governmental health care system was investigated (Mehta et al. 1986). In this study, some 53 basic health workers attached to various primary health centers catering to a population of 470 000 villagers were specially trained for this purpose. In a 1-year period, during their routine house-to-house visits, they examined 39 000 of the estimated 117 000 high-risk group individuals. They detected 20 oral cancers and a large number of precancerous lesions and conditions. The specificity and sensitivity estimates and the predictive values of the diagnosis were found to be within acceptable limits.

The other facet of secondary prevention consists of the management of precancerous lesions aimed at averting their progression to oral cancer. To detect impending malignancy, however, there is a strong need to develop much better techniques than the existing ones.

Interestingly, the World Health Organization's assessment of six approaches on oral cancer control in 1984 showed that preventing people from taking up tobacco habits and helping the current users to stop their habits as well as utilizing paramedical (basic health) workers holds promise as effective methods (WHO 1984).

Summary

Oral cancer is one of the ten most common cancers globally. Certain forms of tobacco use are causally associated with this disease. Oral cancer exhibits notable geographic differences in regard to its occurrence, age, sex, and location distribution. Long-term population-based studies in India demonstrated that in most instances this disease arises from precancerous lesions (nodular leukoplakia) or conditions (submucous fibrosis). Although this disease lends itself to early detection, more often than not a high proportion of patients have lymph node involvement at the time of first diagnosis, tending to a poor prognosis. Encouragingly, however, oral cancer is amenable to prevention.

References

Ahluwalia HS, Dugid JB (1966) Malignant tumors in Malaya. Br J Cancer 20:12–15

Axell T, Holmstrup P, Kramer IRH, Pindborg JJ, Shear M (eds) (1984) International seminar on oral leukoplakia and associated lesions related to tobacco habits. Community Dent Oral Epidemiol 12:145–154

Balendra W (1949) Symposium on oral disease in tropical countries. The effect of betel chewing on the dental and oral tissues and its possible relationship to buccal carcinoma. Br Dent J 87:83–87

Bhonsle RB, Pindborg JJ, Gupta PC, Murti PR, Mehta Fali S (1979) Incidence rate of oral lichen planus among Indian villagers. Acta Derm Venereol (Stockh) 59:255–257

Davis S, Severson RK (1987) Increasing incidence of cancer of the tongue in the United States among young adults. Lancet 2:910–911

Evans SJ, Langdon JD, Rapidis AD, Johnson NW (1982) Prognostic significance of STNMP and velocity of tumor growth in oral cancer. Cancer 49:773–776

Fahmy MS, Sadeghi A, Behmard S (1983) Epidemiologic study of oral cancer in Fars Province, Iran. Community Dent Oral Epidemiol 11:50–58

Fleming M, Shear M, Altini M (1982) Intraoral squamous cell carcinoma in South Africa. J Dent Assoc S Afr 37:541–544

Gupta PC, Mehta FS, Daftary DK et al. (1980) Incidence rates of oral cancer and natural history of oral precancerous lesions in a 10-year follow-up study of Indian villagers. Community Dent Oral Epidemiol 8:287–333

Gupta PC, Mehta FS, Pindborg JJ et al. (1986) Intervention study for primary prevention of oral cancer among 36 000 Indian tobacco users. Lancet 1:1235–1238

Gupta PC, Bhonsle RB, Murti PR et al. (1989) An epidemiologic assessment of cancer risk in oral precancerous lesions in India with special reference to nodular leukoplakia. Cancer 63:2247–2252

Gupta PC, Mehta FS, Pindborg JJ et al. (1990) A primary prevention study of oral cancer among Indian villagers. Eight-year follow-up results. In: Hakama M, Beral V, Cullen JW, Parkin DM (eds) Evaluating the effectiveness of prevention of cancer. International Agency for Research on Cancer, Lyon, pp 149–156

Hakulinen T, Andersen AA, Maiker B, Pukkala E, Schou G, Tulinius H (1986) Trends in cancer incidence in the Nordic countries. Acta Pathol Scand [Suppl] 288:94

Hirayama T (1966) An epidemiological study of oral and pharyngeal cancer in Central and South-East Asia. Bull WHO 34:41–69

Huq SF (1965) Some aspects of site distribution of cancer in East Pakistan. J Pakistan Med Assoc 15:237–245

Indian Council of Medical Research (1989) National Cancer Registry of India. Annual report 1986. Indian Council of Medical Research, New Delhi

Indian Council of Medical Research (1990) National Cancer Registry of India. Annual report 1987. Indian Council of Medical Research, New Delhi

International Agency for Research on Cancer (1985) Tobacco habits other than smoking: betel-quid and areca-nut chewing; and some related nitrosamines. IARC Monogr Eval Carcinog Risk Chem Hum 37

International Agency for Research on Cancer (1986) Tobacco smoking. IARC Monogr Eval Carcinog Risk Chem Hum 38

Johnson NW (1990) Oro-facial neoplasms; global epidemiology. Risk factors and recommendations for research. International Dental Federation. FDI Tech Rep 36

Krolls SO, Hoffman S (1976) Squamous cell carcinoma of the oral soft tissues: a statistical analysis of 14253 cases by age, sex, and race. J Am Dent Assoc 92:571–574

Langdon JD, Harvey POW, Rapidis AD, Patel MF, Johnson NW, Hopps RM (1977) Oral cancer: the behavior and response to treatment of 194 cases. J Maxillofac Surg 5: 221–237

MacFarlane GJ, Boyle P, Scully C (1987) Rising mortality from the cancer of the tongue in young Scottish males. Lancet 2:912

Malaowalla AM, Silverman. S Jr, Mani NJ, Bilimoria KF, Smith LW (1976) Oral cancer in 57 518 industrial workers of Gujarat, India a prevalence and follow-up study. Cancer 37:1882–1886

Mehta FS, Aghi MB, Gupta PC et al. (1982) An intervention study of oral cancer and precancer in rural Indian populations: a preliminary report. Bull WHO 60:441–446

Mehta FS, Gupta PC, Bhonsle RB, Murti PR, Daftary DK, Pindborg JJ (1986) Detection of oral cancer using basic health workers in an area of high oral cancer incidence. Cancer Detect Prev 9:219–225

Mehta FS, Pindborg JJ, Hamner JE III et al. (1971) Report on investigations of oral cancer and precancerous conditions in Indian rural populations, 1966–1969. Munksgaard, Copenhagen

Moller H (1989) Changing incidence of cancer of the tongue, oral cavity, and pharynx in Denmark. J Oral Pathol Med 18:224–229

Murti PR, Bhonsle RB, Pindborg JJ et al. (1985) Malignant transformation rate in oral submucous fibrosis over a 17-year period. Community Dent Oral Epidemiol 13:340–341

Murti PR, Bhonsle RB, Daftary DK et al. (1986) Malignant potential of oral lichen planus: observations in 722 patients from India. J Oral Pathol 15:71–77

Parkin DM, Stejernsward J, Muir CS (1984) Estimates of worldwide frequency of twelve major cancers. Bull WHO 62:163–182

Paymaster JC (1962) Some observations on oral and pharyngeal carcinomas in the State of Bombay. Cancer 15:578–583

Pindborg JJ (1980) Oral cancer and precancer. Wright, Bristol
Piyaratn P (1959) Relative incidence of malignant neoplasms in Thailand. Cancer 12:693–696
Shafer WG, Waldron CA (1975) Erythroplakia of the oral cavity. Cancer 36:1021–1028
Spiro RH, Alfonso AE, Farr H, Strong EW (1974) Cervical node metastasis from epidermoid carcinoma of the oral cavity and oropharynx. Am J Surg 126:562–567
US Department of Health and Human Services (1986) Health implications of smokeless tobacco use. National Institutes of Health, Washington (Consensus Development Conference Statement 6)
US Department of Health and Human Services (1989) Reducing the health consequences of smoking – 25 years of progress: a report of the surgeon general. US Department of Health and Human Services, Washington (DHHS publication no (CDC) 89–8411)
US Public Health Services (1986) The health consequences of using smokeless tobacco. A report of the surgeon general. US Department of Health and Human Services, Washington (NIH publication no 86–874)
Wahi PN, Lahiri B, Kehar U, Arora S (1965) Oral and oropharyngeal cancer in North India. Br J Cancer 19:627–641
Waterhouse J, Muir CS, Shanmugaratnam K, Powel J (eds) (1982) Cancer incidence in five continents, vol 4. International Agency for Research on Cancer, Lyon
WHO Collaborating Reference Center for Oral Precancerous Lesions (1978) Definition of leukoplakia and related lesions: an aid to studies in precancer. Oral Surg 46:517–539
World Health Organization (1984) Control of oral cancer in developing countries. A World Health Organization meeting. Bull WHO 62:817–830
Zaidi SHM, Jafarey NA, Aizaz Ali S (1974) Cancer trends in Karachi. J Pakistan Med Assoc J 24:84–93

Esophageal Cancer:
Problems and Challenges in Early Detection

P.B. DESAI

Introduction

Cancer of the esophagus is a distressing disease to treat as most patients present late and the overall results are poor worldwide, save a very few stray series published (Akiyama et al. 1981, Mathisen et al. 1988). There is little doubt that apart from the generally rapid spread of this cancer, due to the rich lymphatic plexus within the organ and its ramifications in the thorax, abdomen, and neck, the poor results are due to a delayed diagnosis as the disease is asymptomatic in its early stages. Results collected for early T1N0M0 cases show impressive cure rates ranging from 50% to 80% (Yamashita et al. 1972). This clearly indicates that inherently squamous cell carcinoma of the esophagus is not a biologically lethal disease and that concerted attempts to make an early diagnosis may be worthwhile in selected settings.

Esophageal cancer has a distinctive geographic pathology. The incidence is among the highest (165–195 per 100000) (IARC 1988, Dey et al. 1982) in the world around the region of the Caspian Sea in Iran, in the Transkei region of South Africa, and along a belt which extends eastward from Iran into Mongolia and eastwards towards the Linxian areas of China in the northern provinces. Isolated pockets of high incidence in blacks around the Bay region of San Fransisco is also noted (IARC 1988, Dey et al. 1982). In the subcontinent of India it is the third most common cancer in women after that of the uterine cervix and breast (IARC 1988, Dey et al. 1982).

Etiological factors relate to tobacco smoking and chewing in India and deficiency of nutrition and trace elements (vitamin A, zinc, magnesium, and other unknown factors).

Table 1. Correctness of cytologic and tissue diagnosis by endoscopy in esophageal cancer

	Tata Memorial Hospital (1986–1987)	Literature (%)
No. of cases	79	–
BX positive	86.5%	70
Cytology positive	88.1%	90
Both positive	97.0%	95

Premalignant conditions like submucous fibrosis and Plummer–Vinson syndrome in women often predispose them to postcricoid cancers. Hiatus hernia, peptic esophagitis, and Barrett's esophagus with a columnar-lined lower esophagus appear to have a predisposition to squamous neoplasia. Careful surveillance and cytological studies of the lower esophageal mucosa in these group of clinical conditions are therefore worthwhile as one could detect severe dysplasia which may undergo a neoplastic change. The incidence of such changes is reported to be around 5%–7% (Kobayashi and Kasugai 1978) over a period of 10–15 years.

Methods for Early Diagnosis

Cytologic Diagnosis

There is little doubt that cytologic interpretation of exfoliated cells is the method by which diagnosis could be reached in the earliest phase of the disease.

While there have been occasional reports (Winawer et al. 1975, Wu et al. 1982) in which very early diagnosis has been achieved, large scale studies are not found in the literature. This is mainly because most patients are asymptomatic at this stage of the disease, and there is a poor cost-benefit ratio for a survey of the normal population for esophageal cancer, unlike cervical cancer. Routine endoscopy of the normal population is not feasible even under the most affluent conditions.

Our own data indicate that the combination of cytology washings and brush cytology are effective in diagnosing esophageal cancer at very early stages, even when the mucosal changes are minimal and likely to be missed on endoscopy. While the majority of patients present late and pose no problem in diagnosis by routine imaging employing barium swallow and endoscopy, the combination of good endoscopy and cytologic studies yield a diagnostic rate in early and problematic cases up to 98% (Table 1).

Routine Cytology Screening for Esophageal Cancer – Is It Justifiable?

With our own data and that of the literature it is beyond question that cytology interpretation is the most accurate method we have today of diagnosing esophageal cancer at a preclinical stage; however, the routine use of this method as, for example, in the case of uterine cervix cancer diagnosis is neither feasible nor justified. Esophageal cancer is a rare disease except along a particular geographic belt and in the subcontinent of India and parts of South Africa. Early diagnosis by whatever method in these regions may be justified owing to the almost endemic or epidemic proportions the disease has in these regions. A clinical trial in such endemic areas can be considered feasible under the following conditions: A time-bound, well-planned study with adequate statistical support which includes a control group under the aegis of a regional center and supported by national and international study/research groups in an area in which the incidence of esophageal cancer is very high.

No large, well-planned, and controlled study is available in the current literature, although sporadic reports of such studies have been documented.

Routine screening with endoscopy/cytologic studies would therefore be worthwhile in patients with:

1. Chronic esophagitis (reflux esophagitis, hiatus hernia, benign strictures) particularly where there is evidence of dysplasia or atypia of the epithelium. A significant number of these patients undergo a neoplastic change after 10–15 years, and attempts at early diagnosis in this group are entirely feasible and justifiable.
2. Symptomatic patients with heart burn, retrosternal burning, and dysphagia-like symptoms which are often vague.

A rational and multicenter study in a country like India with appropriate planning would be worthwhile in high-risk areas and with a high-risk population.

Imaging Techniques

The advent of modern imaging techniques (CT, MRI, endoscopic ultrasound) does not preclude the importance of a conventional esophagogram for the diagnosis of early esophageal cancer; indeed, modern techniques does not contribute significantly to early diagnosis. While cytology and expert endoscopy are certainly superior in establishing a very early diagnosis, a well done barium swallow with air contrast studies in patients with vague retrosternal symptoms, reflux esophagitis, etc. may reveal cancer limited to the mucosa of the esophagus with minimum mucosal disruption. In many parts of the developing world where esophageal cancer is common and expert cytology and endoscopy are not easily available, this conventional method of diagnosis cannot be totally disregarded; as mentioned earlier, the accuracy of diagnosis with endoscopy, barium swallow, and cytology reaches as high as 98% even for early esophageal cancer.

Endoscopy

The advent of flexible fiberoptic endoscopy has enabled more and more mucosal (T1) lesions to be diagnosed. Complemented with cytology via brushings and washings, the current expertise has reached a very high level of accuracy. Very early mucosal lesions are sometimes difficult to delineate even with endoscopy; nonetheless, they can be diagnosed on accurate cytologic interpretation. These patients undergo total esophagectomy, and the lesion in the operative specimen is discovered only with a negative reaction to Lugol's iodine stain. The cure rates of such lesions in some series as have been reported to be

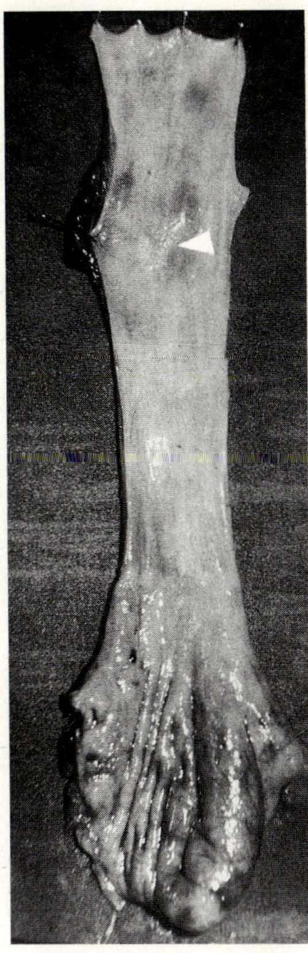

Fig. 1. Operative specimen of total esophagectomy diagnosed by cytology. Preoperative biopsy was inconclusive. The lesion could be identified by a negative staining with Lugol's iodine

upwards of 50% at 5 years. Figure 1 shows one of our patients diagnosed by endoscopy and cytology of esophageal washings. The patient had a negative biopsy result, and it was possible to delineate the lesion in the operative specimen only after Lugol's staining and studying the histology subsequently. The importance of such studies in a high-risk and high-incidence endemic area of esophageal cancers cannot be overemphasized.

Endoscopic Ultrasound for Delineation of Paraesophageal Disease Extension into the Tissues and Lymph Nodes

While not totally relevant to the symposium subject on early diagnosis of esophageal cancer, the advent of ultrasound within the tip of the endoscope has enabled the paraesophageal tissues to be delineated in the mediastinum and para-esophageal nodal disease to be recognized with appropriate echogenic areas. While it adds to our diagnostic technology for obtaining a total disease profile and may help in planning appropriate therapeutic strategy, it has no value in the diagnosis of early esophageal cancer.

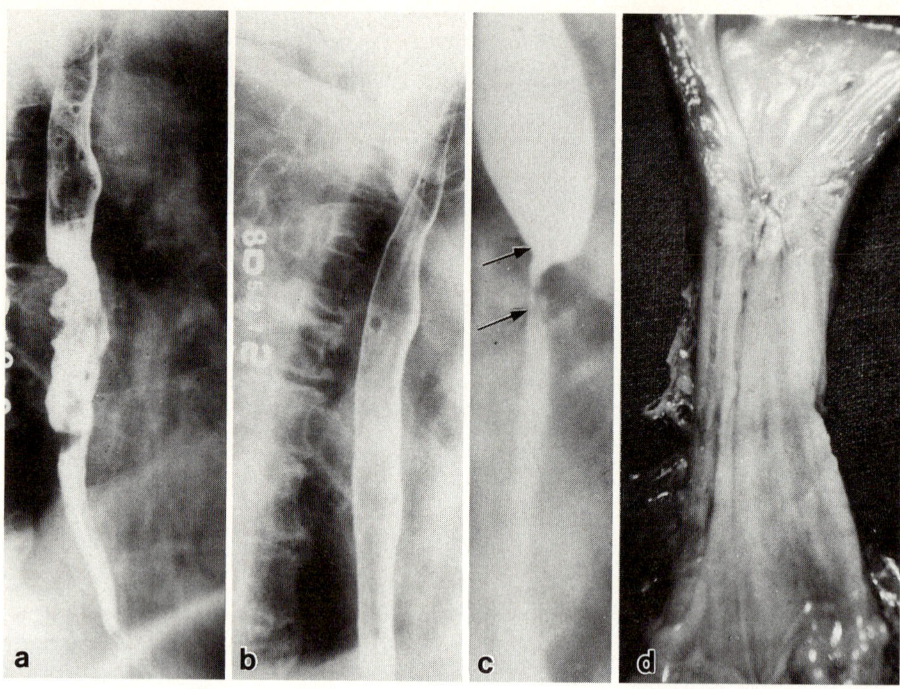

Fig. 2a–d. Pretreatment assessment by endoscopy and barium swallow gives a very good idea of treatment response. **a, b** A large lesions which is proliferative and responds extremely well to radiotherapy/chemotherapy; **c, d** A small lesion which is stenotic and infiltrating and does not respond to radiotherapy/chemotherapy. Operative specimen shows extreme cicatrisation and active cancer after full radiotherapy 4 months ago. This lesion should have had surgery ab initio. Morphologic characteristics of a lesion give a good clinical indication as regards early appropriate therapy which is as important as early diagnosis

In a similar way, the appropriate and early endoscopic diagnosis of the morphology and type of esophageal cancer also helps in planning appropriate initial treatment. Ulcerative and stenotic lesions are best treated early with a surgical approach, while bulky, often noninfiltrative, proliferative lesions, are best treated by radiotherapy and/or chemotherapy to begin with, adding surgical excision as and when needed. Two major morphologic types of esophageal cancers can be identified, ulcerative and proliferative, with many mixed varieties like ulcero-proliferative, nodular-ulcerative, etc. Treatment responses can be predicted by appropriate roentgen and endoscopic evaluations (Fig. 2).

Laboratory Techniques

The current renaissance and studies of the biological approaches to cancer diagnosis and treatment have opened up new inroads in early diagnosis. In the Division of Laboratory Medicine at the Tata Memorial Hospital, which acts as

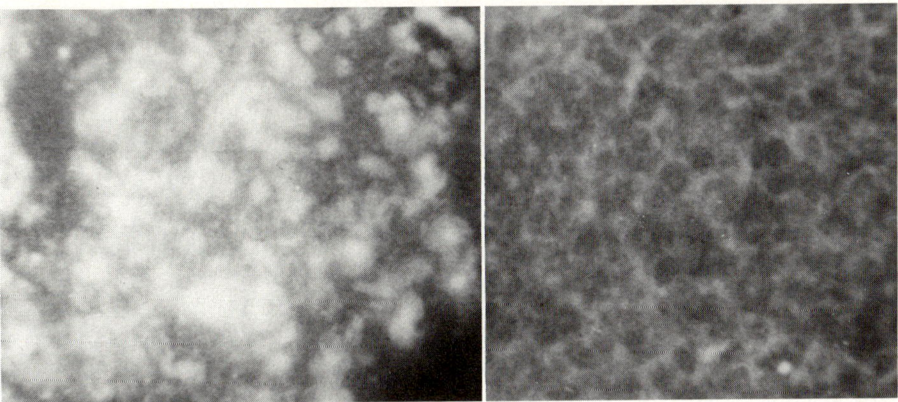

Fig. 3. Immunofluroscence reactivity with 2G3 antibody on a frozen tissue section of esophageal cancer and control (Personal communication)

Table 2. Monoclonal antibody 2G3 tested for reactivity against various established cell lines (Personal communication)

Cancer cell line	Human origin	Immunofluorescence	IP
TE2	Esophagus	+++	+++
T24	Bladder	−	−
HeLa	Cervix	−	−
Sw262	Ovary	−	−
SK-LJ-1	Lung	−	−
HT29	Colon	−	−
Caki-1	Skin	−	−
SAOS-2	Osteogenic sarcoma	−	−
B6Fs	Fibrosarcoma	−	−
IM9	Lymphoma	−	−
RaJI	Burkitt's lymphoma	−	−
HEL	Erythroleukemia	−	−
K562	Erythroleukemia	−	−
CEM	T-all	−	−
Nalm2	B cell line	−	−
T47D	Breast	−	−
ZR75B	Breast	−	−
MC17	Breast	++	++
Drew-B	Breast	−	−
MDA	Breast	−	−
NB2	Rat lymphoma	−	−

an interface between the clinical and theoretical aspects of cancer research, monoclonal antibodies against esophageal cancer have been raised by using the 2G3 antibody, which displays a significant specificity and sensitivity for esophageal cancers in a controlled comparison with a large number of solid tumors studied; mild to moderate reactivity was shown in a few patients with breast cancer (Fig. 3, Table 2; Personal communication).

A specific antigen on an esophageal cancer cell may help not only in raising a specific antibody against esophageal cancer but also in the early laboratory diagnosis of esophageal cancer in a high-risk community; it may also be utilised for targeted drug therapy by tagging the anticancer agent with the specific antibody. These are probable areas of laboratory research in the coming years.

Summary

Esophageal cancer is generally diagnosed late all over the world, save for a very few instances in places where the disease is endemic, and intensive endoscopic/cytology studies have been carried out with a specific aim of an early diagnosis. To date, endoscopy and cytology studies of suspect areas and premalignant lesions of the esophagus remain the only hope for early diagnosis and start of effective therapy for a potentially lethal disease. It is unlikely that the successful experience with cervical cytology for cervix cancer can be repeated for esophageal cancer, due to the logistics and expenditure involved in surveying even a high-risk population by endoscopy, although this may be the only option currently available. Concerted efforts in this direction for screening at least the high-risk populations need to be considered and discussed. Laboratory methods of early detection by raising monoclonal antibodies against esophageal cancer are still in a very preliminary stage and will take quite a while before any breakthrough can be expected for the control and cure of one of the most lethal forms of cancer.

References

Akiyama H, Tsurumuru M, Kawamara T (1981) Principles of surgical treatment for carcinoma of the esophagus: analysis of lymph node involvement. Ann Surg 194:438–446

Day NE, Munoz N (1982) Esophagus. In: Schottenfeld D, Fraumeni JF (eds) Cancer epidemiology and prevention. Saunders, Philadelphia, pp 596–623

International Agency for Research on Cancer (1988) Cancer incidence in five continents, vol 5. IARC, Lyon

Kobayashi S, Kasugai T (1978) Brushing cytology for the diagnosis of gastric cancer involving the cardia of the lower esophagus. Acta Cytol 22:155

Mathisen DJ, Grillo HC, Wilkins EW et al. (1988) Transthoracic esophagectomy: a safe approach to carcinoma of the esophagus. Ann Thorac Surg 45:137–143

Nadkarni JS, Waingankar PR (1991) Personal communication

Winawer SJ, Sherlock P, Belladona JA et al. (1975) Endoscopic brush cytology in esophageal cancer. JAMA 232:1358

Wu YK, Huang GJ, Shao LF et al. (1982) Progress in the study and surgical treatment of cancer of the esophagus in China. J Thorac Cardiovasc Surg 84:325

Yamashita H, Okura J, Yoshioka T, Tanaka Y (1972) Pre-operative irradiation in treatment of cancer of the esophagus. Aust Radiol 16:250

Early Detection of Gastrointestinal Cancers: Recent Progress in Endoscopy and Surgical Results

S. Yoshida, M. Sasako, H. Kato, and N. Moriya

Introduction

Because Japan is a country with a very high risk of gastric cancer, its early detection has been a leading, nationwide project of cancer control. As a result, early diagnosis, particularly that achieved by endoscopy, has developed during the past 3 decades with the extension of a radiographic mass survey. Nowadays, early gastric cancer (EGC) is seen regularly in daily clinical practice (Sakita 1983). The diagnostic advance with EGC also encouraged Japanese endoscopists to detect cases of early cancer in the esophagus and the large intestine. This investigation assesses the efficacy of the anticancer strategy of early detection and early treatment by examining the chronological trend in the diagnostic and surgical results on GI malignancies treated at the National Cancer Center Hospital.

Subjects and Methods

During the period between 1962 and 1989, 5991 patients with gastric, 1113 with esophageal, and 2416 with colorectal cancers had been surgically treated at the National Cancer Center Hospital. These 9520 cases were selected as the subjects of this study. The incidence of early or superficial cancer, the 5-year survival rate as calculated by the Kaplan-Meier method, and their endoscopic appearance were examined chronologically. Early gastric and colorectal cancers were defined as a lesion with invasion limited to the submucosal layer, according to the proposal by the Japanese Gastroenterological Endoscopy Society and the Japanese Research Society of Colorectal Cancer, respectively. As for the esophagus, superficial cancer was defined as a lesion with invasion limited to the submucosal layer and early cancer, as the superficial form without lymph node metastasis, according to the proposal by the Japanese Society for Esophageal Disease.

When the incidence of early cancer or the survival rate were examined chronologically, the period between 1962 and 1989 could be divided into five terms as follows: first (1962–1969), second (1970–1974), third (1975–1979), fourth (1980–1984), and fifth (1985–1989).

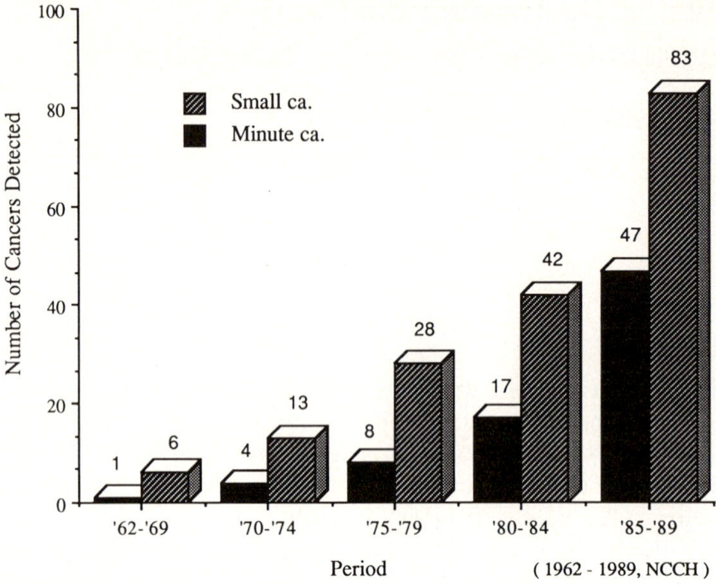

Fig. 1. Number of minute and small gastric cancers (ca.) detected

Table 1. Chronological trend in gastric cancer: incidence of early cancer and 5-year survival rate

Period	No. of cases	Incidence of early cancer (n)	Five-year survival rate (%)
1962–1969	1628	22% (358)	42
1970–1974	1020	32% (325)	56
1975–1979	967	34% (330)	58
1980–1984	1165	43% (502)	65
1985–1989	1211	53% (639)	71

Source of data: National Cancer Center Hospital, Tokyo.

Results

Gastric Cancer

Table 1 shows the incidence of EGC and the 5-year survival rate examined chronologically. The survival rate improved remarkably in recent years proportional to the increase in incidence of EGC, and during the fifth term, the incidence of EGC reached 53% (639/1211), and the 5-year survival rate was calculated as 71%.

Figure 1 shows the chronological trend in number of small and minute gastric cancers detected preoperatively. According to Japanese general under-

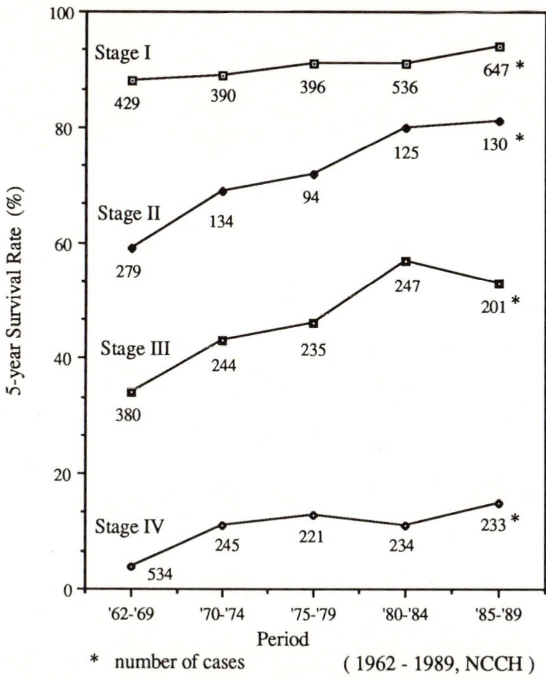

Fig. 2. Chronological trend in 5-year survival rate by stage of gastric cancer

standing, small cancer is defined as cancerous lesions ranging from 6 to 10 mm in size, and the minute one as those less than 5 mm in size. Both types increased in number year by year, and compared with the fourth term, the number of minute cancer cases rapidly increased from 17 to 47 and of the small one from 42 to 83 during the fifth term.

The chronological trend of the 5-year survival rate by stage of gastric cancer is shown in Fig. 2. The 5-year survival rate steadily improved year by year for every stage, except for stage III in 1985–1989, which decreased slightly.

The endoscopic appearance of EGC has also changed over time as shown in Fig. 3, in which EGC was subclassified endoscopically into the following four types: polypoid, ulcerative, gastritis-like, and advanced. The polypoid type is defined as EGC showing protrusion, the ulcerative one as showing ulceration and/or converging folds, the gastritis-like one as showing a superficial, non-ulcerative appearance, and the advanced one as those misdiagnosed as definite advanced cancer preoperatively. The proportion of the gastritis-like type had been increasing since 1980, and it reached 30%–40% during the past 3 years.

Esophageal Cancer

Table 2 shows the incidence of superficial cancer and 5-year survival rate for esophageal cancer examined chronologically. While the incidence of superficial

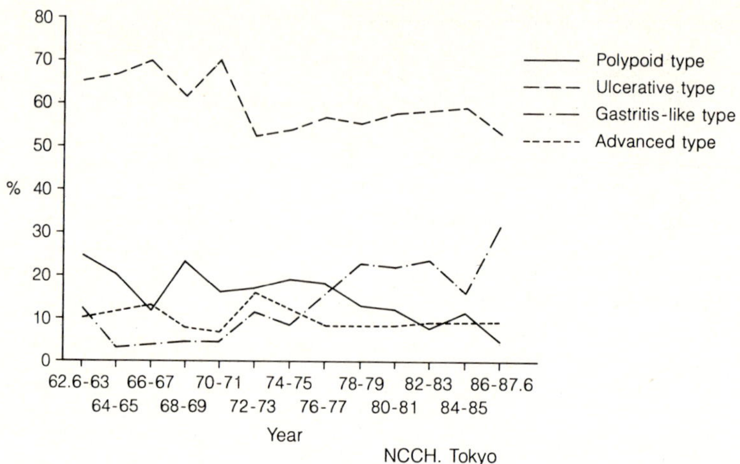

Fig. 3. Chronological trend in endoscopic appearance of early gastric cancer

Table 2. Chronological trend in esophageal cancer: incidence of superficial cancer and 5-year survival rate

Period	No. of cases	Incidence of early cancer (n)	Five-year survival rate (%)
1962–1969	161	8% (12)	17
1970–1974	158	4% (7)	21
1975–1979	191	7% (13)	18
1980–1984	207	14% (28)	23
1985–1989	257	28% (73)	33

Source of data: National Cancer Center Hospital, Tokyo.

cancer was less than 10% during the early period (up to 1979), it increased to 14% (28/207) in the fourth term and to 28% (73/257) in the last term. The 5-year survival rate improved in recent years in proportion to the increase in incidence of superficial cancer, and it reached 33% in the fifth term. The incidence of epithelial and mucosal cancers among the superficial ones is shown chronologically in Table 3. It was 38% (28/73) in the cases detected during the fifth term, whereas it was very low (0%–14%) before 1984. In other words, 82% (28/34) of the epithelial and mucosal cancers was detected during this last term.

Colorectal Cancer

Table 4 shows the incidence of early cancer and the 5-year survival rate of colorectal cancer in each term. Whereas the former had been only 5% during the first term, it increased to 12% during the third and fourth terms and then

Table 3. Chronological trend in epithelial and superficial cancers of the esophagus

Period	No. of superficial ca.	No. of epithelial ca.	Incidence (epith./super.) [%]
1962–1969	12	0	0
1970–1974	7	1	14
1975–1979	13	1	8
1980–1984	28	4	14
1985–1989	73	28	38

Source of data: National Cancer Center Hospital, Tokyo.

Table 4. Chronological trend in colorectal cancer: incidence of early cancer and 5-year survival rate

Period	No. of cases	Incidence of early cancer (n)	Five-year survival rate (%)
1962–1969	357	5% (18)	38
1970–1974	281	10% (28)	51
1975–1979	372	12% (46)	60
1980–1984	570	12% (68)	66
1985–1989	836	17% (142)	67

Source of data: National Cancer Center Hospital, Tokyo.

17% during the last term. The number of early cancer lesions steadily increased throughout these five terms, and its rapid increase during the last 5 years (from 68 cases in the fourth term to 142 cases) is noteworthy. The 5-year survival rate which had been only 38% during the first term, improved year by year in proportion to the increase in incidence of early cancer and became stable at 66%–67% during the fourth and fifth terms.

The chronological trend of the 5-year survival rate by stage of cancer is shown in Fig. 4. The survival rate evidently improved year by year, except for stage I, as about 90% of these cases always survived. Compared with those detected during the first term, the survival rate rose from 60% to 80% with stage II lesions and from 27% to 65% with stage III lesions during the last term.

Discussion

It is not too much to say that early detection in Japan started with the proposal of the definition and endoscopic classification of EGC made by the Japanese Digestive Endoscopy Society in 1962 (Yoshida et al. 1981). In those days, most EGC was identified from the differential diagnosis of ulcerated (type III) or polypoid (type I) lesions, which are easily detected. In the 1970s, early diagnosis progressed, and it became possible to detect an EGC lesion with the

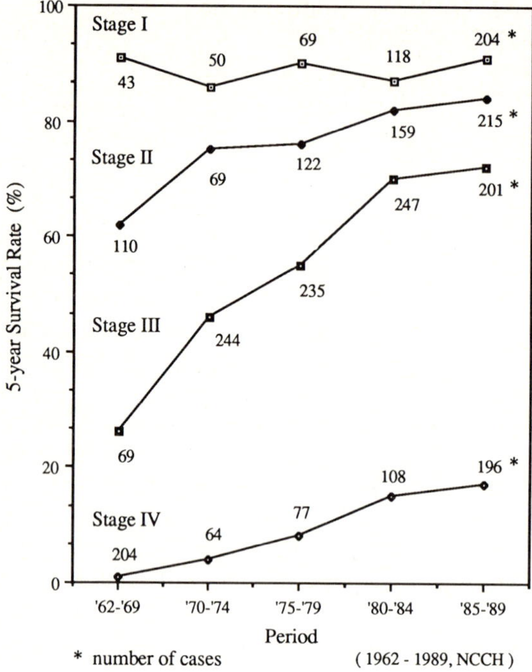

Fig. 4. Chronological trend in 5-year survival rate by stage of colorectal cancer

appearance of an ulcer scar (type IIc) or plateaulike elevation (type IIa). With this advance, early detection of gastric cancer seemed to be mostly complete. In the 1980s, however, retrospective studies of advanced cancer revealed that gastritis-like lesions which could not be diagnosed as malignant by conventional endoscopic criteria rapidly grew into tumorous advanced cancers, indicating the importance of the differential diagnosis of superficial, nonulcerative malignancy (IIb-like type), seen as faint redness, discoloration, and/or unevenness of the gastric mucosa endoscopically (Yoshida et al. 1981). Consequently, nonulcerative and nonpolypoid EGC, namely the gastritis-like type (Yoshida et al. 1984), has increased in incidence during the last decade, and it corresponds now to 30%–40% of EGC diagnosed at the NCCH each year. For diagnosing gastritis-like malignancy, precise endoscopic observation and adequate biopsy are required, and this led to the remarkable increase of detection of minute cancer (less than 5 mm in size).

The diagnostic findings of EGC were firstly applied to the early detection of esophageal and colorectal cancers, because they occur less frequently in Japan. With these cancers, however, "ulcerative cancer" is very rare in the early stage, and mainly polypoid lesions were examined, particularly in the case of colorectal cancer. In the latter half of the 1970s, dye-spraying endoscopy using Lugol's solution (iodine staining; Schiller's test) (Brodmerkel 1971) was applied in cancer detection in Japan, and its diagnostic utility was confirmed for superficial esophageal cancers, which are seen as an unstained area, whose original findings were said to be a faint mucosal irregularity (unevenness) with erythematous or discolored change (Kouzu et al. 1987). With the diffusion of both panendoscopy (esophago-gastro-duodenoscopy) and precise endoscopy revealing the faint mucosal irregularity with the use of iodine staining, superficial esophageal cancers, particularly those with shallow invasion as in epithelial or mucosal cancer, remarkably increased in number during the latter half of the 1980s.

In colorectal cancers, the increase in incidence of early cancer and in 5-year survival rate recently was not so noteworthy as in gastric or esophageal cancer cases, whereas the 5-year survival rate of patients with an advanced stage lesion (stages II, III, and IV) has markedly improved year by year. This may suggest that the early detection of colorectal cancers is still insufficient, even today, whereas the preoperative diagnosis of cancer extension (staging of the disease) has markedly progressed by using computed tomography (CT) and ultrasonography (US) in recent years. A couple of years ago, early invasive cancers of the superficial depressed or flat type began to attract the attention of Japanese endoscopists. These hardly fit the polyp cancer sequence theory by Morson and Dawson (1972), because of their macroscopic appearance and lack of an adenomatous component. Without precise endoscopy they could not be diagnosed, because most of them are small (less than 1 cm) and endoscopically show only a faint, spotty, mucosal irregularity, such as erythematous change, discoloration, and/or slight mucosal deformity (Kudo et al. 1990). Although this new type of early colorectal cancer is not widespread, with less than 100 cases currently in Japan, the number of cases reported certainly increases every year, and the diagnostic progress by precise endoscopy is expected to provide survival benefit in the near future.

In spite of the imperfection of early diagnosis, the results obtained so far indicate the efficacy of an anticancer strategy of early detection and early treatment. Watanabe et al. (1988) statistically examined the data of cancer registration in Japan and found that the discrepancy between incidence and mortality of gastric cancer has markedly increased since 1980, regardless of sex. He and his group estimated that in the twenty-first century in Japan, most gastric cancer patients will not die of the gastric cancer itself. This should be a fruit of the recent progress in early detection.

To make early detection of GI malignancy more accurate, precise endoscopy, particularly aiming at detection of the faint mucosal irregularity, is indispensable, regardless of which organ is involved. The differentiation of mucosal irregularity, however, has a tendency to become more subjective and empirical than that of ulcerative or polypoid lesions. Videoimage endoscopy, in which the optical image is changed into quantitative electronic signals corresponding to color values of red, green, and blue by charged coupled device is expected to become available to make endoscopic diagnosis more objective (Kawai et al. 1988). In the future, the quantification of color and size observed in videoimage endoscopy will make it possible to provide a new objective diagnostic procedure of endoscopy for detecting early cancer.

Summary

The efficacy of the anticancer strategy of early detection and early treatment was assessed in surgical cases of gastrointestinal (GI) malignancies treated at the National Cancer Center Hospital during the period between 1962 and 1989. In the 5991 cases of gastric cancers, the 5-year survival rate was markedly improved recently in proportion to the increase in the incidence of early cancer. In the 1211 cases operated during the latest period of 1985–1989, the incidence of early cancer reached 53% (639/1211), and the 5-year survival rate was calculated as 71% by the Kaplan-Meier method. The progress of early diagnosis could be also evaluated from the remarkable increase in number of small (6–10 mm) and minute (less than 5 mm in diameter) cancers and "gastritis-like" (nonulcerative and nonpolypoid) type of early cancer detected, using precise endoscopy to find a faint mucosal irregularity with discoloration, slight redness, and/or unevenness of its surface structure. An increase in the 5-year survival rate was observed in the recent cases regardless of the stage of the cancer, indicating the progress of early diagnosis in detecting less invasive cancers with a better prognosis.

For the 1113 cases of esophageal and 2416 cases of colorectal cancer, the results obtained were mostly the same as those from gastric cancer, that is to say, an increase in number and incidence of superficial or early cancer detected and in the 5-year survival rate, particularly recently. Malignancy can be confirmed in a faint mucosal irregularity by cancer-specific dye-spraying endoscopy (iodine staining).

With colorectal cancers, the rise in incidence of early cancer and in 5-year survival rate was not so remarkable in those patients surgically treated during the past decade, whereas the 5-year survival rate of those with advanced stage disease (stages II, III, and IV) has increased year by year. A couple of years ago, early cancer of superficial depressed or flat type attracted the attention of Japanese endoscopists. These hardly fit the polyp cancer sequence theory because of their macroscopic appearance and lack of an adenomatous component. They can be diagnosed only by precise endoscopy detecting a shallow depression, discoloration, and/or mucosal deformity.

The recent progress of early detection apparently provides a survival benefit to the GI cancer patients.

References

Brodmerkel GT Jr (1971) Schiller's test, an aid in esophagoscopic diagnosis (Abstr). Gastroenterology 60:813

Kawai M, Yamaguchi Y, Yoshida S, Saito D, Tajiri H, Hijikata A, Miyamoto K, Mukai T, Fujii T, Yamaguchi N, Okazaki H, Tsugiki M, Ishii K, Yoshimori M, Oguro Y (1988) Application of electronic endoscope to colorimeter; an evaluation of clinical utilities (in Japanese). Progress of Digest. Endoscopy 32:69–72

Kouzu T, Yamada H, Onoda S, Isono K (1987) Value of Lugol staining method in diagnosing superficial esophageal cancer (in Japanese). Stomach Intestine 22:1395–1401

Kudo S, Miura K, Takano Y, Bannai H (1990) Detection of colorectal minute cancer (in Japanese). Stomach Intestine 25:801–812

Morson BC, Dawson IMP (1972) The polyp-cancer sequence. In: Morson BC, Dawson IMP (eds) Gastrointestinal pathology. Blackwell, Oxford, pp 542–547

Sakita T (1983) Gastric cancer in Japan – data from the nationwide questionnaire (in Japanese). Gastroenterol Endosc 25:317–343

Watanabe S, Tsugane S, Ohno Y (1988) Prediction of the gastric cancer mortality in 2000 in Japan. Jpn J Cancer Res 79:439–444

Yoshida S, Yoshimori M, Hirashima T, Yamaguchi H, Tajiri H, Nakamura K, Oguro Y, Hirota T (1981) Nonulcerative lesion detected by endoscopy as an early expression of gastric malignancy. Jpn J Clin Oncol 11:493–506

Yoshida S, Yamaguchi Y, Tajiri H, Saito D, Hijikata A, Yoshimori M, Oguro Y, Hirota T (1984) Diagnosis of early gastric cancer seen as less malignant endoscopically. Jpn J Clin Oncol 14:225–241

Detection of Minimal Disease in Hematological Malignancies

W. Wilmanns, H.H. Gerhartz, H. Schmetzer, V. Nüssler, H. Sauer, and C. Clemm

Introduction

Many patients with acute leukemias can be brought into "complete remission" (CR) – a status in which the disease is clinically and morphologically unapparent – by intensive chemotherapy. Nevertheless, the majority ultimately relapse. A method to monitor the residual malignant cell burden would allow the early detection of imminent relapse and thus might influence therapeutic concepts by allowing a response-adapted treatment, bone marrow transplantation included.

Early Detection of Relapse in Acute Myeloid Leukemia

In acute myeloid leukemia (AML) it is possible to demonstrate a myeloid differentiation capacity of blasts by marker studies (Griffin et al. 1983) and by cloning the cells in semisolid media under the influence of colony-stimulating factor (CSF) (Spitzer et al. 1976). Some acute lymphoblastic leukemias are able to express myeloid markers, too (Sobol et al. 1987). Such in vitro culture procedures have some important advantages:

- They measure proliferation, a functional capability of the biologically most important cells
- They are clonal
- They may be much more sensitive than cytological and immunological methods
- Leukemic clones have been found in acute lymphoblastic leukemia (ALL) in some patients who were clinically in "complete remission" (Estrow et al. 1986)

The distinction of normal and leukemic in vitro clones, however, is a problem because both types of progenitors respond, at least partially, to the same growth factors (Vellenga et al. 1987). Cytogenetic methods, e.g., karyotypic analysis, are more precise, but, though applicable to single colony analysis (Dube et al. 1981), they are too time-intensive for routine clinical screening.

We investigated whether normal colonies and leukemic clones are distinguishable by surface markers. Characteristic differences might help to detect even low numbers of residual leukemic clones in remission. For this purpose a method which allowed the analysis of differentiation markers on hundreds of clones in situ was developed by Schmetzer and Gerhartz (1987).

Principals of Methods

Three sources were used for morphological and surface marker analysis:

1. Uncultured bone marrow mononuclear cells (MNC)
2. Suspension cultures
3. Cultured clonogenic cells in agar plugs

After 7 days of culture and stimulation by placenta conditioned medium (PCM) and other sources of CSF, an immunophenotyping using different monoclonal antibodies (MoAb) in a first step and mouse-specific antibody-conjugated alkaline phosphatase in a second step by enzyme immunoassay (EIA) was performed. The suspended cells and the colonies on agar plugs could be stained and analysed cytologically at the same time. Thus, surface markers could be related to morphological phenotypes. The expression of antigens on the cells was affirmed by Western blot analysis.

In some cases cytogenetic anomalies and rearranged bands in Southern blots could be used as clonal markers and be related to the immunological characterization of cells and cultures.

Results

In accordance with other publications investigating surface marker expression of AML (Wouters and Löwenberg 1984), it could be shown that the progenitor cells of AML carry not only early myeloid markers, but also late differentiation antigens, which in most cases are increasingly expressed during culture with growth stimulating factors. Figure 1 gives results obtained with VIM D5 (CD15), a late myeloid differentiation marker (Knapp 1982). The majority of AML cells expressed this antigen to a subnormal degree with a high variability between individual patients. When cultured in vitro with PCM, 16 of 18 cases developed CD15-positive colonies, which demonstrate a partial differentiation in vitro; the relative frequency of CD15-positive clones was lower on average than in myeloid colonies grown from normal BM ($n = 13$). Thus, the CD15 marker is apparently not able to distinguish AML colonies from normal clones.

Different results were obtained with the My10 antibody (CD34, Fig. 2): All but 4 of the 18 AML patients had a 10% or more positive MNC in the bone marrow, whereas this was found in 5 of 13 normal controls only (white bars). The difference was much more evident when the proportion of positive clones was considered (black bars): 15 of 18 AML cases showed positive clones at a rate of 5%–50%, whereas virtually not a single positive colony was found in cultures of 13 normal control marrows. Thus, the My10 antibody appeared to be specific in staining AML clones.

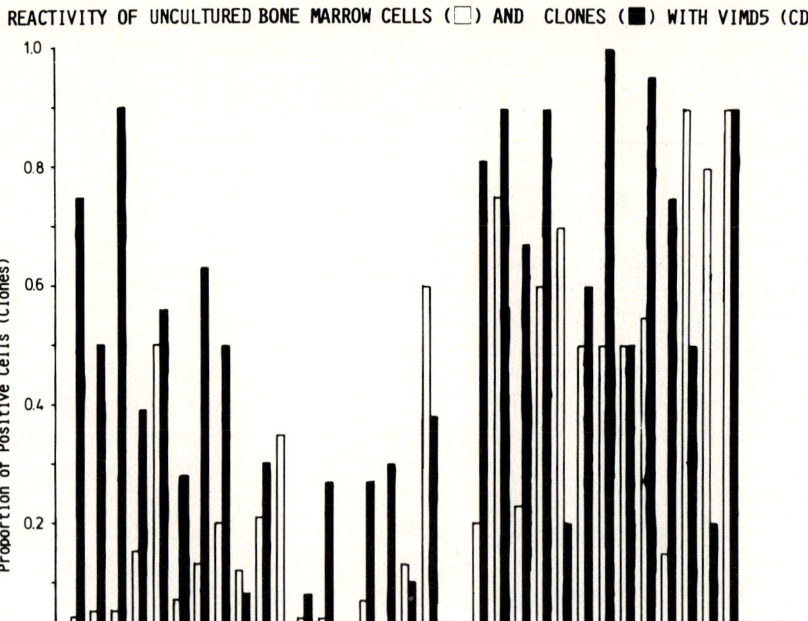

Fig. 1. Reactivity of acute myeloid leukemia (AML) cells and clones as compared with their normal counterparts with VIM D5 (CD15)

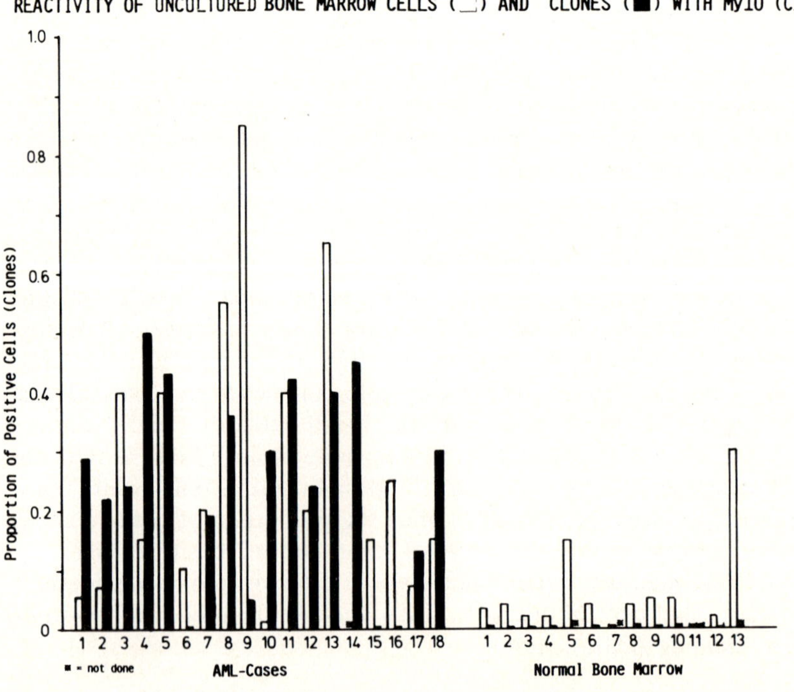

Fig. 2. Reactivity of cells and agar clones with My10 (CD34)

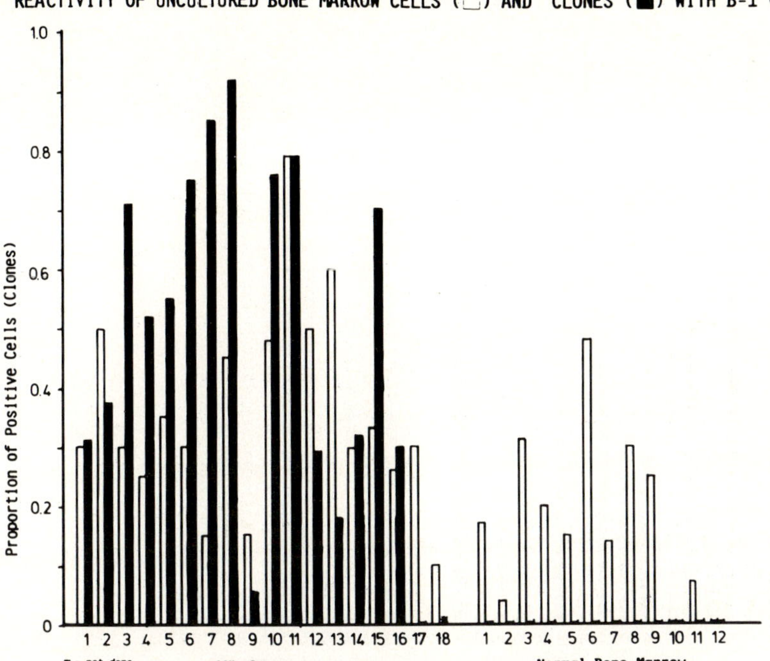

Fig. 3. Reactivity of fresh cells and agar clones with B1 (CD20)

It was an unexpected finding, however, that many AML cells and their clones expressed CD10 (J5) and CD20 (B1) (Fig. 3) determinants because these antigens are thought to be relatively specific for the lymphoid lineage (Nadler et al. 1981). This discrepancy might be explained by the fact that the EIA used in our study is more sensitive than the immunofluorescence methods commonly applied (Pesando et al. 1986). In addition, early lymphatic antigens like CD19 have recently been recognized on AML cells as well (Campos et al. 1987). The results described in Fig. 3 support the view that these antigens may be less lineage-specific as commonly thought and are a characteristic of blasts in general. As is shown in Fig. 3, all 18 AML cases had 10%–50% B1-positive MNC. In normal bone marrow the proportion of B1-positive cells varied between 0% and 48% (white bars). The difference of B1 expression was much more specific when the proportions of positive clones were considered (black bars): All but one of 17 AML cases tested had B1-positive, in vitro clones (5%–90% of all clones), whereas B1-positive clones were absent in all cultures of normal control bone marrow ($n = 12$). Obviously, the B1 antibody has good selectivity and specificity in distinguishing normal and AML clones in vitro. The expression of antigens on the cells was confirmed by Western blots.

An open question was, however, whether the CD15-positive clones in AML marrow originated from the leukemic progenitors or from residual normal stem cells. To investigate this problem, a double marker technique was

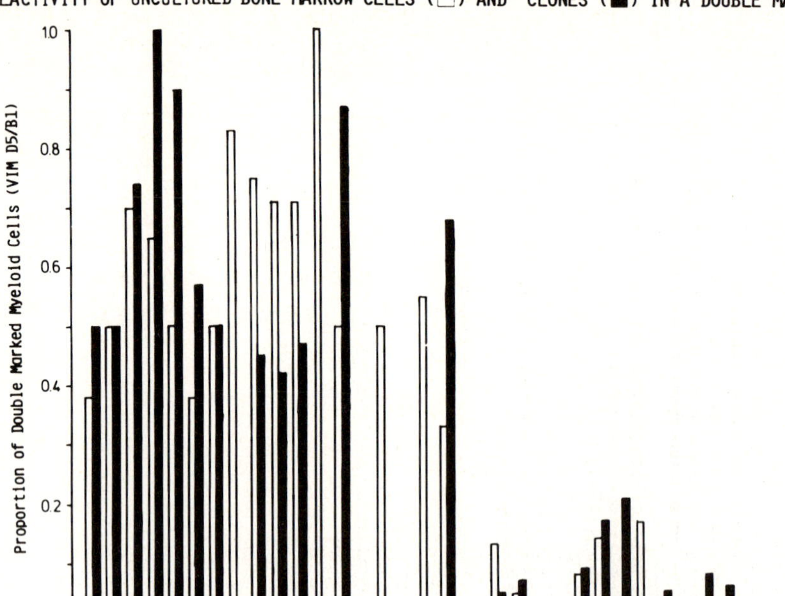

Fig. 4. Proportion of cells positive for VIM D5 (CD15) and B1 (CD20). White bars represent fresh cells, black bars represent cell cultures in suspension for 1 week in the presence of colony stimulating factor

developed which allowed the simultaneous detection of two antigens on the same cells using different color reagents (fast blue and fast red) for the alkaline phosphatase. Specificity of the assay was achieved by an interposed incubation with 2 N HCl which blocked the first enzyme completely. Thus, cells positive for the first antibody were blue, cells positive for the second marker stained red, and cells carrying both antigens could be clearly distinguished by their violet color. For methodological reasons, the double marker studies could be done only with single cell suspensions. By means of this method, it could be demonstrated that early and late differentiation markers were coexpressed on the majority of AML cells, whereas this was not the case in normal bone marrow.

This is shown in Fig. 4, demonstrating the proportions of VIM D5 (CD15)-positive cells which carried, in addition, the CD20 determinant (B1 antibody). In each individual case the respective values are given for uncultured cells (white bars) as well as for cells cultured in suspension in the presence of CSF (black bars). It is evident that all AML cases were characterized by a high degree of coexpression of both CD15 and CD20 determinants, whereas only very low numbers of normal bone marrow cells were stained by both antibodies. Similar results were obtained by analysis using the VIM D5 and J5 antibodies.

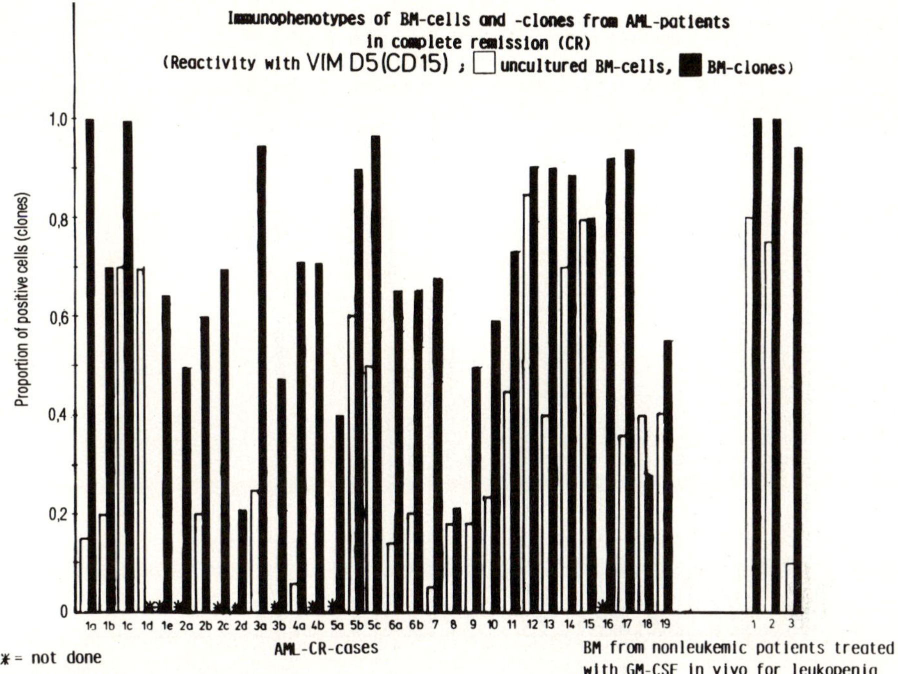

Fig. 5. Reactivity of bone marrow (BM) cells (*white bars*) and clones (*black bars*) with VIM D5 (CD15) of acute myeloid leukemia (AML) patients in complete remission ($n = 19$) as compared with three patients with regenerating normal hematopoiesis

Therefore, it can be concluded that the majority of bone marrow cells in AML expressing VIM D5 (CD15) originated from the leukemic clone. The observation that CD15 was increasingly expressed during culture with CSF demonstrated that AML progenitors can give rise to relatively differentiated myeloid cells. The differentiation capacity of these cells, however, is incomplete because the cells within leukemic colonies continue to express blast markers (CD10, CD20, CD34). It thus appears that the immunological characterization of leukemic clones grown in the presence of specific growth factors by the double marker technique described offers a more sensitive tool for investigating the differentiation capacity of transformed cells than cytological and immunological techniques alone. This approach is very sensitive in distinguishing normal and leukemic clones in culture (Gerhartz and Schmetzer 1988).

Studies During Remission

On the basis of the finding that My10 (CD34)- and B1 (CD20)-positive clones were detectable on AML cells only and not in normal bone marrow, the expression of these markers on colonies grown from 19 patients during complete clinical remission of the disease was studied. Several of these cases were

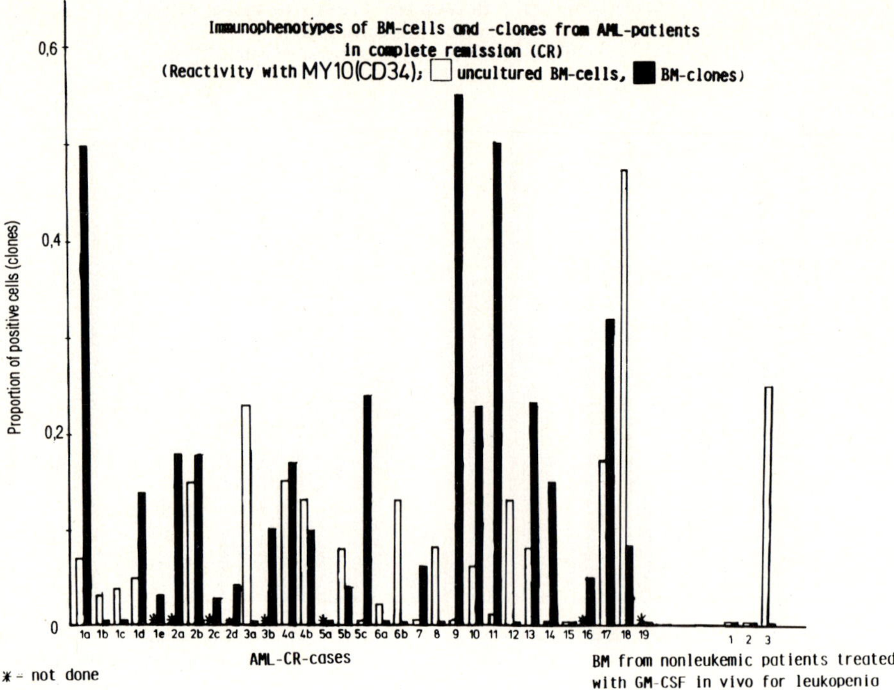

Fig. 6. Reactivity of bone marrow (BM) cells (*white bars*) and clones (*black bars*) of acute myeloid leukemia (AML) patients in complete remission with the My10 antibody (CD34) as compared with three patients with extensively regenerating normal myelopoiesis

investigated repeatedly. The number of clones obtained during complete remission of AML resembled that of normal controls with a plating efficiency of 20–100 (average 40) clones per 2×10^4 seeded MNC.

Figure 5 compares the proportion of VIM D5-positive bone marrow cells (white bars) and of positive agar clones (black bars) of AML patients in CR with those of three patients with carcinomas who received granulocyte macrophage CSF in vivo while recovering from chemotherapy-induced leukopenia. These patients had a heavily regenerating myelopoiesis and therefore were selected as a control with nonmalignant hematopoiesis. All AML cases in CR expressed VIM D5 in the majority of cells and clones. The degree of expression, however, in most patients was lower than in the controls, indicating an impaired myeloid differentiation capability.

Figure 6 gives a corresponding analysis with the My10 (CD34) antibody. It is evident that My10-positive cells were found in AML bone marrow in CR and the controls as well. My10-positive clones, however, were found in AML bone marrow cultures in CR (31 examinations) only at a proportion of 3%–55%.

Similar results were obtained with the antibody CD20 (Fig. 7). The proportion of B1-positive clones remained relatively stable in cases which were investigated repeatedly during the course of CR. These marker-positive clones were

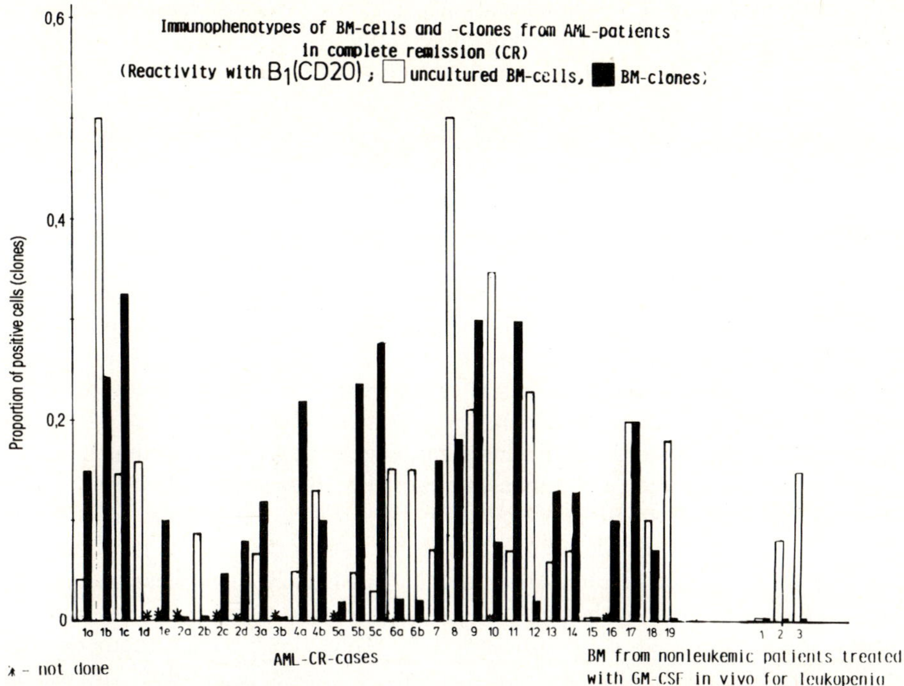

Fig. 7. Reactivity of bone marrow (BM) cells (*white bars*) and clones (*black bars*) using the B1 antibody (CD20) in acute myeloid leukemia (AML) patients in complete remission (*n* = 19) and three controls. *Numbers* indicate individual patients, *lower-case letters* (a, b, . . .) indicate investigations of the same patient at different times

detected in 17 of 19 patients in CR, whereas not a single B1- or My10-positive clone was found in any of the controls. These findings indicate that leukemic progenitor cells persist in the vast majority of patients during "complete" clinical remission of AML (Gerhartz and Schmetzer 1990).

Analysis of Clonality

A formal proof of the leukemic origin of My10- and B1-positive clones in AML bone marrow in CR was possible in 4 cases with a clonal marker. One of the patients had a trisomy 8 in 6 of 16 metaphases from uncultured bone marrow cells analyzed at presentation. During CR 10% of the clones cultured with PCM were My10-positive, and 15% were B1-positive. Cytogenetic analysis performed on single colonies picked from methylcellulose cultures detected the same cytogenetic anomaly, which proves the persistence of the leukemic clone (Gerhartz and Schmetzer 1990).

In three further cases, rearranged bands in Southern blots using the Ig-JH probe were found as clonal marker. Several additional bands in one of these cases indicated an oligoclonal disease. It is known from several studies that AML may have Ig-JH gene rearrangements in 15%–20% of the cases (Rovigatti et al. 1984) and may even differentiate into the cell lineage (Gerhartz et al. 1989). The appearance of several bands with Ig gene rearrangement provides evidence for an oligoclonal disease, a feature which has been described for lymphoblastic leukemia (Raghavachar et al. 1986), but only rarely in AML. In our case, during the course of the disease, some of these subclones obviously proliferated preferentially in the cultures because only some of the bands were detectable.

In the literature, it has already been shown that "clonal remissions" occur in AML by using polymorphisms of the enzyme glucose-6-phosphate dehydrogenase (G6PDH) (Fialkow et al. 1981) or fragment length polymorphism of other X chromosomal enzymes (Fearon et al. 1986). The methods used, however, did not allow detection of a small subpopulation of surviving leukemic cells in an organism which had regenerated with normal hematopoiesis. The advantage of the investigations described here is that they allow the detection of a small subpopulation of surviving leukemic cells in an organism which had regenerated with normal hematopoiesis, even of minimal residual disease. Our results show that the persistence of leukemic clones in clinical CR is the rule rather than the exception, but there is no information about the clonality of differentiated cells. Thus, both DNA methods and culture techniques should be used together to evaluate residual disease in AML.

Prognostic Significance of Leukemic Colonies

It was an obvious question whether the proportion of clones with a leukemic phenotype is prognostically important. Data obtained in 22 patients with clinical follow-ups of 6 months or more were analyzed. A linear regression between the duration of CR and proportion of B1- or My10-positive clones could not be demonstrated since some of those who were investigated repeatedly showed a roughly constant proportion of leukemic clones for periods of up to 2 years (Gerhartz and Schmetzer 1991). However, if the values were compared between the groups of patients relapsing within 6 months following the assay and those who did not, significant differences were found. It appeared that patients with a high proportion of leukemic progenitors (over 40%) relapsed soon (Gerhartz and Schmetzer 1990).

The assay described is useful for clinical investigations in patients treated by experimental protocols. Since maintenance of "CR" is the major problem in AML, this assay may help to investigate the effectivity of new protocols applied during clinical remission as well as the effectivity of bone marrow transplantation and of bone marrow purging methods. It also may help with an early detection of acute leukemia in a state when a diagnosis is not yet possible by morphological examination of the bone marrow.

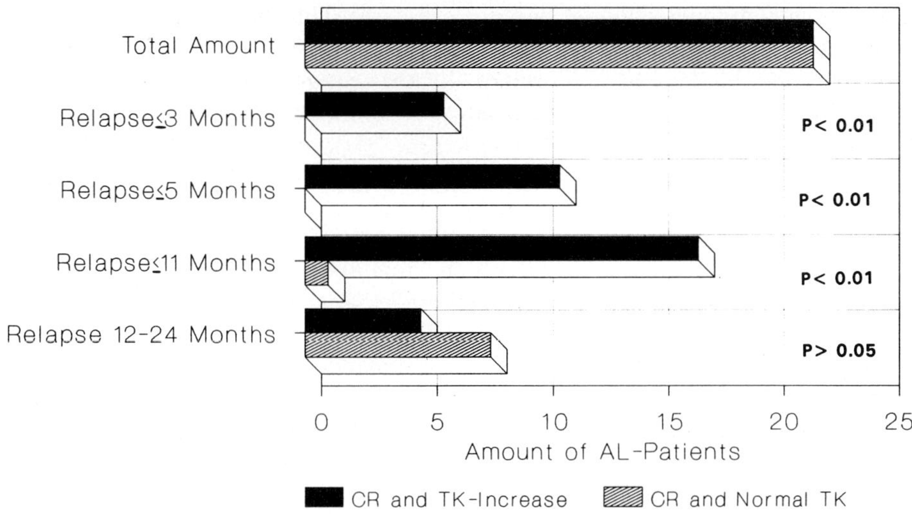

Fig. 8. Prognostic value of thymidine kinase (*TK*) activity in nucleated bone marrow cells during complete remission (*CR*) related to the time to relapse in patients with acute leukemia (*AL*)

Thymidine Kinase as a Marker for the Early Detection of Acute Leukemia and of Imminent Leukemic Relapse During Complete Remission

An increased activity of intracellular thymidine kinase (TK) is a biochemical marker of rapidly proliferating acute leukemia. The assay which was developed in our laboratory can be easily performed and gives quantitatively reproducible results within 2 days. Low enzyme activities were found in the bone marrow cells of smouldering leukemias, even those with a high percentage of blast cells (more than 60%). Thus, TK is an important parameter for distinguishing smouldering and rapidly proliferating variants of acute leukemia (Nüssler et al. 1990). In patients with myelodysplastic syndrome (MDS) a high variation of TK activities – not only related to FAB classification – was found (Wilmanns et al. 1990). An important finding was that untreated MDS patients with an increased TK activity had a higher risk of transformation to AML (median of 13.9 months) compared with patients with normal or decreased TK activity (median transition time of 25.3 months).

Figure 8 demonstrates the prognostic value of TK activity in bone marrow cells in CR of acute leukemia. Of 22 patients with TK increase, 6 (27.3%) developed a relapse within 3 months, 11 (50%) within 5 months, 17 (77.3%) within 11 months, and only 5 patients (22.7%) between 12 and 24 months. For 22 patients with normal TK activity there was no relapse within 5 months.

Thus, the control of TK activity in bone marrow cells during remission is of high prognostic value concerning the risk of relapse within 3–11 months and probably for the detection of minimal disease. This has to be proved by comparison of TK activities with the results of surface marker analysis in cultured cells. An increased TK activity during remission at least should be an indication for morphological bone marrow examination at short intervals.

Summary

AML clones can differentiate partially in vitro under the influence of colony stimulating factors. This differentiation remains as indicated by the persistence of early markers (CD10, CD20, CD34). "Complete remission" of AML is not an eradication of the disease but rather a balance of normal and leukemic hematopoiesis. Increase of leukemic clones to more than 40% of CFUs and/or increase of TK precede clinical relapse by 2–6 months.

References

Campos L, Gyotat D, Gentilhomme C, Treille D, Fiere D, Germain D (1987) Expression of a B-lymphoid differentiation antigen (CD19) on acute nonlymphocytic leukemia cells. Eur J Hematol 38:220–224

Dube JD, Eaves CJ, Kalousek DK, Eaves AC (1981) A method for obtaining high quality chromosome preparations from single hemopoetic colonies on a routine basis. Cancer Genet Cytogenet 4:157–168

Estrow Z, Grunberger T, Bube JD, Wang YP, Freedman MH (1986) Detection of residual acute lymphoblastic leukemia cells in cultures of bone marrow obtained during remission. N Engl J Med 315:538–542

Fearon ER, Burke PY, Schiffer CA, Zehnbauer BA, Vogelstein B (1986) Differentiation of leukemia cells to polymorphonuclear leukocytes in patients with acute nonlymphoycytic leukemia. N Engl J Med 315:15–24

Fialkow PJ, Singer JW, Adamson JW, Vaidya K, Dow LW, Ochs J, Moohr JW (1981) Acute nonlymphocytic leukemia; heterogeneity of stem cell origin. Blood 57:1068–1073

Gerhartz HH, Schmetzer H (1988) Verteilung früher und später Differenzierungsantigene auf normalen und Leukämiezell-Kolonien. In: Wilms K, Rückle H, Meyer P (eds) Diagnostische und therapeutische Entwicklungen in der Hämatologie und Onkologie. Zuckschwerdt, Munich, pp 67–77

Gerhartz HH, Schmetzer H (1990) Detection of minimal residual disease in acute myeloid leukemia. Leukemia 4(7):508–516

Gerhartz HH, Schmetzer H (1991) Minimal residual disease in acute leukemia (Letter). Eur J Cancer 27:809–810

Gerhartz HH, Bartram CR, Schmetzer H, Clemm C, Wilmanns W, Thiel E (1989) Spontaneous Epstein-Barr virus transformed B cell line sharing the identical immunoglobulin gene rearrangements with acute myeloid leukemia. Blood 73:684–687

Griffin JD, Meyer RJ, Weinstein HJ, Rosenthal DS, Coral FS, Beveridge RP, Schlossmann SF (1983) Surface marker analysis of acute myeloblastic leukemia: identification of differentiation associated phenotypes. Blood 62:557–563

Knapp W (1982) Monoclonal antibodies against differentiation antigens of myelopoiesis. Blut 45:301–308

Nadler LM, Stashenko P, Ritz J, Hardy R, Pesando JM, Schlossman SF (1981) A unique cell surface antigen, identifying lymphoid malignancies of B cell origin. J Clin Invest 67: 134–140

Nüssler V, Sauer H, Pelka-Fleischer R, Hoelzel D, Wilmanns W (1990) Clinical, biochemical and cytokinetic parameters for distinguishing smoldering and rapidly proliferating variants of acute leukemia. Eur J Haematol 45:19–25

Pesando JM, Hoffman P, Martin N, Conrad T (1986) Anti-CALLA antibodies identify unique antigens on lymphoid cells and granulocytes. Blood 67:558–591

Raghavachar A, Bartram CR, Ganser A, Heil G, Kleihauer E, Kubanek B (1986) Acute undifferentiated leukemia: implication for cellular origin and clonality suggested by analysis of surface markers and immunoglobulin gene rearrangement. Blood 68(3): 658–662

Rovigatti U, Mirro J, Kitchingman G, Dahl G, Ochs J, Murphy S, Stass S (1984) Heavy chain immunoglobulin gene rearrangement in acute nonlymphocytic leukemia. Blood 63:1023–1027

Sobol RE, Mick R, Royston I, Davey FR, Ellison RR, Newman R, Cuttner J, Griffin JD, Collins H, Nelson DA, Bloomfield CD (1987) Clinical importance of myeloid antigen expression in adult acute lymphoblastic leukemia. N Engl J Med 316:1111–1117

Spitzer G, Dicke KA, Gehan EA, Smith T, McCredie KB, Barlogie B, Freireich EJ (1976) A simplified in vitro classification for prognosis in adult acute leukemia: the application of in vitro results in remission-predictive models. Blood 48:795–807

Schmetzer H, Gerhartz HH (1987) Immunological phenotyping in situ of myeloid colonies in agar cultures. Exp Hematol 15:877–882

Vellenga E, Dewel HR, Touw IP, Löwenberg B (1987) Patterns of acute myeloid leukemia colony growth in response to recombinant granulocyte-macrophage colony-stimulating factor (GM-CSF). Exp Hematol 15:652–656

Wilmanns W, Nüssler V, Sauer H, Pelka-Fleischer R (1990) DNA synthesis in bone marrow cells as a basis for rational treatment of myelodysplastic syndromes (MDS) (Abstr). Blood 10 [Suppl 1]:337a

Wouters R, Löwenberg B (1984) On the maturation order of AML cells: a distinction on the basis of self-renewal properties and immunologic phenotypes. Blood 63:684–689

Summary of Discussion: Session 1

B. Dörken

E.G. Jung reported on skin cancer and melanoma. The discussion of his presentation focused mainly on the remarkably high incidence of skin tumors in immunosuppressed patients after renal transplantation. There is, in general, substantial evidence for a strong correlation between UV irradiation of the skin and skin carcinogenesis. According to E.G. Jung, immune surveillance is an important control mechanism for the elimination of oncogenic cells before they reach an invasive stage. In immunocompromised patients, the lag phase between UV radiation and the appearance of skin tumors is shortened. It was then commented that lymphomas in particular occur frequently in organ allograft recipients and that the majority of these tumors are associated with the Epstein-Barr virus, representing a spectrum of disease ranging from benign reactive polyclonal B-cell hyperplasia to monoclonal malignant lymphoma. In response to a question, Prof. Jung answered that there was no evidence to date that virus infection plays a role in the development of skin tumors in allograft recipients.

In his presentation on cancer of the oral cavity, D.K. Daftary displayed impressive slides demonstrating that certain forms of tobacco use were causally associated with this disease. A.B. Miller asked about the methods used for primary prevention. D.K. Daftary answered that in his experience personal communication is superior to posters or films in persuading people to give up their tobacco habit. We found that, especially in children and adolescents, the tobacco habit had declined as a result of the family prevention programs. D.K. Daftary was then asked if poor oral hygiene was an important factor in the development of oral carcinoma. He answered that teeth are not particularly decayed in heavy smokers, leading him to think that there is no correlation, as had been thought in previous studies. E.G. Jung asked about the role of sunlight as a cofactor in the development of oral carcinoma, giving as an example the development of squamous cell carcinoma on the tip of the tongue in patients with xeroderma pigmentosum. According to D.K. Daftary, epidemiological studies show carcinoma of the tip of the tongue to be very rare. An interesting obervation is that oral pigmentation is very common, perhaps as a result of tobacco chewing. However, there was no correlation between the pigmentation and the development of oral cancer. H. Weidauer stated that in Germany patients often present with lymph-node metastases and asked why this was not the case in D.K. Daftary's series. He answered that in earlier studies lymph-node metastases at the time of presentation were very common, but since the introduction of the secondary prevention programs by health workers, the carcinomas were now picked up at a much earlier stage. In addition, P.B. Desai commented that, especially in carcinoma of the buccal mucosa, the disease is only locally invasive and thus lymph-node metastases occur at a late stage. V. Diehl asked about the role of viruses. D.K. Daftary said that this would be a subject for future studies, and that the papilloma virus would be an important candidate. The next question was with regard to the role of cytology in the early detection of oral cancer. D.K. Daftary made reference to a large study of 50 000 patients in which the correlation between cytology and histology was very poor. Therefore, he stressed the necessity for a punch biopsy which can be easily carried out, even in the field.

H. Weidauer then reported on carcinoma of the oropharynx and larynx. With regard to lymph-node metastases he was asked, firstly, how metastases were detected, secondly, whether the primary tumor was still in situ, and thirdly, whether chemotherapy had been given. H. Weidauer answered, that several methods were used to diagnose these secondary manifestations, such as ultrasound and radiology. Many patients present very late with T3 and T4 tumors, and primary chemotherapy is then necessary to avoid a mutilating operation. H. Weidauer was then asked whether tumor markers were of value in the assessment of the completeness of removal of the tumor. The so-called squamous cell carcinoma antigen was quoted as an example. In H. Weidauer's experience, tumor markers have not been found to be useful, and therefore scanning techniques such as CT remain important. D.K. Daftary then asked whether alcohol alone is a significant risk factor or whether the effect is purely synergistic with tobacco. H. Weidauer answered that alcohol is an independent risk factor, but of a much lower order than the combination of alcohol and tobacco. H. Weidauer mentioned that there was no correlation between the percentage of alcohol (whisky vs. beer) and the development of oral cancer. P.B. Desai asked about the value of modern endoscopic techniques in comparison to conventional methods such as indirect laryngoscopy in the early detection of carcinoma. H. Weidauer answered that, with the exception of specific sites of tumor involvement, there are no significant advantages with the newer methods. It was pointed out that the accessability of the oral cavity and the oropharynx should facilitate early detection. H. Weidauer agreed and stressed that high risk groups should be regularly examined. In this context, D.K. Daftary mentioned the important role of the dental surgeon. Prof. Wilmans asked whether there was a difference between cigarette and pipe smokers, and whether the length of time that the patient had smoked was of importance. According to H. Weidauer, the highest risk is in cigarette smokers. The risk appears to be directly correlated with the number of cigarettes smoked; the risk is particularly high after having smoked more than 20 cigarettes daily for more than 10 years. In cigar smokers who do not inhale smoke deeply, cancer of the oral cavity is more common than cancer of the oropharynx and larynx. It was then pointed out that poor motivation is the major problem in cancer prevention programs. According to V. Diehl, about 13 persons per 100 000 per year developed cancer of the oropharynx/larynx and

5.6 per 100 000 per year die from it. This figure is much too high for developed countries such as Germany, and improvement of these figures is an educational problem. One has to consider whether patients who neglect their health should be made to contribute to paying for the costs of their illness, and V. Diehl asked A.B. Miller about the opinion of the WHO in this matter. A.B. Miller stated that if early detection is regarded as being beneficial in a particular condition, then it must be done in the context of an organized program; otherwise, those at the highest risk will not attend for a screening. There is, however, evidence that people do change their habits, as can be seen in the reduction of smoking in North America compared to Europe. Prof. Diehl added that reducing tobacco advertising is against government policy because of the strength of the tobacco lobby. A.B. Miller commented that it is better for a government to allow smoking, firstly to maintain revenue, and secondly, because premature death reduces the costs of social insurance. He stressed the importance of obtaining the support of the public in order to get governments to act, such as was done by the cancer societies in the United States. The combination of public education and the action of municipal governments to ban smoking in public places was of particular importance in North America.

P.B. Desai spoke about the problems and challenges in early detection of esophageal cancer. During discussion of his presentation, the point was raised that there are several areas in the world with an increased incidence of esophageal carcinoma: China, Iran, Britanny, and Transkai in South Africa. This suggests that risk factors must exist, but these are not known to date. In contrast to oropharyngeal carcinoma, smoking is not known to be a risk factor for esophageal carcinoma. There are studies indicating that human papilloma virus may be a risk factor. In China, using the relatively simple so-called balloon technique, it is possible to diagnose carcinoma in situ, which can be easily excised, and this can be life saving. P.B. Desai replied that, disappointingly, superficial lesions which can be detected by balloon cytology were often multicentric and therefore had a poorer prognosis. Biological behavior would appear more important than tumor size for survival.

S. Yoshida then spoke about the early detection of gastrointestinal cancers, in particular about recent progress of endoscopy. A.B. Miller asked how patients were selected for endoscopy and whether an increase in sensitivity has been associated with a decrease in specificity. The following methods for selecting patients for endoscopy were mentioned by S. Yoshida: self-presentation by the patient, radiology screening programs (which S. Yoshida regarded to be insufficient), biochemical methods such as tumor markers, and finally computer programs to characterize a high risk profile of a given patient. According to S. Yoshida, the Japanese method of screening is efficient but very expensive. In reply to a question regarding the value of dye spraying endoscopy in the diagnosis of gastric carcinoma, S. Yoshida stated that in contrast to esophageal carcinoma this technique is of no value due to the lack of glycogen in the gastric mucosa. It was then commented that carcinoma of the colon is less common than in Western countries, and S. Yoshida was asked whether, in his experience, the sequence of development of carcinoma was mainly from a flat carcinoma in situ or from an adenomatous polyp according to the usual concept. S. Yoshida stressed than in his opinion both sequences can lead to the development of carcinoma of the colon.

W. Wilmanns reported on detection of minimal disease in hematological malignancies. He was asked whether the results which he had presented should lead to the redefinition of complete remission. W. Wilmanns answered that, at the moment, the significance of detection of leukemic clones is still uncertain and that conventional criteria should still be applied in the definition of a complete remission. It was then commented that in nearly all cases marker expression, at first thought to be solely a characteristic of leukemic cells, had subsequently also been found in normal cells. W. Wilmanns was, therefore, asked whether normal myeloid cells also express the CD20 antigen which has been characterized as a B-lineage specific molecule. He answered that a very small percentage of normal myeloid cells express CD20 but cannot be cloned.

In his concluding remarks, V. Diehl stated that sensitive techniques for the detection of early cancer are certainly important, but that even more important are appropriate therapeutic strategies. There is no advantage, for example, in detecting clonogenic cells in acute myeloid leukemia with ever more sensitive techniques if more effective treatment is not available.

Clinical Aspects II

Chairman: G. BASTERT

Early Detection of Carcinoma
of the Prostate and Transitional Cell Carcinoma:
Current Aspects*

B.J. Schmitz-Dräger, T. Ebert, and R. Ackermann

Introduction

Symptoms of genitourinary tumors are usually unspecific and occur, in most cases, only in the more advanced stages of disease. Therefore, only screening programs can improve the detection of localized and potentially curable tumors. Besides patient motivation and efficacy, the cost/benefit ratio remains a crucial problem of screening programs. It therefore remains to be determined which population should be examined and how the screening should be performed. The aim of this presentation is to analyze recent techniques for their potential value as diagnostic measures in future screening programs in the detection of carcinoma of the prostate (CaP) and transitional cell carcinoma (TCC).

Carcinoma of the Prostate

According to the 1987 figures reported by Hoffmeister, CaP ranks second among the most common malignant diseases in the former Federal Republic of Germany (Schön et al. 1987). Until today, the diagnosis of the early tumor lesion remains a domain of the digital rectal examination (DRE). There are some specific features related to the early detection of CaP that should be mentioned.

It is known from large autopsy studies done by Franks (1954), Schmalhorst and Halpert (1964), and Rullis et al. (1975) that incidental tumor foci can be observed in the prostates of approximately 50% of men older than 70 years. This contrasts to a reported incidence of 400/100000 men in this age group and a mortality of 200/100000 in these men in the former FRG (Schön et al. 1987). From these data it must be concluded that (a) less than 1% of all tumors will be diagnosed and (b) even fewer tumors will become symptomatic.

To estimate the sensitivity and specificity of a given diagnostic modality, the findings of this technique have to be compared with those of histopathology. This information cannot be obtained from screening examinations. Staging in patients subsequently undergoing radical surgery, however, may provide an

* Supported in part by grant 01 GA 8701/7 of the Bundesministerium für Forschung und Technologie der Bundesrepublik Deutschland.

idea about the value of a modality in the diagnosis of prostate cancer. Tumor extension and localization appear to be suitable parameters for this type of analysis.

The accuracy of DRE in the clinical staging of CaP has been examined in several prospective trials in patients subsequently undergoing radical prostatectomy (RP). Salo et al. (1987a) reported on the correlation of clinical tumor stages obtained by DRE with the pathohistological stage after RP. They observed understaging by DRE in 47% of 32 patients. Recent results by Ebert et al. (1991), who investigated 62 patients prior to RP, yielded a correct local tumor stage in only 21%, while understaging was observed in 77%. Similar correlations were observed by other investigators (Catalona and Stein 1982; Cordes et al. 1987; Palken et al. 1990). These results underscore the poor sensitivity of DRE. It therefore has to be asked whether or not modern imaging modalities might be superior in the diagnosis of CaP to DRE.

Since real-time transrectal ultrasonography (TRUS) was introduced in the diagnosis of CaP by Watanabe et al. (1975), numerous investigations have been performed in order to determine the value of this technique in the diagnosis and evaluation of the extent of malignant lesions. Initial reports on the diagnostic accuracy were as high as 80%. These reports have been followed by others which found this technique to be of only limited value (Andriole et al. 1988; Clements et al. 1988; Dähnert et al. 1986; Denis et al. 1980; Friedman et al. 1988; Fujino and Scardino 1985; Pontes et al. 1985; Resnick et al. 1980; Salo et al. 1987a).

Important observations were reported by Dähnert et al. (1986) who performed an ex vivo study on 64 prostates immediately after RP. Using a 5-MHz linear array transducer, they found that 38 glands (59%) had echopenic or hypoechoic lesions which were subsequently identified to be tumors. Tumor areas were isoechoic in the remaining 26 specimens. In contrast, Salo et al. (1987b) reported 30% hyperechoic tumor lesions in 20 RP specimens examined ex vivo by TRUS, while 40% were found to be hypoechoic. The conclusion from these studies is that a 60% sensitivity represents the upper limit of TRUS in the detection of CaP.

Initial results of TRUS examination prior to RP were reported by Resnick et al. (1980). They investigated 23 patients with localized CaP. The extent of the lesion and seminal vesical infiltration were recognized by TRUS in all patients. Pontes et al. (1985) evaluated 31 patients with clinically localized CaP by TRUS prior to RP. Capsular and seminal involvement were predicted with a 89% and 100% sensitivity, respectively. More recent studies yielded less favorable results. Salo et al. (1987a) were able to uncover tumor invasion beyond the capsule or seminal vesicle infiltration in 14 out of 21 (67%) patients. Andriole et al. (1988) detected extracapsular tumor extension with TRUS in 4 out of 7 (57%) cases. Cordes et al. (1987) reported a sensitivity of 54% in the prediction of extracapsular and seminal vesicle infiltration in 13 patients. Similar results were obtained by Ebert et al. (1991). They detected extracapsular tumor growth in 16 out of 30 patients (53%) with TRUS. Summarizing these findings, capsular penetration was predicted in most trials with approxi-

Table 1. Screening for carcinoma of the prostate by digital rectal examination (DRE): *diagnostic costs based on BMÄ figures (1990)* (modified after Torp-Pedersen et al. 1988)

DRE in 784 volunteers à DM 6.50	DM 5,096.–
29 biopsies and histological examination à DM 70.–	DM 2,030.–
Total screening costs	DM 7,126.–
1. Costs per cancer ($n = 10$)	DM 713.–
2. Costs per early cancer ($n = 7$)	DM 1,018.–
3. Costs per early cancer saved from progression:	
I. $n = 7 - (10 \times 0.6)$	DM 7,126.–
II. $n = 7 - (10 \times 0.2)$	DM 1,425.–

Table 2. Screening for carcinoma of the prostate transrectal ultrasound (TRUS): *diagnostic costs based on BMÄ figures (1990)* (modified after Torp-Pedersen et al. 1988)

TRUS in 784 volunteers à DM 40.–	DM 31,360.–
64 biopsies and histological examination à DM 70.–	DM 4,480.–
Total screening costs	DM 35,840.–
1. Costs per cancer ($n = 20$)	DM 1,792.–
2. Costs per early cancer ($n = 17$)	DM 2,108.–
3. Costs per early cancer saved from progression:	
I. $n = 17 - (20 \times 0.6)$	DM 7,168.–
II. $n = 17 - (20 \times 0.2)$	DM 2,757.–

mately a 60% sensitivity. It should be mentioned, however, that false-positive findings of capsular penetration were also observed in some investigations (Ebert et al. 1991; Pontes et al. 1985; Salo et al. 1987a).

While most authors detect tumor invasion beyond the capsule with TRUS with a 60%–85% sensitivity, there are remarkably conflicting results concerning the sensitivity of detecting seminal vesicle involvement. While Resnick et al. (1980) reported a 100% sensitivity, other investigations yielded a sensitivity of less than 30% (Ebert et al. 1991; Pontes et al. 1985; Salo et al. 1987a).

Besides sensitivity and specificity, cost effectiveness is another important parameter which must be considered in the setting up of screening programs. This question has been recently addressed by Torp-Pedersen et al. (1988) who performed a screening trial in 784 men using DRE and TRUS. Based on TRUS findings, 64 men underwent needle biopsy. In 20 (31%) CaP was diagnosed; 17 of these patients had an early lesion confined to the prostate. Only 29 men were found to have a palpable nodule by DRE and were referred for biopsy. In 10 (34%) CaP was diagnosed; 7 of these patients had a clinically localized CaP.

Based on the data reported by Torp-Pedersen et al. (1988) the costs for this screening program were calculated using the German reimbursement system BMÄ (Tables 1, 2). The higher number of suspicious lesions detected by TRUS led to a higher number of biopsies, thus further increasing the costs of the TRUS screening program resulting in a 5:1 cost ratio as compared with

DRE. Due to the fact that twice as many cancers were diagnosed by TRUS the cost ratio changed to approximately 2.5:1 per cancer case detected. Looking at the costs per early cancer diagnosed by these two modalities, TRUS was only twice as expensive as DRE. Since a certain amount of early tumors will be diagnosed even without screening programs, the costs per localized cancer saved from progression by the screening program is the most important figure. This figure depends largely upon the incidence of early CaP among those patients diagnosed without a screening program. Currently, no precise data on this issue are available for the FRG. However, from the data presented in Tables 1 and 2, it can be calculated that DRE would be the more economical, but not more efficient, screening method in the detection of early cancers, if the portion of incidentally diagnosed early lesions does not exceed 60%.

Summarizing these considerations, TRUS appears to be a sensitive but not very specific examination in the diagnosis of CaP. Since a decreased specificity will influence the positive predictive value of an examination, TRUS may be of interest predominantly in the screening of patient populations with a high tumor incidence. It has to be kept in mind, however, that particularly in CaP the value of early tumor diagnosis remains unclear, since the vast majority of lesions will never become clinically relevant. The search for prognostic factors predicting the outcome of the disease, therefore, appears to be even more important than the development of measures increasing the sensitivity of tumor diagnosis.

Transitional Cell Carcinoma

The high risk for patients with a history of TCC of the bladder of developing a tumor recurrence is well documented (Barnes et al. 1977; Lutzeyer et al. 1982; National Bladder Cancer Collaborative Group A 1977). Barnes et al. (1977) reported a recurrence rate of 52% in 375 patients within 5 years after trans-urethral bladder tumor resection. Tumor recurrence in these patients was associated with an increase in the tumor stage in 22%. This underlines the importance of careful follow-up investigations. Presently, cystoscopy and urinary cytology are the basic diagnostic tools in the follow-up of patients with bladder tumors. Cystoscopy, however, is an invasive procedure which may be painful, especially in male patients. Despite the high specificity of voided urine cytology, the value of this method is limited by its low sensitivity, particularly with low-grade tumors (National Bladder Cancer Collaborative Group A 1977; Dubernard et al. 1982; Esposti et al. 1970; Koss et al. 1985; Zein et al. 1984). The development of sensitive and noninvasive techniques would allow more frequent examinations of patients at risk and thus might improve the efficiency of follow-up investigations. Flow cytometry and immunocytology are new methods which must prove their clinical value in routine diagnosis. The ability of MoAbs to visualize molecular changes should allow recognition of cell transformation even before morphological changes become evident. Based on this hypothesis, several attempts have been made to generate MoAbs directed against TCC. So far, none of these mAbs can be regarded as tumor-specific (Bander 1987). Some of them show cross-reactions with morphologically normal urothelial cells (Decken et al. 1991; Arndt et al. 1987). This does not necessarily exclude them from being utilized in immunocytology, but the staining of some morphologically normal urothelial cells must be anticipated. Based on this consideration Huland and coworkers introduced quantitative evaluation of the specimens and the arbitrary definition of a cut-off value (Huland et al. 1987, 1988).

There are only a few reports of the use of MoAbs in the cytological diagnosis of TCC. In most of them bladder wash specimens were used. Chopin et al. (1985) were the first to report on the use of MoAbs in cytology. Using MoAbs G 4 and E 7 they observed positive results in 14 out of 18 specimens obtained from patients with TCC. In 13 out of 15 specimens derived from control patients no positive cells were observed.

Huland et al. (1987, 1988) investigated 104 specimens by quantitative immunocytology using MoAb 486 P 3/12. Since the antigen recognized by this MoAb is preferably expressed by bladder tumor cells but is also present on normal urothelial cells (Arndt et al. 1987), a cut-off value of 30% was used to discriminate between normal and pathological results. Using this approach, they found a sensitivity of 87% (60 out of 69). A simultaneous cytological investigation yielded a sensitivity of 54%. No correlation between sensitivity and tumor grade was observed. The specificity was investigated in 35 specimens from patients with diseases not related to TCC. Positive findings were obtained by immunocytology and by cytology in 3 and 4 cases, respectively. The specificity was 91% for immunocytology and 89% for conventional cytology.

Sheinfeld et al. (1990) investigated 129 bladder barbotage specimens simultaneously by conventional cytology and immunocytology. Using the monoclonal Lewis X-specific antibody P-12 they reported a sensitivity of 88% in 76 patients with histologically proven TCC and a specificity of 85% in 40 control patients. Interestingly, in 5 out of 8 specimens derived from patients with prostate carcinoma, Lewis X-positive urothelial cells were observed. This corresponds to the observation made by Schmitz-Dräger et al. (1991) that the control patient with the highest number of immunocytologically positive cells also suffered from prostatic carcinoma.

Recently, Walker et al. (1989) reported preliminary results on the use of voided urine as a source for immunocytology. They investigated 8 samples from patients with advanced TCC of the bladder by immunocytology. Using MoAb BLCA-8, antigen-positive urothelial cells were found in all specimens. Since only a limited number of specimens derived from patients with advanced high grade tumors were evaluated, the clinical value of this assay must be defined in further investigations.

Schmitz-Dräger et al. (1991) reported on the prospective investigation of 74 specimens from patients with TCC and 60 specimens obtained from patients without clinical evidence of TCC using MoAb Due ABC 3. Evaluation was possible with conventional cytology in 126 (94%) and with immunocytology in 100 (74%) specimens. An insufficient number of urothelial cells, cellular

Table 3. Sensitivity and specificity of conventional cytology and immunocytology using monoclonal antibody Due ABC 3 in the evaluation of 74 specimens derived from patients with TCC and 60 control patients

Method	Transitional cell carcinoma ($n = 74$) Correct positive (%)	Control group ($n = 60$) Correct negative (%)
Conventional cytology	35/74 (47)	55/60 (92)
Immunocytology	49/74 (66)	35/60 (58)
Conventional cytology and/or immunocytology	56/74 (76)	53/60 (88)

degeneration, and severe pyuria prevented a quantitation of antigen-positive urothelial cells in 34 immunocytological specimens. Of 74 specimens (66%) 49 derived from patients with TCC were correctly classified by immunocytology (Table 3). A correct diagnosis was made by conventional cytology in 35 (47%) of these specimens. All 55 out of 60 samples derived from control patients evaluable by conventional cytology were classified as normal, resulting in a specificity of 92%. The immunocytological examination showed an increased amount of antigen-positive cells in 7 samples. As 18 of the 60 samples could not be evaluated with this method, a specificity of 58% was calculated.

The sensitivity of cytology was found to correlate with tumor grade. In only 3 of 21 (14%) specimens obtained from patients with low grade malignancy tumor cells were detected. A sensitivity of 42% (8/19) in grade 2 lesions and 71% (24/34) in high grade TCC was observed. The sensitivity of immuno-cytology was similar in grade 1 and 2 lesions (57% and 53%, respectively) and was 79% in grade 3 tumors.

The sensitivity of cytology and immunocytology was improved by combining the results obtained with the two techniques (Tables 3, 4). Altogether, 56 of the 74 tumor specimens (76%) were positive on either cytology or immunocytology. The combined specificity was 88% (53/60).

Comparing the results obtained by Schmitz-Dräger et al. (1991) to those reported by Huland et al. (1988) and to those reported by Sheinfeld et al. (1990), it appears that the differences could be related to the high number of immunocytological specimens that could not be evaluated in this study. No information concerning the frequency of appropriate specimens for evaluation has been obtained from the literature. However, it seems likely that the use of voided urine in the study of Schmitz-Dräger et al. (1991) accounts for at least a part of this problem. Nevertheless, immunocytology has been shown to be a valuable adjunct to conventional cytology in the diagnosis of TCC. The results indicate that this method might be of particular value in low grade tumors.

A possible application of immunocytology could be the follow-up of patients with a history of TCC. It is conceivable that high-risk patients with a negative cytology ought to be examined by immunocytology. Those patients with a positive test could then undergo further examinations, such as cysto-

Table 4. Sensitivity of conventional cytology and immunocytology using monoclonal antibody Due ABC 3 in the diagnosis of transitional cell carcinoma according to tumor grade

Method	Sensitivity (%)		
	Grade 1	Grade 2	Grade 3/4
Conventional cytology	3/21 (14)	8/19 (42)	24/34 (71)
Immunocytology	12/21 (57)	10/19 (53)	27/34 (79)
Conventional cytology and/or immunocytology	12/21 (57)	10/19 (53)	33/34 (97)

scopy and mucosal biopsy. The efficiency of this concept, however, still has to be proven by prospective trials.

Summary

The correlation between early detection with subsequent therapy and disease prognosis is well established for genitourinary tumors. The investigation of new techniques for their clinical value in the early diagnosis of genitourinary tumors represents an important aspect of urological cancer research.

Since real-time transrectal ultrasonography (TRUS) was introduced in the diagnosis of prostate carcinoma (CaP) by Watanabe and coworkers, numerous studies have investigated the value of this technique in the localization and evaluation of the extent of malignant lesions. Initial reports on the diagnostic accuracy were as high as 80%. These reports have been followed by others which found this technique to be of only limited value. Torp-Pedersen and coworkers investigated the efficacy and costs of TRUS and digital rectal examination (DRE) in the detection of CaP. The higher sensitivity of TRUS as compared with DRE was found to result in significantly higher costs per diagnosed cancer. Since more early CaPs were detected by TRUS, however, the authors concluded that the additional costs were justified.

The high risk for patients with a history of transitional cell carcinoma (TCC) of the bladder of developing a tumor recurrence is well documented. The development of sensitive and noninvasive techniques would allow more frequent examinations of patients at risk and thus might improve the efficiency of follow-up investigations. Flow cytometry and immunocytology are new methods which must prove their clinical value in routine diagnosis.

The ability of monoclonal antibodies (MoAbs) to visualize molecular changes should allow recognition of cell transformation even before morphological changes become evident. So far, there are only a few reports on the use of MoAbs in the cytological diagnosis of TCC. Huland and coworkers investigated 104 bladder wash specimens by quantitative immunology. They reported a sensitivity of 87% as compared with 54% with cytology. The specificity was 91% for immunocytology and 89% for conventional cytology. Similar results were reported by Sheinfeld and coworkers. Schmitz-Dräger and coworkers reported less favorable results in a prospective trial using MoAb Due ABC 3 in voided urine specimens obtained from 74 patients with TCC and 60 control patients. Comparing the results with those reported by Huland and coworkers and by Sheinfeld and coworkers, it seems likely that the use of voided urine specimens accounts for at least a part of this discrepancy. In all trials immunocytology was found to be a valuable adjunct to conventional cytology in the diagnosis of TCC. The results indicate that this method might be of particular value with low grade tumors. Its noninvasiveness allows unlimited application according to the clinical requirements. These advantages should be of special value in the follow-up of patients with previous TCC.

References

Andriole GL, Kavoussi LR, Torrence RJ, Lepor H, Catalona WJ (1988) Transrectal ultrasonography in the diagnosis and staging of carcinoma of the prostate. J Urol 140:758–760

Arndt R, Dürkopf H, Huland H, Donn F, Loening T, Kalthoff H (1987) Monoclonal antibodies for characterization of the heterogeneity of normal and malignant transitional cells. J Urol 137:758–763

Bander NH (1987) Monoclonal antibodies: state of art. J Urol 137:603–607

Barnes RW, Dick AL, Hadley HL, Johnston QL (1977) Survival following transurethral resection of bladder carcinoma. Cancer Res 37:2895–2896

Catalona WJ, Stein AJ (1982) Staging errors in clinically localized prostatic cancer. J Urol 127:452–456

Chopin DK, deKernion JB, Rosenthal DL, Fahey JL (1985) Monoclonal antibodies against transitional cell carcinoma for detection of malignant urothelial cells in bladder washing. J Urol 134:260–262

Clements R, Griffith GJ, Peeling WB, Roberts EE, Evans KT (1988) How accurate is the index finger? A comparison of digital and ultrasound examination of the prostatic nodule. Clin Radiol 39:87–89

Cordes M, Tunn UW, Neidl K, Haasner E (1987) Prostatakarzinom. Stadieneinteilung durch transrektale Prostatasonographie und Computertomographie mit histopathologischer Korrelation. ROFO 146:412–414

Dähnert WF, Hamper UM, Eggleston JC, Walsh PC, Sanders RC (1986) Prostatic evaluation by transrectal sonography with histopathologic correlation: the echopenic appearance of early carcinoma. Radiology 158:97–102

Decken K, Schmitz-Dräger BJ, Rohde D, Nakamura S, Ebert T, Ackermann R (1992) Monoclonal antibody Due ABC 3 directed against transitional cell carcinoma. I. Production, specificity analysis and preliminary characterization of the antigen. J Urol 147:235–241

Denis L, Appel L, Broos J, Declerq G (1980) Evaluation of prostatic cancer by transrectal ultrasonotomography and CT scan. Acta Urol Belg 48:71–77

Dubernard JM, Devonec M, Amiel J, Bouvier R, Fontaniere B, Faucon M (1982) Correlation between cytology and cystoscopy in the follow-up of patients with bladder tumours. Eur Urol 8:5–8

Ebert T, Schmitz-Dräger BJ, Bürrig K-F, Miller S, Pauli N, Kahn T, Ackermann R (1991) Accuracy of imaging modalities in staging the local extent of prostate cancer. Clin Urol North Am 18:453–458

Esposti PL, Moberger G, Zajicek J (1970) The cytologic diagnosis of transitional cell tumors of the urinary bladder and its histologic basis. A study of 567 cases of urinary-tract disorder including 170 untreated and 182 irradiated bladder tumors. Acta Cytol 11: 145–152

Franks LM (1954) Latent carcinoma of the prostate. J Path Bact 68:603–616

Friedman AC, Seidmon EJ, Redecki PD, Lev-Toaff A, Caroline DF (1988) Relative merits of MRI, transrectal endosonography and CT in diagnosis and staging of carcinoma of prostate. Urology 31:530–537

Fujino A, Scardino PT (1985) Transrectal ultrasonography for prostatic cancer: its value in staging and monitoring the response to radiotherapy and chemotherapy. J Urol 133:806–810

Huland E, Huland H, Arndt R, Baisch H, Klöppel G (1988) Urindiagnostik oberflächlicher Harnblasentumoren durch Zytologie, Immunzytologie und Flowzytometrie: Ergebnisse einer prospektiven vergleichenden Studie an 104 Patienten. Aktuel Urol 19:13–17

Huland H, Arndt R, Huland E, Loening TE, Steffens M (1987) Monoclonal antibody 486 P 3/12: a valuable bladder carcinoma marker for immunocytology. J Urol 137:654–659

Koss LG, Deitch D, Ramanathan R, Sherman AB (1985) Diagnostic value of cytology of voided urine. Acta Cytol 29:810–816

Lutzeyer W, Rübben H, Dahm H (1982) Prognostic parameters in superficial bladder cancer: an analysis of 315 cases. J Urol 127:250–252

National Bladder Cancer Collaborative Group A (1977) Cytology and histopathology of bladder cancer cases in a prospective longitudinal study. Cancer Res 37:2911–2915

Palken M, Cobb OE, Warren BH, Hoak DC (1990) Prostate cancer: correlation of digital rectal examination, transrectal ultrasound and prostate specific antigen levels with tumor volumes in radical prostatectomy specimens. J Urol 143:115–119

Pontes JE, Eisenkraft S, Watanabe H, Ohe H, Saitoh M, Murphy GP (1985) Preoperative evaluation of localized prostatic carcinoma by transrectal ultrasonography. J Urol 134:289–291

Resnick MI, Willard JW, Boyce WH (1980) Transrectal ultrasonography in the evaluation of patients with prostatic carcinoma. J Urol 124:482–484

Rullis I, Shaeffer JA, Lilien OM (1975) Incidence of prostatic carcinoma in the elderly. Urology 6:295–297

Salo JO, Kivisari L, Rannikko S, Lehtonen T (1987a) Computerized tomography and transrectal ultrasound in the assessment of local extension of prostatic cancer before radical retropubic prostatectomy. J Urol 137:435–438

Salo JO, Ranniko S, Makinen J, Lehtonen T (1987b) Echogenic structure of prostatic cancer imaged on radical prostatectomy specimens. Prostate 10:1–9

Schmalhorst R, Halpert B (1964) Carcinoma of the prostate gland in patients more than 80 years old. J Clin Pathol 42:170

Schmitz-Dräger BJ, Nakamura S, Decken K, Pfitzer P, Rottmann-Ickler C, Ebert T, Ackermann R (1991) Monoclonal antibody Due ABC 3 directed against transitional cell carcinoma. II. Prospective trial on the diagnostic value of immunocytology. J Urol 146: 1521–1524

Schön D, Bertz J, Hoffmeister H (1987) Schlußfolgerungen und Ausblick. In: Hoffmeister H (ed) Bevölkerungsbezogene Krebsregister in der Bundesrepublik Deutschland. MMV Medizin, Munich, pp 170–180

Sheinfeld J, Reuter VE, Melamed MR, Fair WR, Morse M, Sogani PC, Herr HW, Whitmore WF, Cordon-Cardo C (1990) Enhanced bladder cancer detection with the Lewis X antigen as a marker of neoplastic transformation. J Urol 143:285–287

Torp-Pedersen ST, Littrup PJ, Lee F, Mettlin C (1988) Early prostate cancer: diagnostic costs of screening transrectal US and digital rectal examination. Radiology 169:351–354

Walker KZ, Russell PJ, Kingsley EA, Philips J, Raghavan D (1989) Detection of malignant cells in voider urine from patients with bladder cancer, a novel monoclonal assay. J Urol 142:1578–1582

Watanabe H, Igari D, Tanahashi Y, Harada K, Saitoh M (1975) Transrectal ultrasonotomography of the prostate. J Urol 114:734–739

Zein T, Wajsman Z, Englander LS, Gamarra M, Lopez C, Huben RP, Pontes JE (1984) Evaluation of bladder washings and urine cytology in the diagnosis of bladder cancer and its correlation with selected biopsies of the bladder mucosa. J Urol 132:670–672

Problems in the Early Detection of Cervical Cancer

G. KINDERMANN

Introduction

It is more than half a century since George Papanicolaou reported the chance finding of cancer cells in vaginal smears from patients with cancer of the uterine cervix. It is more than 70 years since Hans Hínselmann reported the possibility of looking at the surface of the ectocervix under magnification. Those creative observations led to the development of cervical cytology and colposcopy. The development of both ideas created the base for the early diagnosis and treatment of clinically unsuspected cervical cancer and its precursors. Today, both methods are used for screening the female adult population, but in a different way and with a different value for the clinician. Both methods can and should be used in combination to obtain the best results, but worldwide only cytology screening is widespread, with the aim to reduce the mortality from cervical cancer. From a theoretical point of view it could be expected that mortality from cervical cancer will be virtually eliminated. However, this expectation has not been fulfilled. Although many reports have indicated a significant impact on the overall incidence of the disease itself, others have shown an increased incidence in certain age groups (Bonett et al. 1989). Therefore, I would like to present critical clinical aspects to the problems (Table 1) in the early detection of cervical cancer. In many countries, such as the FRG or the USA, a critical analysis of the reasons for the failure of cervical cancer screening has been done and attention has been drawn (Koss 1989) to several causal factors. The success of a cervical cancer detection programme implies the diagnosis and successful treatment of all precancerous lesions and all early invasive carcinomas. It is based on a complex series of social, epidemiological, medical and laboratory factors, and in each of these areas any weak point can lead to the failure of the programme itself. In Table 1, I want to show some main reasons for the problems in the early detection of cervical cancer. First, there are several limitations to the actual screening programme in most countries. Secondly, there is a relatively high false-negative result rate for a single smear. This is related to the adequacy of the smear itself, the sampling from the patient, the preparing of material on the slide, and last but not least the inaccuracy of the cytological interpretation. Additionally, the false-negative rate may be influenced by the inadequate use of cytology in patients with clinical cancer.

Third, there is some support for the hypothesis of a rapid-onset type of cancer that may be missed by presently established screening intervals. This should be discussed briefly. Those failures in the established protocols for the management of a pathological smear or colposcopy finding may be the result of the wrong choice of histological evaluation.

The Screening System

The organisation, protocols and concepts of cervical screening programmes vary considerably around the world. There are highly centralised programmes, such as in British Columbia (Andersen et al. 1988) or Iceland (Sigurdsson et al. 1989), where an efficient call and recall system notifies the patient that she is due to present for a Papanicolaou smear. More commonly, as in the FRG or USA, the responsibility for regular smear screening is left with the patient herself. The impact of the centralised systems on the overall incidence of the disease is impressive. The incidence of invasive cervical cancer in British Columbia has fallen by 78% since the programme began. In our self-responsibility system the rate of participation in the programme is too low (Fig. 1). And it is disappointing that the rate is decreasing during the period of establishing the programme. Furthermore, there are important indications that we possibly screen the wrong group, for the proportion of the high-risk patients for cervical cancer is low. For instance, it seems clear that older women, particularly from the epidemiologically recognisable high-risk groups, should be targetted for greater attendance at screening programmes. We have to identify the reasons, why (Fig. 2) the older women seem to be little interested in participating. This figure from Mitchell and Medley (1987) shows the experience in Australia. Several factors have been significant variables for the attendance of women for cytology: the availability of female physicians or nurses to perform the tests, the perceived attitude of the doctor, and the socioeconomic situation of the patient. In addition, the prevailing attitude towards cervical cancer as a sexually transmitted disease tends to dissuade some women from attending a screening programme (Dickenson et al. 1988). The chance to decrease the actual limitations is to increase the attendance! Wain and Hacker (1990) believe that screening the entire population at least once each decade probably would have a greater impact on cervical cancer mortality than would the annual screening of a committed minority.

The Problem of Accuracy

The problem of the false-negative smear has received much attention. It seems reasonable to define the false-negative smear as one in which the histological diagnosis is at least two-thirds worse than the cytological prediction within 6 months of the smear. Factors contributing to the false-negative result rate, such as quality control of cytology laboratories and accuracy of the cervical sampling, have loomed large recently in the literature. Approximately two-

Table 1. Problems in the early detection of cervical cancer

---

1. Limitations to the actual screening programs in most countries
2. The accuracy: relatively high false-negative rate for a single smear
3. Is there a rapid-onset type of cancer missed by presently established screening intervals?
4. Failures in the established protocols for the management of a pathological smear or colposcopy finding

---

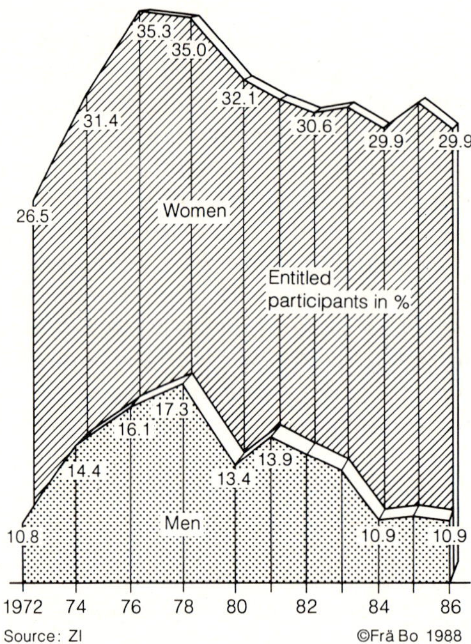

Fig. 1. Participation in the cost-free screening programme for genital cancer, for the male (*below*) and female German population. The figure shows the low attendance, with a decreasing tendency in the last period observed (from 1980 to 1986)

thirds of false-negative smears are related to the failure of cervical sampling and one-third, to the failure of the cytology technicians to detect abnormal cells present on the slide (Wain and Hacker 1990). A third factor causing false-negative smears is the inappropriate use of the test in symptomatic women, those with clinical findings. The Papanicolaou smear is a screening test for asymptomatic women, who have a macroscopically normal cervix. Patients who have an abnormal cervix should undergo a biopsy, whereas patients with abnormal bleeding require uterine curettage or colposcopy-directed biopsy, regardless of the Papanicolaou smear report. Because of hemorrhage and necrosis in the tumor, the false-negative result rates for Papanicolaou smears in the presence of invasive cancer is about 50%.

Recently, assessing the adequacy of cervical sampling has focused on the presence of absence of endocervical cells in the smear. The identification of endocervical cells generally has come to be considered as a measure of the adequacy of sampling of the squamocolumnar junction: the absence of these cells generally is thought to be an indication that the examination should be

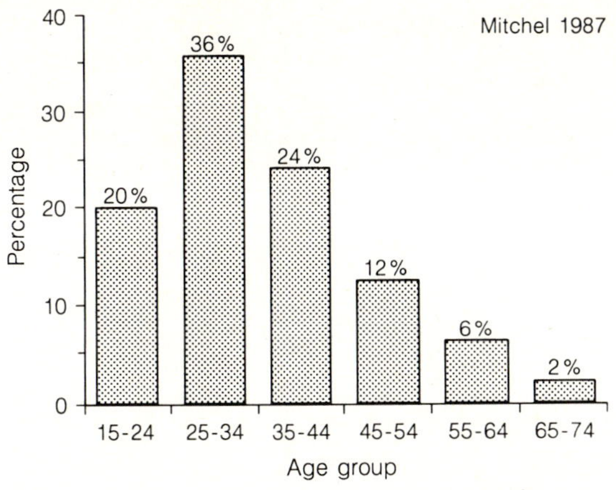

Fig. 2. Age distribution of Pap smears in Australia from 1984 to 1986 (from Mitchel and Medley 1987)

repeated. Additionally, the increasing proportion of adenocarcinomas and adenosquamous carcinomas in recent reports underlines the need for deliberate cervical sampling in all patients. Whereas adenocarcinomas accounted for about 5% of several cancers 20 years ago, they now represent up to 20% of cases (Wain and Hacker 1990).

Rapid-Onset Cervical Cancer

A significant concern for cervical screening programmes relates to the possibility that the rapid-onset type of cancer may be increasing in frequency. Whereas it generally has been assumed that the natural history of cervical cancer has a long preclinical phase, with gradual progression from preinvasive epithelial abnormalities to frankly invasive malignancy, there is some evidence to support the concept of a rapid-onset type of cancer that may not be detected by currently recommended screening intervals. Further studies have to prove whether there is a genuinely increasing incidence of those forms of cervical neoplasia.

In conclusion, the cytology screening test could detect the precancerous lesion or microinvasive cancer of the cervix. Therefore, it should be possible to eliminate frankly invasive cervical cancer from the population. This goal has not been achieved because most women remain unscreened each year. The cytology smears are sometimes taken inappropriately or read ineffectively. Clinicians do not always follow recommended guidelines for the management of patients with normal smears.

Problems in the Histological Evaluation

Histological diagnostic procedures should be safe, simple and representative for the underlying lesion. The following (Table 2) diagnostic procedures have

Table 2. Diagnostic histological procedures with high reliability

	Non-mutilating techniques
Conization/endocervical curettage (ECC)	Portio scraping (PS)/endocervical curettage (ECC) Colposcopy-directed biopsies/endocervical curettage (ECC)

Table 3. Indications for portio scraping/endocervical curettage

Cytology:	Recurring group III_D Group III Group $IV_{a\ and\ b}$ Group V
Colposcopy:	Abnormal finding, with endocervical abnormal cytology

been accepted around the world because of their high reliability. In the FRG and Eastern European countries, conization is the method of choice and has the highest popularity. However, worldwide the non-mutilating techniques are widespread and preferred. Meanwhile, more and more young women have the diagnosis of a pathological Pap smear; it must become a challenge for us to develop diagnostic alternatives to conization, equally safe and with better accuracy but less radical and without the morbidity. There are two methods.

Since 1963 I have used the colposcopy-directed biopsy only in selected cases. Among the acceptable alternatives of non-mutilating methods, personal experience (Egger et al. 1975; Kindermann 1979, 1981) with ectocervical scraping and endocervical curettage (ECC) will be reported here. The indications (Table 3) for portio scraping (PS)/ECC are pathological findings in cytology of groups III and IV with demonstrated variations, meaning exclusively the preclinical cases. We do not recommend the procedure to confirm clinical cancer; here, a biopsy is adequate.

Technique

Some brief remarks to the technique. The procedure is started with a Schiller iodine test. This simple procedure should be the first step to mark suspicious areas of the ectocervix. The iodine-negative surface of the ectocervix has to be scraped especially carefully. It is mandatory to combine this technique of PS with ECC. The material is then collected thoroughly, because it is small in volume and mixed with blood and mucus. It must be cleaned and separated out. This can then be embedded in paraffin and examined by histological step-sections. The amount of work in the histological laboratory is low compared with that necessary for cone evaluation.

Table 4. Reliability of portio scraping/endocervical curettage (Erlangen 1963–1978, Berlin 1979–1987)

Pretherapeutical histological diagnosis	Cases	Posttherapeutical evaluation		
		Agreement	Disagreement	
			with importance for treatment	without importance for treatment
		(%)	(%)	(%)
CIN II–III	1028	987 (96.1)	6 (0.5)	35 (3.4)
Microcarcinoma	71	58 (82.0)	3 (4.2)	10 (14.0)
Macrocarcinoma	66	60 (91.0)	6 (9.0)	0
	1165	1105 (94.8)	15 (1.3)	45 (3.9)

Table 5. Accuracy of portio scraping/endocervical curettage in 1165 patients (1963–1987)

Pre-and posttherapeutical histological diagnosis:	Agreement in 94.8%	(1105)
	Disagreement in 5.2%	(60)
Clinically important disagreement:	1.3%	(15)
	Primary overtreatment: 0.7%	(8)
	Primary undertreatment: 0.6%	(7)

Results

The results from 1963 to 1987 are given in Table 4. In 24 years the procedure has been performed with 1165 patients. The pretherapeutical histological diagnosis from PS/ECC is compared with the postsurgical histological evaluation of the specimens (in some cases cones, mostly hysterectomy specimens or a few Wertheim specimens). Pre- and posttherapeutic agreement is presented in the second row of Table 4, related to CIN lesions, microcarcinomata and frank cancer. On the right side, the disagreement is demonstrated and differentiated into cases with or without clinical importance. The definition "clinically important" should be explained in more detail (Table 5). The overall agreement was 94.8%. Disagreement was found in 5.2%, but in these 60 patients the histological difference between pretherapeutical and postsurgical statements was important for only 15, that is, 1.3%.

Unnecessary primary overtreatment was the clinical consequence in 0.7%. Here, a Wertheim procedure was performed, as more than microcarcinoma was expected in the primary histological diagnosis. Postsurgically the disease had to be classified as only microcarcinoma. The primary undertreatment in 7 patients (0.6%) has to be considered of greater clinical importance for the patients involved. The disease was underestimated primarily and a hysterectomy performed; this operation was for them insufficiently radical because of stage Ib cancer in the hysterectomy specimens.

Table 6. Advantages of portio scraping/endocervical curettage
in pretherapeutical diagnostic procedure

1. High accuracy
2. Simple technical procedure
3. No perioperative mortality and morbidity
4. No negative influence on fertility
5. No negative influence for the following treatment
6. Inexpensive

In summary, ectocervical scraping and endocervical curettage (PS/ECC) has proven a diagnostic histological procedure with high reliability in the histological evaluation of pathological findings in cytology or colposcopy. For the overwhelming majority of CIN cases, especially in young women, the procedure is very advantageous (Table 6). The pretherapeutical histological diagnosis is made with high accuracy. It is a simple technical procedure. No perioperative mortality or morbidity could be found. No negative influence on fertility and reproductive function has been seen. There was no negative influence for subsequent necessary treatment of the underlying lesion. These conditions play an essential role in recommending non-mutilating procedures in the early detection of cervical cancer. Last but not least, compared with other procedures it is inexpensive.

Summary

From a theoretical point of view the problem of early diagnosis of cervical cancer seems to be solved. The instruments of early detection of preclinical cervical cancer in the preinvasive or early invasive stage were developed some decades ago. Screening programmes are well-established in many countries around the world. From the practical point of view the problem of the early diagnosis of cervical cancer is still unsolved, mainly because of the low acceptance of the screening programmes by the female population. Other problems concern the accuracy of cytology and colposcopy findings with histological evaluation.

Because pathological Pap smears are encountered more and more in the very young female population, nonmutilating procedures should be preferred for histological classification in these cases. There are two diagnostic alternatives to the less cervix-conserving conization: the colposcopically directed biopsy plus endocervical curettage and the ectocervical (portio) scraping plus endocervical curettage (PS/ECC). Ectocervical scraping and endocervical curettage have proven to be a diagnostic method of high accuracy and reliability in the histological evaluation of pathological cytology or abnormal colposcopy. The indications are discussed in the paper.

The technique of PS is described. It is mandatory to combine the procedure with an ECC. Personal examination results from 1963 to 1987 are given. The pretherapeutical histological diagnosis and postsurgical histological findings in the specimens (cone/uterus/Wertheim specimen) are compared. Pre- and posttherapeutical agreement was found for CIN lesions, microcarcinomata and macrocancer (stage Ib). The agreement can be considered highly acceptable and is comparable with conization in a randomized prospective study of PS/ECC versus conization. The overall agreement was 94.8%. Disagreement was found in 5.2%, but in these 60 cases the histological difference between pretherapeutical and postsurgical statements was important for only 15 patients. These 1.3% of the total received primary overtreatment (0.7%) or undertreatment (0.6%).

The clinical advantages of PS/ECC are mainfold. It is a simple technical procedure. No perioperative mortality or major morbidity was found in 1165 patients so treated. No negative influence on later fertility and reproductive function is expected and could be seen. No negative influence for a subsequent necessary treatment could be seen. Compared with alternative procedures, it is inexpensive.

References

Anderson GH, Boyes DA, Benedet JL, Le Riche J, Matisic JP, Sven KC, Worth JA, Millner A, Bennett OM (1988) Organisation and results of the cervical cytology screening program in British Columbia, 1955–1985. Br Med J 296:957–958

Bonett A, Davy M, Roder D (1989) Cervical cancer in South Australia: trends in incidence mortality and case survival. Aust N Z J Obstet Gynecol 29:193–196

Dickenson JA, Leeder SR, Sanson-Fisher RW (1988) Frequency of cervical smear-tests among patients of general practitioners. Med J Aust 148:128–131

Egger H, Kindermann G, Michalzik K (1975) Portioabschabung und Cervixcurettage–eine Alternative zur Konisation bei positiver Zytologie. Geburtshilfe Frauenheilkd 35: 913–918

Kindermann G (1979) Konisation versus Portioabschabung/Cervixcurettage. Arch Gynecol 227:267–270

Kindermann G (1981) Operatives Vorgehen bei cytologischen und kolposkopischen Verdachtshinweisen. Arch Gynecol 232:102–105

Kindermann G (1988) Voraussetzungen und Möglichkeiten der Funktionserhaltung bei intraepithelialer Neoplasie und Mikrokarzinom der Cervix uteri. Gynäkologe 21: 298–301

Koss LG (1989) The Papanicolaou test for cervical cancer detection: a triumph and a tragedy. JAMA 261:737–743

Mitchell, Medley (1987) Community Health Stud 11:183–185

Sigurdsson K, Adalsteinsson S, Tulinius H, Ragnarsson J (1989) The value of screening as an approach to cervical cancer control in Iceland, 1964–1986. Int J Cancer 43:1–5

Wain GV, Hacker NF (1990) Pitfalls in the screening and early diagnosis of cervical cancer. Curr Opin Obstet Gynecol 2:74–79

Breast Cancer Screening

D. von Fournier, H.-W. Anton, H. Junkermann, and G. Bastert

Introduction

The evidence supporting breast cancer screening can be based on two controlled randomized trials in which population screening by mammography (and in one by clinical examination) was offered on a random basis (HIP: Shapiro et al. 1982; Four-County: Tabar et al. 1985), and two case-control studies in which the screening history of women dying from breast cancer was compared with that of healthy controls (Nijmegen: Verbeek et al. 1984; DOM: Collette et al. 1984). The question is whether breast cancer is always systemic or whether it is sometimes localized in cases of smaller tumors, in which case early detection should improve survival.

The updates of the HIP (Health Insurance Plan, New York: Shapiro et al. 1988; Fig. 1) and the Two-County Trial, a randomized trial in Sweden (Tabar et al. 1989), support the hypothesis that mammographic screening has many more advantages than disadvantages. Therefore, the German Mammographic Study was set up in June 1989 in four centers: Cologne (Hoeffken), Hamburg (Frischbier), Heidelberg (von Fournier), and Esslingen (Barth), with the epidemiologic center in Hannover (Robra) and a quality control center in Berlin (Friedrich). Many scientific societies and medical societies in the FRG are involved in this study. It is financed by the German Ministry for Research and Technology.

Screening Procedure

Probands are women in the age group 40–70 years who are apparently free of symptoms. In the first round, 2-view mammography is performed followed 1 and 2 years later, in the second and third rounds, by 1-oblique-view mammography. A clinical examination is carried out on each person before mammography.

If further investigations of abnormalities are necessary, the centers carry out magnification views, ultrasonography, fine needle aspiration, stereotaxic localization, and as required a surgical biopsy. Each center is made up of a multidisciplinary team with the necessary experience in radiodiagnosis, surgery, pathology, and radio-oncology. Since 1990, in a second step each of the centers has become a kind of "reference center for the decentralization" of screening. The Screening is performed in private practice by radiologists, who have had experience in mammography.

The first experience was that approx. 30%–50% of the women had already had mammographies. In fact, in the FRG screening mammographies carried out at least every 2 years have already been established in many women groups, depending on various factors such as social status and the number of experienced doctors available. The gynecologists mostly invite the women to undergo a screening every 2 years.

Reasons and Current Understanding of Screening

In the FRG (population ca. 80 million) there are 33000–40000 new cases of breast cancer each year. Some 200000 women live with breast disease, and 70% of them will at some time die as a result. Breast cancer is the number one cause of death in German women in the age group 38–58 years. To illustrate the problem, in the USA 57000 died during the Vietnam War, while 330000 women died at the same time from breast cancer (Washington Post, 21 January 1990). It is accepted that breast cancer is, in most cases, a "systemic disease." Even 30 years and more after first treatment, patients still die from metastatic disease (Brinkley and Haybittle 1984; Rutqvist and Wallgren 1985). The 30% of "survivors" from breast cancer may die because of other reasons, before the slow-growing metastases become evident (personal cure). In a meta-analysis of 28000 women (61 randomized trials), the EBCTCG (Early Breast Cancer Trialists' Collaborative Group 1988) could show that systemic treatment following operation (chemotherapy or antiestrogen) is able to prolong relapse-free survival and the overall lifetime (in the range of about 10%). The BCDDP Study in the USA showed that 22% of all detected cancers during the first 5 years were noninfiltrating (Shapiro et al. 1982), 10% of the infiltrating cancers were less than 1 cm in size, and about 75% showed free axillary lymph nodes. It is known that noninfiltrating cancer does not metastasize, and if detected, the patient is cured. It is also agreed that the overall survival increases the smaller the tumor is at first treatment (Duncan and Kerr 1984; Fig. 2).

It is now accepted that breast conserving therapy shows the same survival (during the first 15 years at least) compared with mastectomy. More and more patients request and doctors accept "breast conserving therapy," which now is standard therapy in our clinic in about two-thirds of these patients.

Carter et al. (1989) showed that for invasive cancer less than 1 cm in diameter the incidence of positive axillary lymph nodes was less than 20%, and the 5-year survival was over 95%. The 5-year survival for all breast cancers was less than 60%.

A breast cancer 1 cm in size contains 1 billion cancer cells. If the estimated tumor volume doubling time ranges between 2–5 months, it would take 15 years from a single cell (10 µm) to 1 cm.

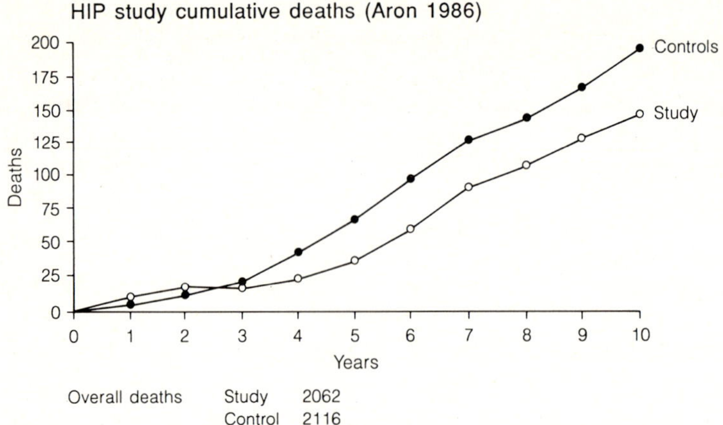

Fig. 1. Cumulative deaths in the study and control groups of the Health Insurance Plan (HIP) trial

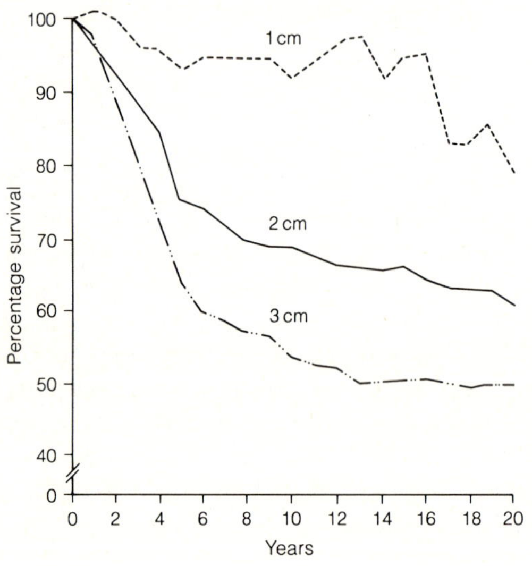

Fig. 2. Age-corrected survival rates for women treated for breast cancer up to 3.0 cm in diameter (Duncan and Kerr 1976)

Natural Growth Rate and Its Effect on Screening

For example, a fast-growing tumor was missed at the first screening interval and the patient came 1/2 year later with a so-called "interval cancer". In its "sojourn" period the breast cancer growth is in a pre-clinical asymptomatic phase. The fast-growing cases can be missed by mammographic screening, whereas the slow-growing cases may be detected at a earlier stage.

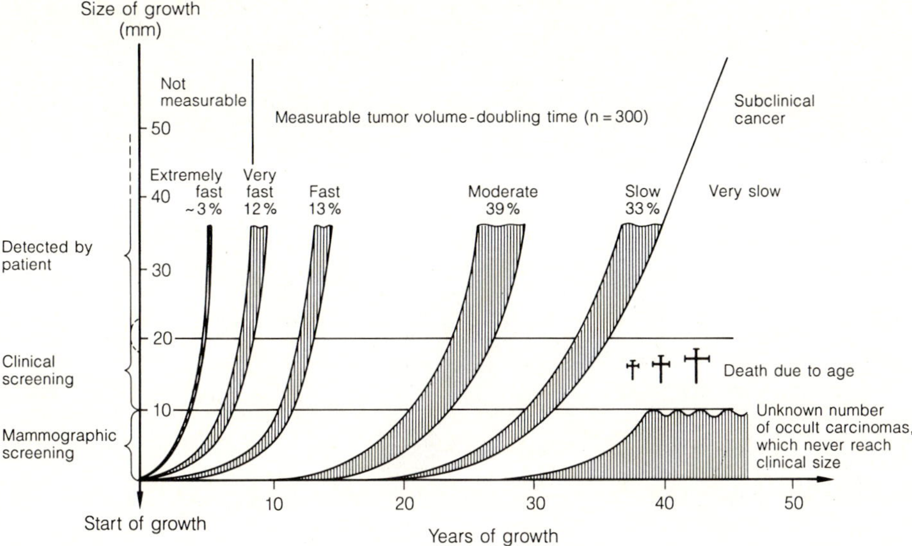

Fig. 3. Proportion of tumors with different growth rates and their clinical relevance (von Fournier et al. 1989)

In another case a standstill in the growth of a tumor could be observed for 2 years; then, the invasive carcinoma was confirmed by operation. These cancer types sometimes never reach a clinically relevant size.

Figure 3 shows the speed of growth with the variations in the natural speed of growth in clinical breast cancers. We observed 28% extremely or very fast-growing tumors. Moderate growth was observed in 39% and slow growth in 33% of the cases.

The curve on the extreme right of Figure 3 shows there is an unknown number of tumors growing so slowly that they never reach a palpable size. According to that, Andersen et al. (1989) found that 25% of all Danish women have breast cancer cells in the breast at some time in their lives, but only 7% develop "clinical" cancer. So detection of some non-infiltrating breast cancers has no clinical benefit for the patient (in 18% out of 25% of all women).

Figure 4 shows the growth time and growth behavior in breast cancer. Beginning with the first tumor cell, it can be calculated that 21 volume doublings are needed to achieve a size of 5 mm. It takes the tumor half its whole life to reach this 5 mm. To reach 1 cm it needs over 25 doublings. After 42–45 doublings the tumor burden kills the patient. The curve on top shows mammographic efficiency. Today this may reach 50%, when the tumor becomes 1 cm in size (von Fournier et al. 1989).

Table 1 lists the case control studies of screening together with the number of cases, type of mammography, clinical examinatio, age at entry, etc. All showed a reduction in mortality. In a most recent analysis, the DOM study, which used both 2-view mammography and clinical examination, showed the greatest reduction in mortality (Tables 2, 3).

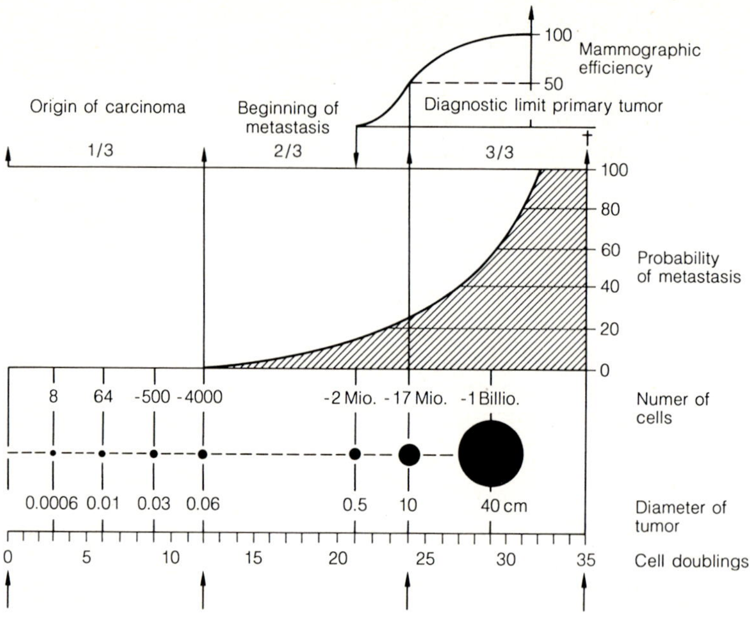

Fig. 4. Model of tumor growth behavior based on constant volume doubling times

Table 1. Four randomized trials of breast screening: design of the trials

Study	Age (years)	Mammography (no. of views)	Clinical examination	Intervals	Study group	Control group	Follow-up (years)	Reference
HIP	40–64	2-view	Yes	1 year × 4	31 000	31 000	18	Shapiro et al. (1982)
Two-County	>40	1-view	No	2–3 years	78 085	56 782	7	Tabar et al. (1985)
Edinburgh	45–64	2-view	Alternate	2 years	23 194	127 117	7	UK Trial (1988)
Guildford	45–64	1-view	Alternate	2 years	22 647	127 117	7	UK Trial (1988)
Malmo	>45	2-view	No	1.5–2 years	21 088	21 195	8	Andersson et al. (1988)

Table 2. Breast cancer cases and mortality in randomized trials of screening

Study	Age (years)	Breast cancer incidence		Breast cancer deaths		Relative risk (95% CI)	Reference
		Study	Control	Study	Control		
HIP	<50	151	145	61	77	0.79	Shapiro et al.
	>50	220	226	92	119	0.77	(1982)
Two-County	<50	222	123	25	18	1.26 (0.56–2.86)	Tabar et al.
	>50	1073	645	180	135	0.61 (0.44–0.84)	(1985)
UK trial		748	1472	102	362	0.54 (0.36–0.81)	UK Trial (1988)
Malmo	<55	123	91	28	22	1.29 (0.74–2.25)	Andersson et al.
	>55	457	356	35	44	0.79 (0.51–1.24)	(1988)

Table 3. Results of case control studies of screening

Study	No. of cases	Mammography (no. of views)	Clinical examination	Relative risk (95% CI)	Reference
Nijmegen	62 000	1-view	Yes	0.48 (0.23–1.0)	Verbeek et al. (1984)
DOM	20 555	2-view	Yes	0.3 (0.13–0.7)	Collette et al. (1984)
Florence	24 813	2-view	No	0.53 (0.29–0.95)	Palli et al. (1986)

Extent of Benefit in Screening

In the trials since 1963 we observed:

1. Reduction in mortality ranging between no reduction and 50% especially in women older than 50 years.
2. The Malmo trial (Andersson et al. 1988) showed a reduction in size from 2.8 cm in controls to 1.3 cm in the screening group on average.
3. Reduction of involved axillary lymph nodes: The Breast Cancer Detection and Demonstration Project (BCDDP: Wright 1985) showed a reduction in involved axillary lymph nodes to less than 30%.
4. The correct interpretation of mammographies increased, especially when combined with palpation: The rate of "interval cancers" within 1 year was 42% in the HIP Study, starting with 1963 (Shapiro et al. 1982). This fell to 10% in the Nijmegen Study (Verbeek et al. 1984).

Improvement in mammographic efficiency can also be shown by comparing the older HIP Study with 60% of cancer being diagnosed by clinical palpation alone with 25% in the following BCDDP Study. Nowadays, 75% were detected by mammography alone. The improvement in the younger age group of 40–49-year-old women became obvious.

Dissent with Screening

Neither the Malmo Trial nor the Edinburgh Trial (randomized trials) nor the British Cooperative Trial of Early Detection of Breast Cancer showed a significant mortality advantage (Andersson et al. 1988; UK Trial of Early Detection of Breast Cancer Group 1988; Roberts et al. 1990). The power of the statistics in the Malmo and Edinburgh Trials has been questioned, as the UK-TEDBCG was not randomized (Forrest 1991). The HIP Study showed after 18 years a 23% reduction in breast cancer mortality. After 18 years the study shows a benefit for women under 50 years of age at entry. It revealed that benefits from screening by means of mortality reduction do not emerge until the 5 or 7 years' follow-up.

Table 4. Screening pick-up rates for breast cancer in several studies

Study	Prevalent rate per 1000 cases	Reference
HIP	2.7	Shapiro et al. (1982)
Two-County	5.6	Tabar et al. (1985)
Nijmegen	3.9	Verbeek et al. (1984)
DOM	2.5	Collette et al. (1984)
CSPO	3.2	Palli et al. (1986)
Edinburgh	2.5	UK Trial (1988)
Guildford	2.6	UK Trial (1988)

Table 5. Interval cancers, diagnosed between two screenings

Study	No. of cases	Percentage of all cancers	Reference
HIP	92	42	Shapiro et al. (1982)
Two-County	261	22	Tabar et al. (1985)
Nijmegen	31	10	Verbeek et al. (1984)
DOM	17	24	Collette et al. (1984)
CSPO	11	39	Palli et al. (1986)
Edinburgh	47	13	UK Trial (1988)
Guildford	68	18	UK Trial (1988)
Malmo	100	17	Andersson et al. (1988)

Figure 1 shows the cumulative death in the study and control groups of the HIP trial during the first ten years.

Acceptance Rate

The highest acceptance rate was achieved in Sweden. By the fourth round of screening the greatest proportion still attending was 70%, reported in the Malmo Trial. Pick-up rates for breast cancer in the first prevalent screen ranged between 2.5 and 5.6 cancer cases among 1000 women (Table 4). The interval cancers within 1 year reached 42% in the HIP, but this fell to 10% in the Nijmegen Study (Table 5).

Radiation Risk

The reduced radiation dosage per mammography is now between 0.4–0.1 cGy (or 0.1 rad). The cumulative dosage for 10 screenings would be 1 cGy or 1 rad. This low dose is unlikely to lead to a significant increase in radiation-induced cancer. It has been calculated that a breast dose of 0.1 rad would lead to 4 cancers per million women screened after a 10-year latency period. This has been described as a similiar risk to a 10-mile car journey.

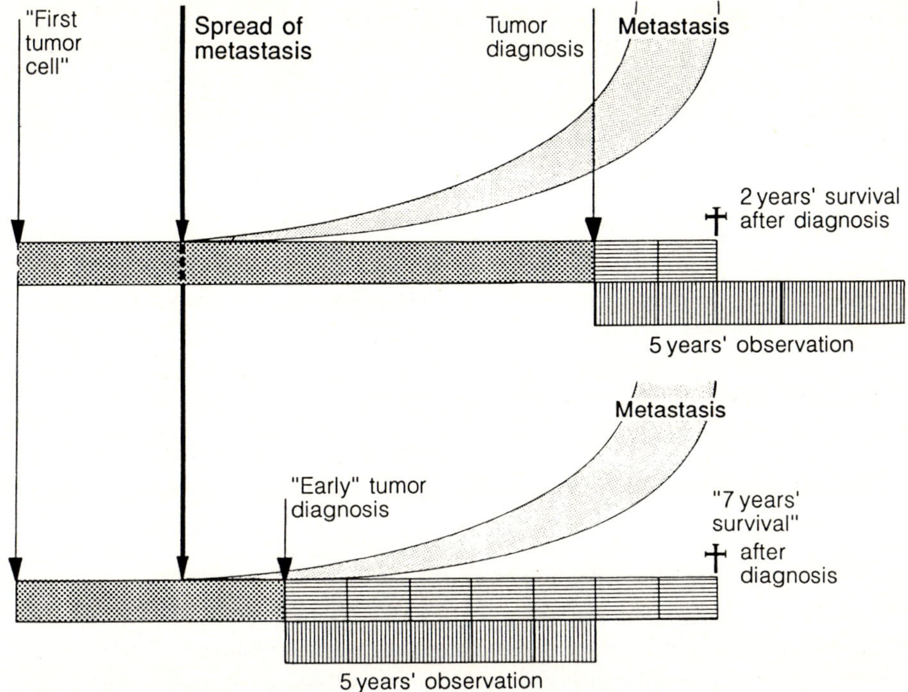

Fig. 5. Effect of so-called early diagnosis in some cases: lead-time bias

Breast Self-examination

A recent overview (Hill et al. 1988) of breast self-examination (BSE) studies
have shown that there may be a very small benefit. The UK trials in Nottingham
and Huddersfield do not suggest a benefit for mortality (Hill et al. 1988). The
interval cancer rate in mammography screening trials now ranges between 10%
and 20%. Therefore, BSE will have to be introduced as a part of screening
trials to detect interval cancers as early as possible.

Further Problems

Further problems and dissent with screening include: lead-time bias, length-
time bias, nonrelevant cancers, interval cancers and elevation of the biopsy
rate.

The Lead-Time Bias. Figure 5 demonstrates the lead-time bias: If metastases
arise before the first screening, the patient has seemingly no benefit in the risk
for mortality. The lead-time problem may occur in a certain precentage of
patients.

Detection of Nonrelevant Cancers. As shown above, Anderson et al. (1989)
report an incidence of 25% carcinomas of the breast in all women in Denmark.

The life-long incidence of clinically relevant cancers was 7%. The remaining 18% of histological cancers are therefore "nonrelevant" cancers. These cancers cause a problem because of unnecessary biopsies and unnecessary cancer treatment.

Interval Cancers. As mentioned above, the rate of interval cancers fell to 10%–20% in the new trials.

Elevation of the Biopsy Rate. In the first year of the BCDDP study, 9600 biopsies (100%) were performed, and 1400 cancers (15%) were detected. The 85% of biopsies with negative results were in many cases "unnecessary surgery" (Wright 1985). If benign biopsy represents "harm," that is, unnecessary surgery, then the harm: benefit ratio was 5.6:1. Nowadays, this ratio has dropped in the new trials (Malmo Trial) and in our clinic is 1.4:1.

The Malmo Trial as well as the Canadian Trial (Miller, this volume) surprisingly showed a higher breast cancer rate and a higher death rate from breast cancer in the screening group compared with the control group. In the screening group in most trials the detection rate of negative lymph nodes was much higher. It is suspected that in many cases the "negative" lymph nodes were a false-negative diagnosis. In an earlier stage, lymph node metastases are very small and can be missed by the average pathological work-up. Those false-negative lymph node patients did not receive adjuvant therapy (CHT or hormonal). Therefore, it has been discussed (Miller, personal communication) that in future cases with negative lymph node results combined with "unfavorable prognostic parameters" should undergo systemic adjuvant therapy.

Summary

1. Screening intervals (according to Tabar et al.) of 1 year in women younger than 50 years in order to minimize "interval cancers" and of 2 years in women older than 50 years.
2. Mammographic views (according to Lundgren 1988) should be 2 at first round and 1 oblique in the following, yearly rounds. All women at risk should attend screening. The identification of useful "high-risk groups" has not been established. Palpation is recommended at each screening, as is self-examination.
3. Prescription of adjuvant therapy should not depend on lymph node status when screening cancer cases. It should depend rather on clinical and histological "prognostic factors."

References

Andersen JA, Nielsen JM, Ottesen GL, Thomsen JL (1989) In situ carcinoma of the female breast: frequency, growth pattern and biologic significance. In: Kubli F, von Fournier D (eds) Breast disease. Springer, Berlin Heidelberg New York, pp 513–522

Andersson I, Aspergen K, Janzon L et al. (1988) Mammographic screening and mortality from breast cancer: the Malmo mammographic screening trial. Br Med J 207:943–948

Bringkely D, Haybittle JL (1984) Long-term survival of women with breast cancer. Lancet 1:118

Carter CL, Allen C, Henson DE (1989) Relation of tumor site, lymph node status and survival in 24 740 breast cancer cases. Cancer 63:181–187

Collette HJA, Day NE, Rombach JJ, DeWaard F (1984) Evaluation of screening for breast cancer in a non-randomised study (the DOM project) by means of a case-control study. Lancet 1:1224–1226

Duncan W, Kerr GR (1976) The curability of breast cancer. Br Med J 42:781–783

Early Breast Cancer Trialists' Colloborative Group (1988) Effects of adjuvant tamoxifen and of cytotoxic therapy on mortality in early breast cancer. An overview of 61 randomized trials among 28 896 women. N Engl J Med 319:1681–1691

Fentiman IS (ed) (1990) Detection and treatment of early breast cancer. Dunitz, London, pp 58–72

Friedrich M, von Fournier D, Hoeffken W (1989) The value of diagnostic methods: mammography, screening and other imaging techniques. In: Kubli F, von Fournier D (eds) Breast disease. Springer, Berlin Heidelberg New York, pp 112–128

Hill D, White V, Jolley D Mapperson K (1988) Self examination of the breast: is it beneficial? Meta-analysis of studies investigating breast self examination and extent of disease in breast cancer. Br Med J 297:271–275

Lundgren B (1988) Breast screening in Britain and Sweden. Br Med J 297:1266

Palli D, del Turco MR, Buiatli E et al. (1986) A case-control study of the efficacy of a non-randomised breast cancer screening program in Florence (Italy). Int J Cancer 38: 501–504

Roberts MM, Alexander FE, Anderson TJ et al. (1990) The Edinburgh trial of screening for breast cancer. Lancet 335:241–246

Rutqvist LE, Wallgren A (1985) Long-term survival of 458 young breast cancer patients. Cancer 55:658–665

Shapiro S, Venet W, Strax P et al. (1982) Ten-to-fourteen-year effect of screening on breast cancer mortality. JNCI 69:349–355

Shapiro S, Venet W, Strax P, Venet L (1988) Periodic screening for breast cancer. The Health Insurance Plan Project and its sequelae 1963–1986. Johns Hopkins University Press, Baltimore

Spitalier JM, Kurtz JM, Amalric R, Brandone H, Ayme Y, Bressac C, Hans D (1989) Long-term survival following breast-conserving therapy in comparison to radical surgical treatment: an overview. In: Kubli F, von Fournier D (eds) Breast disease. Springer, Berlin Heidelberg New York, pp 276–284

Tabar L, Fagerberg CJG, Gad A et al. (1985) Reduction in mortality from breast cancer after mass screening with mammography. Randomised trial from the Breast Cancer Screening Working Group of the Swedish National Board of Health and Welfare. Lancet 1:829–832

Tabar L, Fagerberg G, Fuffy SW, Day NE (1989) The Swedish two-county trial of mammographic screening for breast cancer: recent results and calculation of benefit. J Epidemiol Community Health 43:107–114

UK Trial of Early Detection of Breast Cancer Group (1988) First results on mortality reduction in the UK trial of early detection on breast cancer. Lancet 2:411–415

Verbeek ALM, Hendricks JHCL, Holland R et al. (1984) Reduction of breast cancer mortality through mass screening with modern mammography: first results of the Nijmegen project, 1975–1981. Lancet 1:1222–1224

Veronesi U, Luini A, del Vecchio M (1989) Local recurrence and new primary ipsilateral carcinomas after conservative treatment of breast carcinoma. In: Kubli F, von Fournier D (eds) Breast disease. Springer, Berlin Heidelberg New York, pp 301–307

Von Fournier D, Hoeffken W, Friedrich M (1989) Natural growth rate of primary breast cancer and its metastases. In: Kubli F, von Fournier D (eds) Breast disease. Springer, Berlin Heidelberg New York, pp 78–96

Washington Post, 21. Jan. 1990

Wright CJ (1985) Breast cancer screening: a different look at the evidence. Surgery 100: 594–598

Summary of Discussion: Session 2

M. KAUFMANN

The three presentations of this session dealt with clinical problems of early detection of carcinoma of the prostate (CaP) and transitional cell carcinoma (TCC), cervical cancer and breast cancer. All three papers demonstrated the great hope placed in screening programmes for early cancer detection, and prevention trials for these types of malignancies have also been discussed.

For the three cancer localizations general as well as selective screening programmes have been presented. In detail, proposals and statements included the questions of which populations (age groups, certain risk groups) should be screened, which methods should be used and which are the best methods, also with regard to cost-benefit analyses? This includes clinical examinations, which always have to be compared with technical facilities.

For *CaP* it was obvious that only few small prospective studies analysed the sensitivity and specificity of screening programmes using various methods like digital rectal examination or transrectal ultrasonography. It was also mentioned that there are no relevant screening programmes in Germany. Finally, discussion concentrated on the fact that for CaP the value of early tumour diagnosis really remains unclear, since in the vast majority of men this type of cancer never will become clinically symptomatic and relevant. Therefore risk groups remain to be defined.

In *TCC*, cystoscopy and urinary cytology are the diagnostic techniques. New tools like flow cytometry and immunocytology show early promise, and the data were discussed in detail. However, the few data presented so far do not allow one to draw final conclusions on screening programmes. Immunocytology seems an appropriate method for follow-up examinations in patients with a history of TCC, which show a high rate of tumor recurrence.

Cervical cytology and colposcopy are well established tools for early detection of *cervical cancer* and its possible precursor lesions. Screening programmes are well established all over the world. The acceptance of the programmes is still low, and further information and advertisement are necessary. However, there is again a small trend toward a better acceptance rate in Germany.

For the histological classification of pathological Pap smears a nonmutilating procedure to replace conization of the cervix was described and discussed. This new procedure comprises ectocervical scraping (PS) combined with endocervical curettage (ECC). Data on more than 1000 patients treated from 1963 to 1987 using this simple, effective and inexpensive technique were presented. Histological findings differed from PS/ECC results only in 5.2% of cases, and only in 1.3% of the patients was the difference important. In 0.7% there was overtreatment and in 0.6% there was untertreatment. In general, it was stated in the discussion that the cost-benefit ratio of PS/ECC seems significantly better than that of today's standard procedures. It is hoped that this new procedure will come to have wider application in clinical practice.

The objective of *breast cancer* screening is to detect small invasive cancers. However, it is not known whether it is of any benefit to detect or even treat subclinical in situ lesions of the breast.

It is generally accepted that breast cancer screening is mammographic screening. Updates on several worldwide randomized and non-randomized trials of population screening by mammography and by clinical examination were presented and discussed. This overview included the German Mammography Study, which finally was set up in 1989. Evidently no information for the situation in Germany is yet available due to the late onset of this non-randomized study. However, this study may result in some benefit in quality control of mammography, which is widely conducted in this country.

Screening has the potential to reduce the mortality from breast cancer. In the discussion it was clearly seen that the extent of benefit in screening is not homogeneous; indeed, benefit seems to be confined to subgroups of patients. It was concluded in a statement by A.B. Miller, Toronto, that "Screening for breast cancer by mammography every 1–3 years can reduce breast cancer mortality substantially in women age 50–60. In women under age 50 there is little evidence of a benefit, at least in the first 10 years after initiation of screening" (UICC Project on Evaluation of Screening for Cancer, 1990). However, the age limitation was not accepted by all.

Further progress will be achieved only by high-quality mammography, better education on physical examination and breast self-examination and higher compliance with screening invitations. Breast self-examination must be taught and trained; after negative mammography, breast self-examination should be started. Here, especially, selective screening of high-risk women seems to have a major impact on mortality.

After this session it was evident that, especially in Germany, there are far too few efficient cancer screening programmes, and worldwide further prospective randomized trials are necessary to yield more reliable data to use in deciding whom to screen or to define high-risk patients for different cancer types.

Tumor Markers

Chairman: R. Lamerz

Introductory Remarks

R. Lamerz

Concerning the early detection of cancer, the use of circulating tumor markers (TM) has been one of the most intriguing designs because of its little harm for the patient, the use of high technology of epitope-specific monoclonal antibodies, highly sensitive determination by radio- or enzyme, fluorescent or luminescent immunoassays (detection limit 1ng–1pg/ml), the availability of commercial kits, and cost-effective automization for high numbers of determinations in a very short time of 1–3h. Yet these theoretical and practical advantages are in sharp contrast to the manifold disadvantages precluding TM from use in the early detection of cancer.

First, the least tumor mass that can be detected by TM comprises more than 10^5 or 10^6 tumor cells and is still dependent on TM expression, synthesis, release, catabolism, excretion, as well as the tumor's blood supply. This means that a TM relevant for a special tumor may only be partially expressed and synthesized, expressed but not released, incorrectly elevated in serum because of a disturbed catabolism (e.g., liver insufficiency) or excretion (e.g., renal insufficiency), or not elevated because of insufficient blood supply.

Second, all established circulating TM are not tumor-specific but may be elevated transiently or often maintained in the low pathologic range in different or counterpart benign diseases of the tumor in question, thus leading to lower specificity (about 80%–90%). Most of them are also not organ-specific but may be found elevated in several diseases except for some organ-specific markers (PSA/PAP for prostatic cancer or thyroglobulin in the serum of patients following total thyroidectomy because of differentiated or papillary thyroid carcinoma).

Third, circulating TM are correlated by definition with tumor mass, thus exhibiting often exponentially increasing serum levels with follow-up. This means that early stages of cancer show only a low sensitivity of TM (between 10% and 30%), whereas progressive and metastatic disease may account for >50%–90% of sensitivity. Therefore, the main indication of all established circulating TM is monitoring of the course of the disease and response to therapy rather than diagnosis or prognosis and even less so screening.

Cancer screening in its strict sense is looking for cancer in a normal population without clinical symptoms, eventually restricted by sex or age. In this situation, no established TM has proven valuable because of its too low sensitivity (s) and specificity (sp) in early cancer and a too low incidence of cancer in the distinctive sample (prevalence <1‰), leading to a low predictive value (pv+) of TM. This has been shown, e.g., for carcinoembryonic antigen (CEA) in colorectal (s = 40%, sp = 90% in Dukes' stages A/B; prevalence about 1‰ in an asymptomatic normal population) or breast cancer (s = 30%, sp = 90%; prevalence in women aged 49–59 years 260/100000). In colorectal cancer (Fletcher 1986), 60% of developing tumors would be missed (test-negative) in contrast to 250 false-positive tests seen for one true-positive patient with cancer (pv+ = 0.4%). In breast cancer (Tondini et al. 1989), 70% would be test-negative and 125 false-positive patients found for 1 true-positive patient with cancer (pv+ = 0.8%). In this respect, mammography (s = 95%, sp = 99.5%) is by far superior, yielding a positive predictive value of 34% (one-third of test-positive women has cancer).

The only TM of screening quality in asymptomatic candidates with a higher prevalence is the determination of calcitonin in relatives of patients with hereditary medullary thyroid cancer (MEN II) to whom thyroidectomy is offered upon a positive test. A further TM with screening ability, prostate-specific antigen (PSA), has quite recently been recommended in combination with rectal examination and ultrasonography (Catalona et al. 1991).

During transition from an asymptomatic to symptomatic state or by choosing a defined patient group at risk for certain cancers, a higher prevalence of cancer is noted; in this situation TM may be used as an adjunct together with imaging or endoscopic methods to facilitate an earlier detection of cancer (e.g., CA 125 and ultrasound in ovarian cancer, alpha-fetoprotein (AFP) and human chorionic gonadotropin (HCG) in testicular cancer, AFP and sonography in patients with liver cirrhosis for detection of hepatocellular cancer (Regan 1989), CA 19-9 in patients with pain in the upper abdomen and weight loss for detection of pancreatic cancer (Richter et al. 1989), CEA in patients with changing diarrhea/obstipation and a positive fecal blood test result for detection of colorectal cancer).

A further possibility of using circulating TM is in the early detection of recurrence or changing response to therapy as has been shown by numerous studies for CEA in colorectal cancer, AFP and HCG in testicular cancer, CA 15-3 in breast cancer, and some others. This indication is highly dependent on a still feasible treatment, which often limits its usefulness. Further improvement is effected by monitoring TM kinetics following operation or other treatment modalities by calculating TM half-life and/or TM doubling rates or an e-functional calculation of TM production time (in days) (Horwich and Peckham 1984, Price et al. 1990). A half-life longer than physiological (e.g., HCG 1–2 days, AFP 5 days, CA 125 6 days, CEA 4–8 days) with normal liver/kidney function is highly predictive of residual disease, thus influencing earlier treatment planning by, e.g., a more aggressive therapy (Toner et al. 1990, Hunter et al. 1990). Significantly rising TM serum levels are incompatible with tumor remission and may lead to earlier discovery of therapy failures thus requiring a change of therapy or even earlier withdrawal of an ineffective chemotherapy (Price et al. 1990).

In summary, the usefulness of TM monitoring for early cancer detection is rather restricted because of biological and technical limitations and more concerned with early recurrence of cancer than with its first detection. At the moment, it is unknown whether more specific TM or more refined detection methods might be developed and overcome the restrictions, although their ease of determination and noninvasiveness for the patient are still attractive for screening purposes.

References

Catalona WJ, Smith DS, Ratcliff TL, Dodds KM, Coplen DE, Yuan JJJ, Petros JA, Andriole GL (1991) Measurement of prostate-specific antigen in serum as a screening test for prostate cancer. N Engl J Med 324:1156–1161

Fletcher RH (1986) Carcinoembryonic antigen. Ann Intern Med 104:66–73

Horwich A, Peckham MJ (1984) Serum tumor marker regression rate following chemotherapy for malignant teratoma. Eur J Cancer Clin Oncol 20:1463–1470

Hunter VJ, Daly L, Helms M, Soper JT, Berchuck A, Clarke-Pearson DL, Bast RC (1990) The prognostic significance of CA 125 half-life in patients with ovarian cancer who have received primary chemotherapy after surgical cytoreduction. Am J Obstet Gynecol 163: 1164–1167

Price P, Hogan SJ, Horwich A (1990) The growth rate of metastatic non-seminomatous germ cell tumours measured by marker production doubling time. I. Theoretical basis and practical application. Eur J Cancer 26:450–453

Price P, Hogan SJ, Bliss JM, Horwich A (1990) The growth rate of metastatic non-seminomatous germ cell testicular tumours measured by marker production doubling time. II. Prognostic significance in patients treated by chemotherapy. Eur J Cancer 26: 453–457

Regan LS (1989) Screening for hepatocellular carcinoma in high risk individuals. Arch Intern Med 149:1741–1744

Richter JM, Christensen MR, Rusky AK, Silverstein MD (1989) The clinical utility of the CA 19-9 radioimmunoassay for the diagnosis of pancreatic cancer presenting with pain and weight loss. Arch Intern Med 149:2292–2297

Tondini C, Hayes DF, Kufe DW (1989) Circulating tumor markers in breast cancer. Hematol Oncol Clin North Am 3:653–674

Toner GC, Geller NL, Tan C, Nisselbaum J, Bosl GJ (1990) Serum tumor marker half-life during chemotherapy allows early prediction of complete response and survival in nonseminomatous germ cell tumors. Cancer Res 50:5904–5910

Circulating Tumour Markers in Clinical Practice for the Early Detection of Cancer

G.J.S. Rustin

Introduction

This paper critically examines those situations in which circulating tumour markers can be used in the early detection of primary or recurrent cancer. Other uses such as confirming the diagnosis, assessment of adequate surgical resection, indicator of prognosis, and monitoring of therapy will not be discussed. Many "cancer tests" have been produced which aim at indicating the presence of an early occult cancer (Table 1). Unfortunately, to date these tests have all suffered from either not being reproducible by investigators other than their discoverer or not being sufficiently sensitive or specific. It is unlikely that non-invasive or benign tumours will produce a factor in sufficient quantity that it can be measured in the circulation. However, once we know more about the transformation from a benign to a malignant tumour, compounds such as specific enzymes might be found to be increased in association with cancer cell invasion. Despite there not being a universal cancer test, there are several tumour markers currently used for the early detection of specific cancers.

Human Chorionic Gonadotropin

Human chorionic gonadotropin (HCG) produced by trophoblast cells comes closest to being the "ideal" tumour marker. Evaluation of its use in the early detection of persistent or recurrent trophoblastic tumour demonstrates the potential uses and pitfalls of the "ideal" marker. Elevated serum levels are found with as few as 10^5 trophoblast cells. The smallest number of cells detectable by clinical examination or on chest X-radiograph is over 10^9 cells, whilst modern CT scanners can detect about 10^7 cells. Although HCG is a sensitive marker, it is not specific for trophoblastic tumours, as it is also elevated in normal pregnancy, and slightly elevated levels are found in patients with a variety of tumours. The best method of diagnosing hydatidiform mole is by ultrasound examination. A patient who has had a hydatidiform mole has a 7% chance of requiring chemotherapy for invasive mole or choriocarcinoma (Rustin and Bagshawe 1984).

In 1972, the first and still the best national screening programme for any cancer was set up by the Royal College of Obstetricians and Gynaecologists in the UK. Following a hydatidiform mole patients are registered at the Charing Cross Hospital, in Sheffield or in Dundee. The patient then receives requests for aliquots of an early morning urine sample which they send in a box, with prepaid postage on a reversible lid. One side of the lid has the patient's, and the other side the assay laboratory's name and address. Tumour markers measured in urine sent from home is very "consumer" friendly, which is essential for large scale screening. An automated follow-up service sends requests at regular intervals, and a serum sample is requested once the urine level is within the normal range (<24 U/l). Patients whose HCG falls to the normal range within 8 weeks, as confirmed by a serum sample, are followed for just 6 months; the remaining patients are followed for 2 years. All patients are requested to send further samples 3 weeks and 3 months after all future pregnancies.

The indications for requiring chemotherapy depends greatly on HCG measurements and are: very high ($>40\,000$ IU/24 h) urine HCG at 4–6 weeks, elevated HCG at 5–6 months, rising HCG on three consecutive samples, persistent uterine haemorrhage or pulmonary metastases which are associated with elevated HCG, central nervous system, gastrointestinal or hepatic metastases.

The value of this follow-up system is proved by the results. Between 1973 and 1978 there were 8302 women registered with hydatidiform mole at the Charing Cross Hospital, which was 77% of all registrations in the UK. Despite there being over 600 women requiring chemotherapy, only two deaths have occurred due to drug-resistant choriocarcinoma. There have been six additional deaths possibly related to gestational trophoblastic tumours, such as amniotic fluid emboli, infection and bleeding, and eight unrelated deaths.

The patients whose gestational trophoblastic tumours follow a term delivery or abortion are not entered into a screening programme for choriocarcinoma as this sequel is uncommon, occurring in less than 1 in 10 000 non-mole pregnancies. However, if choriocarcinoma was considered earlier in the differential diagnosis of women presenting usually with irregular vaginal bleeding or chest symptoms, an HCG estimation could lead to a quick diagnosis and high chance of cure by chemotherapy.

There are several lessons to be learnt from examining the use of HCG and the mole follow-up service.

1. In the ideal situation of an invasive tumour whose cells naturally secrete HCG, a minimum of 10^5 tumour cells are required before elevated levels can be detected. Unless tumour cells naturally produce a hormone, it is unlikely that they would produce circulating markers leading to such sensitivity.
2. Even the "ideal" marker is only specific for trophoblastic disease in certain situations, e.g. outside pregnancy. There are likely to be situations with most markers in which non-malignant conditions lead to elevated levels.
3. A screening programme is most cost effective in a high-risk population, i.e. post-molar.

Table 1. Tests for "malignancy"

Macrophage electrophoretic mobility
Malignin-specific antibodies
B5 antibody erythrocyte test
Erythrocyte oleic/linoleic acid ratio
Plasma magnetic resonance spectroscopy
Serum procoagulant activity

---

4. For large-scale screening to be accepted by the general public on a regular
    basis, it is necessary for the marker to be measurable in urine or other
    easily obtained fluid such as saliva.
5. Early diagnosis is only of value if it leads to improved survival.

Screening for Neuroblastoma

The only other national screening programme using a circulating tumour
marker was set up in Japan in 1985. Since then, urine samples from children 6 months old are screened for increased levels of catecholamines
(vanillylmandelic acid, VMA, and homovanillic acid HVA). Of 337 children
with neuroblastoma detected in Japan by mass screening up to 1988, 328 (97%)
are alive after aggressive therapy. However, there are no population-based
data from controlled studies showing any reduction in overall mortality due to
the screening. It is possible that the cases detected by screening are in the
groups with a favourable prognosis, and patients presenting over the age of 12
months with tumours that arose after the screen usually have a poor prognosis
(Murphy et al. 1991).

Germ Cell Tumours

Although over 80% of germ cell tumours produce HCG and/or AFP, less than
60% of localised stage I tumours are associated with elevated markers. These
markers can help in confirming the diagnosis but are of limited value for early
detection. Their main value for detecting early disease is in patients who are
on surveillance, having had an orchidectomy for stage I disease. With early
recognition and treatment of testicular tumours, an increasing number of
patients have no metastases following orchidectomy. With a policy of close
surveillance, almost 75% will never require any further therapy (Freedman
et al. 1987). The 25%–30% of patients who relapse, need close follow-up by
clinical examination, tumour markers and chest X-radiography, and at least
one CT scan 3 months after orchidectomy. If surveillance is adequate, the
relapse will be detected early, and virtually all patients will be cured.

The frequency of HCG and AFP estimations depends on the importance of an elevated marker and how fast they can rise. The degree of elevation of HCG has been shown in many studies to be the most powerful prognostic indicator (Rustin 1986). Recent studies suggest that patients with HCG > 10 000 IU/l and/or AFP > 1000 kU/l should be treated as having a poor prognosis (personal communication from the Medical Research Council).

It has been shown that markers for germ cell tumours have the potential to double in less than 1 week. If tumour marker tests are performed monthly, it is usually 6 weeks before a rise can be acted upon. In a retrospective study we found almost 25% of a group of patients had tumour marker doubling times that would have resulted in HCG levels >1000 IU/l and/or AFP levels >500 kU/l if the doubling rate was maintained (we intervened before that was possible). It was calculated that if monthly examination of markers was performed with patients on surveillance, 1 per 400 patients would be likely to die due to having high tumour marker levels and therefore a poor prognosis at the start of chemotherapy (Seckl et al. 1990). It is suggested that these patients have 2-weekly markers estimates for the first 6 months of surveillance.

In addition to their value in the surveillance of patients with stage I disease, AFP and HCG as well as isoenzyme 1 and 2 of lactate dehydrogenase can be useful in the early detection of relapse following chemotherapy.

Hepatocellular Cancer

Over 80% of black or Chinese patients with hepatocellular carcinoma have AFP levels >10 kU/l at presentation, with a smaller percentage of Caucasian patients having an elevated AFP level. Almost 65% of those tumours detected by AFP screening are small; many are resectable. In patients who are Hbs Ag-positive or cirrhotic, regular AFP estimations and ultrasound examinations are indicated (Oka et al. 1990). Patients who have solitary tumours detected by screening and undergo successful resection have a high chance of surviving in the long term without development of a further tumour.

Ovarian Cancer

CA 125 is the only commercially available, commonly used tumour marker for ovarian cancer. Although its level is elevated in over 95% of patients with advanced ovarian carcinoma, raised concentrations are found in less than 50% of patients with stage I disease (Bast et al. 1983). Despite the knowledge that about 50% of early cancers would be missed, large screening studies have been performed in the hope of at least detecting a large minority of stage I tumours which are the only ones that are potentially curable. Over 20 000 post-menopausal, well women have been screened at the London Hospital (Oram et al. 1990). Those women who had CA 125 levels >30 U/ml underwent pelvic

Table 2. Preliminary results of London Hospital Ovary Screening Clinic (modified from Oram et al. 1990)

	CA 125 (U/ml)	Ultrasound	No. of patients
Screen negative	<30	Not done	19 719
	>30	Normal	258
False negative (incomplete follow-up)			3
True positive	>30	Abnormal (Stage I,3; II,1; III,5; IV,2)	11
False positive		Abnormal	11

ultrasound, and if that was positive a laparotomy was performed (Table 2). As this was the first screen, it was not surprising that only 3 of the 11 cancers detected were stage I. One would hope that on the second screen the proportion of stage I tumours would be higher.

A long follow-up is required of this and other screening studies to determine whether the screen-detected cancers are cured by simple surgery. This uncertainty plus the extra years of anxiety without any survival benefit if cancers of stages II–IV are diagnosed suggest that such screening should only take place in a research setting at present. The United Kingdom Co-ordinating Committee on Cancer Research has firmly stated that screening with CA 125 should not be offered outside a clinical trial. The fact that it costs over £100 000 to detect each stage I cancer by such screening also needs addressing.

Once a patient has been diagnosed as having ovarian carcinoma, early detection of tumour progression or recurrence by serial CA 125 levels could be beneficial through avoidance of ineffective chemotherapy and other more expensive investigations. Van der Burg et al. (1990) have shown that an increase in CA 125 levels occurs before any other evidence of progression in 63% of cases, with lead times in excess of 6 months in 18%. We have recently studied this in more detail to determine firstly the optimal definition for progression and then the potential benefits of performing serial CA 125 measurements on patients receiving first-line treatment for ovarian carcinoma (Rustin et al. 1992). Among 71 patients, 20 relapsed on treatment. The optimal definition for progression was either two values >100 U/ml which had decreased by less than 50% over a minimum of 56 days, or a rise of 25% between successive samples plus a confirmatory sample. This definition gave 12 true-positives, one false-positive (who 1 month later was shown to be positive on scans but has remained symptom-free for 3 more years), 8 false-negatives and 50 true-negatives. Using this definition in the same patient group, we retrospectively evaluated what benefits could have been obtained if the CA 125 results had been acted upon. These amounted to 11 ultrasound scans, 4 CT scans, 1 bone scan and 22 courses of Carboplatin, which cost £7970. The cost of 7 CA 125 assays on all 21 patients during therapy was £5467. This shows how a tumour marker test can be both useful and cost effective.

Breast Cancer

There are several polymorphic epithelial mucin assays that are now commercially available, with most data available on the CA 15-3 assay. Although elevated levels are found in 55%–100% of patients with advanced disease, elevated levels were only found in 10%–46% of patients with primary breast cancer (Kenemans et al. 1988). As 2%–20% of patients with benign breast disease have elevated levels, too, it is clear that mucin assays are both lacking in sensitivity and specificity as a screening tool. There are currently no other serological candidates for breast cancer screening.

The observation that over 60% of patients who develop recurrent breast cancer have raised levels of CA 15-3 suggests a potential value in the early detection of recurrence. Before all women have serial mucin assays performed following mastectomy, some important questions need answering. Foremost is whether earlier detection of recurrence will alter survival. Even if the answer to this question is no, there may be other benefits from detecting recurrence earlier; the patient is likely to be fitter and have less advanced disease. They might therefore require less intensive therapy and less time in hospital. Studies are required to answer these questions.

Gastrointestinal Malignancies

No tumour markers are sensitive enough for screening of oesophageal, gastric or pancreatic carcinomas. Markers such as CA 19.9 and pancreatic oncofecal antigen (POA) are elevated in over 50% of patients with pancreatic cancer, but by the time the marker is elevated, the tumour is already incurable by surgery in most cases. CEA and CA 19.9 are elevated in 50%–70% of patients with metastatic colorectal cancer but in less than 30% of patients with Dukes stage A or B tumours. They are therefore of no value in screening asymptomatic patients and are even too insensitive for screening high-risk patients such as those with polyposis coli or ulcerative colitis (Begent and Rustin 1989).

Raised serum CEA values indicate recurrence of colorectal cancer on an average 4–6 months before it is clinically evident in about one-third of cases. The value of surgery, with a view to resection of recurrence performed when serum CEA levels start to rise, has been advocated by some groups who suggest that prolonged survival can result. The available studies strongly suggest that survival may be prolonged by resection under these circumstances, but randomised trials are needed to determine whether the benefits outweigh the surgical morbidity and mortality and the disturbance of regular serum CEA monitoring. A multi-centre trial of this type is in progress under the auspices of the Cancer Research Campaign Clinical Trial Centre at Kings College Hospital.

Prostate Cancer

Prostate specific antigen (PSA) is now widely accepted as the tumour marker of choice for monitoring men suspected of having prostatic cancer as it is more sensitive and more specific than prostatic acid phosphatase. Although PSA is elevated (>4 mg/l) in about 65% of men with localized stage A prostatic cancer, from 30% to 50% of patients with benign prostatic hypertrophy also have elevated levels (Beastall et al. 1990). Despite a low predictive value, the combination of rectal examination and PSA determination with prostatic ultrasonography in patients with abnormal findings appears the best method at present of detecting early prostatic cancer. Unfortunately, many screen-detected cancers will already have spread outside the prostate. In one study of healthy men who had cancer found at screening, 59% of those with PSA levels 4.0–9.9 mg/l and only 13% with levels $\geq$10 mg/l had localized cancer on surgical staging (Catalona et al. 1991). Until we have the results of the large-scale studies which are about to start, it will remain unclear whether screening can reduce the death rate from prostate cancers, and it cannot therefore be recommended.

Other Cancers

Monoclonal immunoglobulins detectable by serum electrophoresis (M proteins) occur in the serum and/or urine of 98% of patients with myeloma. Although the presence of M proteins is highly suggestive of the presence of myeloma, radiological bone lesions and marrow infiltration by plasma cells are required to confirm the diagnosis. This is due to M proteins being found in patients with other B-cell neoplasms and in 0.9% of asymptomatic adults over the age of 25 years, and their prevelance increases with age. The findings of an M protein can lead to the diagnosis of a solitary plasmacytoma which can be cured by radiotherapy or surgery.

There are several tumours of endocrine tissue that can be diagnosed and whose therapy can be monitored through the measurement of their eutopically produced hormones which are increased following malignant transformation. Measurement of calcitonin after provocation is used in the screening of families with medullary carcinoma of the thyroid. Phaeochromocytomas and the 50% of adrenal cortical carcinomas that are functional are other examples of endocrine tumours producing eutopic hormones. There are many different gastrointestinal endocrine tumours such as VIPomas, gastrinomas and glucagonomas which may be diagnosed through the finding of elevation of a specific gut polypeptide. Although carcinoid tumours may be monitored by measurement in the urine of the serotonin metabolite, 5-hydroxyindole acetic acid, it is unusual for isolated resectable tumours to be associated with elevated levels.

Summary

There are only two tumour markers that are currently used in national screening programmes for the early detection of cancer. Regular measurement of serum or urine HCG in women who have had a hydatidiform mole should result in fewer than 1/2000 screened women dying from choriocarcinoma. It is unclear as yet whether measurement of urine catecholamines in 6-month-old infants reduces overall mortality from neuroblastoma. Screening programmes using AFP and HbAg are being set up, as regular AFP estimations in populations at high risk of hepatocellular carcinoma results in successful resection of solitary tumours. Other tumour markers are too insensitive for screening but can be of value in the early detection of recurrent or progressive disease. These include HCG, AFP and LDH for germ cell tumours, CA 125 for ovarian cancer, polymorphic epithelial mucins for breast cancer and PSA for prostatic cancer. Of these, only the use of markers for early detection of relapsed germ cell tumours are at present likely to have an impact on survival.

Acknowledgements. I am funded by the Cancer Research Campaign and had support from the Department of Health for the completion of some of these studies. I am grateful to Breda Simmons for typing the manuscript.

References

Bast RC Jr, Klug TL, St John E et al. (1983) A radioimmunoassay using a monoclonal antibody to monitor the course of epithelial ovarian cancer. N Engl J Med 308:883–887

Beastall GH, Cook B, Rustin GJS, Jennings J (1990) A review of the role of established tumour markers. Ann Clin Biochem 28:5–18

Begent R, Rustin GJ (1989) Tumour markers: from carcinoembryonic antigen to products of hybridoma technology. ICRF Cancer Surv 8:107–121

Catalona WJ, Smith DS, Ratliff TL, Dodds KM, Coplen DE, Yuan JJJ, Petros JA, Andriole GL (1991) Measurement of prostate-specific antigen in serum as a screening test for prostate cancer. N Engl J Med 324:1156–1161

Freedman LS, Parkinson MC, Jones W, Oliver TD, Peckham MJ, Read G, Newlands E, Williams CJ (1987) Histopathology in the prediction of relapse of patients with stage I testicular teratoma treated by orchidectomy alone: a Medical Research Council Collaborative Study. Lancet 2:294–297

Kenemans P, Bast RCJ, Yedema CA, Price MR, Hilgen J (1988) CA 125 and polymorphic epithelial mucin as serum tumour markers. Cancer Rev 11/12:119–144

Murphy SB, Cohen SL, Craft AW, Woods WG, Sawada T, Castleberry RP, Levy HL, Prorok PC, Hammond GD (1991) Do children benefit from mass screening for neuroblastoma? Lancet 337:344–346

Oka H, Kurioka N, Kim K, Kanno T, Kuroki T, Mizoquochi Y, Kobavashi K (1990) Prospective study of early detection of hepatocellular carcinoma in patients with cirrhosis. Hepatology 12:680–687

Oram DH, Jacobs J, Brady L, Prys-Davies A (1990) Early diagnosis of ovarian cancer. Br J Hosp Med 44:320–324

Rustin GJS (1986) Tumour markers in germ cell tumours. Br Med J 292:713–714

Rustin GJS, Bagshawe KD (1984) Gestational trophoblastic tumours. CRC Crit Rev Oncol Haematol 3:103–141

Rustin GJS, Nelstrop A, Stilwell J, Lambert HE (1992) Benefits obtained by CA 125 measurements during therapy for ovarian carcinoma. Eur J Cancer 281:79–82
Seckl MJ, Rustin GJS, Bagshawe KD (1990) Frequency of serum tumour marker monitoring in patients with non-seminomatous germ cell tumours. Br J Cancer 61:916–918
van der Burg MEL, Lammer FB, Verweij J (1990) The role of CA 125 in the early diagnosis of progressive disease in ovarian cancer. Ann Oncol 1:301–302

Summary of Discussion: Session 3

S. MEUER

The question arose whether serologic tumor markers can help to define patients at high risk of developing recurrent disease. There was an agreement that, at present, costs for large-scale screening programs would not justify their general recommendation since the predictive value of this type of analysis is limited. Moreover, analysis of tumor markers alone is less efficient than its combination with other methods such as sonography, X-radiography, endoscopy, etc.

Nevertheless, longitudinal studies have produced evidence that the shorter the doubling time of tumor markers or their e-functionally calculated tumor marker production time, the worse is the prognosis and, in a reciprocal fashion, that a slower than physiologic decay rate of markers such as human chorionic gonadotropin (HCG) and α-fetoprotein (AFP) may require more aggressive therapy.

Early cancer detection can be performed at the level of single cells by looking at chromosome breaks (which is not a method for routine screening). In addition, monoclonal antibodies reactive with epithelial cells have most recently turned out to be quite useful in detecting early metastasis in bone marrow aspirates of patients with, e.g., breast and colorectal cancer. Preliminary evidence supports the notion that those patients who are antibody-positive have a worse prognosis than antibody-negative ones. This, however, would support, e.g., in breast cancer patients, the need for adjuvant hormone or chemotherapy, the benefit of which has still to be demonstrated by randomized clinical trials. Furthermore, investigating older men for prostatic cancer cells may provide information on the question of how early bone marrow metastasis occurs prior to a clinically symptomatic tumor.

Finally, the observation was put forward that through the use of more refined methods and more regular investigations (e.g., ultrasound in patients with benign gastrointestinal diseases) an increasing rate of marker-negative and often smaller tumors is detected (e.g., AFP-negative hepatocellular cancer, CA 19-9-negative pancreatic cancer). This observation stresses the importance of multiple clinical tools for early cancer detection, e.g., endoscopy, ultrasound, endoscopic retrograde cholangiopancreatography, computer tomography, magnetic resonance imaging, scintigraphy, immunoscintigraphy, etc.

SESSION 4

Imaging Procedures

Chairman: M.F. WANNENMACHER

Contributions of Ultrasonography
to Early Cancer Diagnosis

G. van Kaick

Introduction

Ultrasonography (US) has some advantages compared with other imaging procedures: It is generally available, noninvasive, repeatable, and of relative low expense. US therefore can influence the early detection of cancer through the screening of asymptomatic patients, by more rapid clarification of ambiguous clinical symptoms, and by follow-up of curatively treated tumor patients. For staging and treatment planning, CT and MRI are superior.

In parenchymal organs, lesions of 1–2 cm and in superficial areas, of 0.5 cm can be readily diagnosed. The sensitivity for the detection of a lesion depends on the contrast of the tumor echo-pattern compared with the surrounding tissue, the experience of the examiner, and the quality of the ultrasound unit. A differentiation of benign and malignant lesions in principle is not possible. However, cytopathologic classification can be obtained with the help of sonographically guided fine-needle biopsy.

In the following, I shall consider the contribution of US to the early detection of cancer concerning the different organs.

Liver

Hepatocellular carcinoma has a variable echo-pattern; small tumors are commonly hypoechoic (Fig. 1), whereas larger lesions, caused by secondary tissue alterations like fibrosis, fatty degeneration, etc., often present as an irregular isoechoic or hyperechoic lesion.

In Japan where there is a high incidence of liver cancer, US was used as a screening method (Tanaka et al. 1990). Periodic check-up by US was conducted on patients with chronic liver diseases. A total of 2000 examinations were performed on 660 patients (with liver cirrhosis and with chronic hepatitis, younger than 70 years old). In all, 22 hepatocellular carcinomas (3.3%) were detected and finally diagnosed. By the periodic check-up, 15 small, single nodules less than 2 cm in size were detected. Twelve surgical resections of the tumor were performed.

Similar results were 'reported also in Europe (Cottone et al. 1988, Tremolda et al. 1989). US was more sensitive than alpha-fetoprotein for the diagnosis of hepatocellular carcinoma.

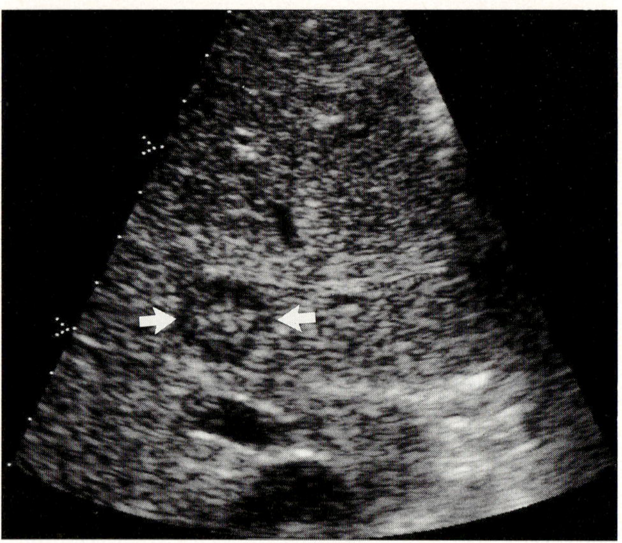

Fig. 1. Sonographic cross-section of the left hepatic lobe in a 64-year-old Thorotrast patient. Ultrasound examination was performed as part of the screening program of the German Cancer Research Center. An echo-poor rim in the liver (*arrows*) was detected. The 2-cm-sized tumor could be removed by Prof. Dr. P. Schlag, University Hospital of Surgery, Heidelberg. Pathohistological examination result was cholangiocarcinoma of the liver 2 cm in diameter

Our own experience in this field is focused on the fate of the so-called Thorotrast patients (Van Kaick et al. 1989). Thorotrast was the trade name of an X-radiography contrast medium consisting of a 25% colloidal solution of thorium dioxide. About 60% of the intravascularly injected thorium dioxide is stored lifelong in the liver, giving a high radiation burden to the organ. The risk of developing primary liver tumors proved to depend on the mean α-dose rate to the liver. The German Thorotrast Study comprises 2360 Thorotrast patients. We offer to the living Thorotrast patients reexaminations every 2 years including US and computed tomography (CT) and if necessary magnetic resonance imaging (MRI). We give advice to the family physicians to repeat US and laboratory tests every 4–6 months. The results of our US examinations were evaluated by Layer et al. (1991). Out of the 1536 evaluated studies, 53 patients showed a suspected liver lesion which was confirmed by surgery, biopsy, clinical course, or autopsy. In another 10 patients, a positive sonographic finding was not confirmed. In the 10-year examination period, only 4 confirmed liver lesions were not detected by US. Five additional liver tumors may have been missed as those patients died within a year after the US study due to malignant liver lesions. However, these 5 lesions were also not detectable by CT at the same time of examination. Even considering those cases as false-negative, US still has a high sensitivity of 85% and a very high sensitivity (99%) due to the large number of examinations.

Gall Bladder

The gall bladder is easily visualized by US. Carcinoma of the gall bladder presents with different echographic findings: Weak echoes fill the extended gall bladder and thickening of the wall, often combined with invasion of the liver. It is difficult to discriminate between benign lesions and a carcinoma in an early stage (Hederstrom and Forsberg 1987, Kersjes et al. 1990). In former times, tumors of the gall bladder could preoperatively be detected in less than 10%! This figure is now about 70%; however, no improvement in the diagnosis of *early* carcinomas was achieved! In a series of 60 patients with carcinoma of the gall bladder, Frank et al. (1989) reported on preoperative tumor diagnosis by US in 70%, but 98.5% of the tumors were in an advanced stage.

Pancreas

Pancreatic carcinoma usually is hypoechoic relative to the normal pancreatic parenchyma. It is often recognized because of contour bulging or the presence of a dilated pancreatic duct. US remains the primary approach in the evaluation of the jaundiced patient. It will reveal bile duct dilatation, the presence of any liver metastases, or enlarged lymph nodes. US visualizes the tumor unless it is very small, being quite good for lesions of the head and body, but less accurate for lesions of the tail. However, pancreatic cancer is at present virtually incurable. Apart from the occasional tumor at the papilla vateri, metastases usually have occurred before there are any symptoms. The role of US imaging is to help make a rapid diagnosis (Damascelli et al. 1989).

Kidneys

Renal carcinoma presents as a echogenic mass compared with the renal parenchyma; however, sometimes it could also be hypoechoic and almost cystic-looking. As both kidneys can be visualized very easily, renal masses are sometimes discovered as incidental findings.

Abdominal US screening of patients clinically asymptomatic for abdominal disease was performed in 5720 persons by Kremer et al. (1984). Pathological findings were reported in 47% of all persons, but these mostly were without clinical relevance like fatty degeneration of the liver, cholelithiasis, cystic lesions of the kidney, and the liver. Asymptomatic malignant abdominal tumors were detected in 0.2% (13 patients). Ten of these tumors were renal cell carcinomas (mean age of the patients 54 years; mean diameter of the lesion 5.4 cm).

Similar results were published by a Japanese group (Tereda et al. 1989). A total of 7800 persons with a mean age of 48.7 years underwent renal US during a screening by the Health Service. Of these subjects, 29 were suspected of having solid masses in the kidneys. Further examinations disclosed 6 malignant renal tumors which were treated by a radical nephrectomy. There were no clinical signs or symptoms referable to renal cell carcinoma. The size of the tumors measured 3–7 cm in longest axis.

Patients with incidentally diagnosed renal cell carcinomas ($n = 16$) were compared with a group of symptomatic patients ($n = 39$). The incidentally diagnosed renal carcinomas represented a lower tumor stage and grade, offering a much better prognosis as compared with symptomatic ones (Rauschmaier 1986).

Hollerweger et al. (1990) reported on their results of abdominal US screening in 18 700 patients. Out of 64 renal cell carcinomas 35 were asymptomatic and incidentally disclosed. Mean diameter of the tumors ranged between 4 and 5 cm.

Some critical remarks should be added. US has the advantage of being employable as a screening method for kidney cancer. The sensitivity and specificity of contrast-enhanced CT, however, are clearly superior compared with US. Therefore, it is often necessary to clarify US findings by contrast CT (Fig. 2).

Adrenal Glands

Unlike CT, US is not able to visualize normal adrenal glands with high reliability. Space-occupying lesions can be detected measuring more than 2 cm on the right side and more than 3 cm on the left side. Therefore, US is not the method of choice for the early detection of small primary or secondary malignant tumors of the adrenals.

Lymphatic System

In the early detection of malignant lymphomas, US is the first method to reveal an enlarged spleen and/or circumscribed, echo-poor splenic lesions and enlarged retroperitoneal lymph nodes (>1.5 cm). US can also be used for the early detection of recurrences in cases of curatively treated malignant lymphomas. However, one must be careful in the interpretation of the findings basing on the size of a lymph node, as tiny metastatic lesions can be overlooked and reactively enlarged nodes may lead to false-positive results.

Breast

Using US for screening of breast cancer was a concept which could never be realized. Automatic scanning systems were developed in different countries. However, up to now there have been no convincing results for using automated US units for breast cancer screening (Kaplain et al. 1990, Kimme-Smith et al. 1988).

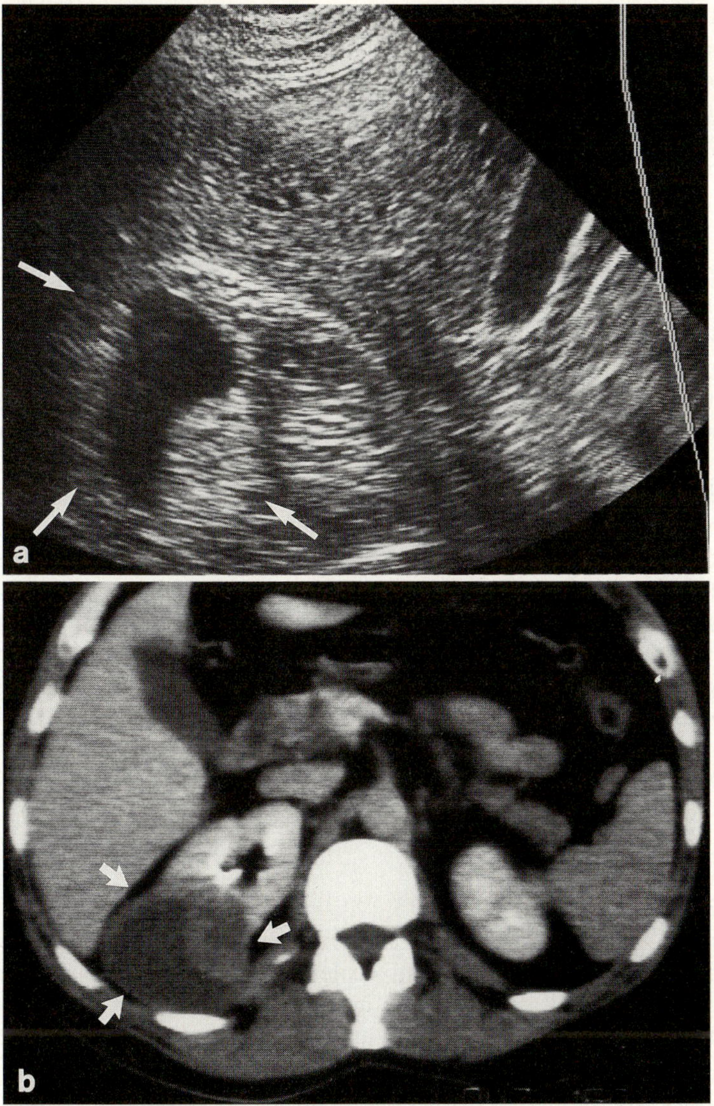

Fig. 2. a Sonographic cross-section of the right liver and the right kidney. Space occupying lesion (*arrows*) at the right side of the kidney composed of a liquid center and a solid thick capsule. The tumor was sonographically detected by chance. **b** CT cross-section of the same region after contrast enhancement. Liquid and solid areas of the tumor can be clearly differentiated. Pathohistological result was renal cell cancer. Four years after surgery, the 40-year-old patient is free of recurrence or metastases

Early clinical investigations of the value of US for breast cancer detection showed results approaching those of mammography. However, these clinical studies included many patients who were symptomatic, and the carcinomas generally were larger than those found in a screening population (Basset and

Kimme-Smith 1991). Later investigators reported poor results for US compared with state-of-the-art mammography in the screening of asymptomatic women. In a prospective study comprising 1000 women, Sickles et al. (1983) sonographically detected only 58% of 64 pathologically proved cancers, compared with 97% detected by mammography.

Real-time, hand-held breast US has come into widespread use. Teubner et al. (1985) evaluated the diagnostic value of mammasonography using real-time technique in a prospective study based on the experience of 452 pathomorphologically confirmed sonographic results. Large cysts (more than 1 cm) were correctly classified in 97%, while cysts smaller than 1 cm were recognized in 84%. Only 50% of in situ carcinomas and carcinomas smaller 1 cm were recognized, while 97% of the carcinomas larger than 1 cm were demonstrated. Out of 102 malignant breast lesions 79% were evaluated as malignant. However, 22% were classified as probably benign or equivocal, or no lesion could be detected.

In principal, the US findings are unspecific, and malignant and benign lesions sometimes imitate each other. The typical US pattern of a cirrhotic carcinoma is the shadowing behind the tumor, which, for example, may be caused also by calcification in a fibroadenoma. On the other hand, the normal fibroadenoma is characterized by an echo-enhancement behind the lesion and a lateral shadow sign. Medullary carcinoma of the breast can present with the same echographic characteristics. Therefore, the major indications for sonography are the differential diagnosis of cystic versus solid lesions, differentiation of a palpable or mammographically detected lesion, and sonographically guided needle aspiration.

Thyroid

The echo-pattern of the normal thyroid is homogenously hyperechoic. Malignant tumors appear as a hypoechoic or mixed lesion. The borderline can be smooth or irregular. US as a screening method for thyroid cancer is handicapped by the fact that benign lesions are frequent, and thyroid carcinomas are seldom. Benign lesions sometimes can be discriminated by a "halo" surrounding the lesion; however, they often present a similar aspect to malignant ones.

Mass screening for thyroid cancer using US was performed by Omata and Iguchi (1986). Echo-guided aspiration cytology was carried out in 1169 persons; 71 were found to have carcinomas including 40 cases of small papillary carcinomas less than 10 mm in largest diameter.

Diagnosis of *medullary thyroid carcinoma* is often delayed as a consequence of its rarity. Calcitonin measurement and fine-needle aspiration biopsies provide an acurate preoperative diagnosis. After removal of all tumoral cervicothoracic tissue by total thyroidectomy and a careful node excision, follow-up examination includes basal and pentagastrin-stimulated calcitonin measurements. An abnormal level necessitates the search for the tumoral site by US and, if a mediastinal location is suspected, by CT and as necessary also by selective venous catheterization. In cases of recurrence or distant metastases, surgical excision has to be considered first.

Lorenz et al. (in preparation) examined 96 patients suffering from medullary thyroid carcinoma. In total, 386 US examinations were performed. Based on the results of surgery and/or calcitonin measurement, they were able to evaluate the accuracy of the US examination. The sensitivity for the detection of recurrences of medullary thyroid carcinoma was 84% and the specificity, 80%. The smallest lesion measured 4 mm in diameter.

Head and Neck

US proved also to be an effective imaging method for the early detection of recurrent head and neck tumors. Mende et al. (1991) evaluated the results of 140 patients who underwent US examinations because of the clinical suspicion of a relapse. In 136 patients the US suspected neoplastic process was histologically confirmed. Some 60% of the patients had a recurrent tumor with or without affected lymph nodes, and 19% of the patients developed a second primary tumor. The important message of this study is that in 20% of these patients clinical examination had not given evidence of a recurrence or a second primary, which were only disclosed by US. US screening in the case of post-therapeutic care provides the necessary data for planning and monitoring an adequate relapse therapy.

Testis

Though space-occupying lesions of the testis easily can be detected by palpation, US has contributed to minimizing the time delay between first symptoms and surgical therapy. It should be mentioned that Csapo et al. (1987) described the application of US in the early detection of nonpalpable, second primary, testicular tumors. The 91 patients were examined 1–6 times in 18 months following radical orchiectomy for testicular germ-cell tumors. In addition to the usual routine checks, US of the residual testicles also formed part of the established follow-up protocol. Among these patients, US had identified in residual testicles 4 testicular tumors which had escaped detection on palpation. In all instances, the second lesion was different from the first tumor in histology.

US examination is also particularly useful for evaluating a normally sized testicle when metastasis is the first manifestation of an occult primary testicular neoplasm.

Prostate

Prostatic carcinoma in its early stages is usually peripheral and hypoechoic. However, its echogenicity is variable. The transabdominal approach through the filled bladder is adequate to evaluate prostatic size and urinary tract obstruction but not for tissue characterization. *Transrectal US* performed with high frequency transducers allows a very accurate visualization of the parenchymal texture as well as of the capsule integrity. With transrectal US guidance it is also possible to perform very accurate fine-needle aspiration biopsy of very small suspicious areas.

Several clinical studies were performed comparing transrectal US and digital rectal examination for screening (Chodak 1989, Dershaw et al. 1990, Hernandez and Smith 1990, Nesbitt et al. 1989). Encouraging results were reported by Lee et al. (1988, 1989). The authors examined 484 self-referred men over 60 years of age. Biopsies were performed in 77 cases, and 22 cancers were detected: 20 with transrectal US and 10 at digital examination. Overall detection rate for prostatic cancer with transrectal US was two times higher than that with digital examination (2.6%/1.3%). Transrectal US demonstrated 100% (17 of 17) of the tumors with the most favorable prognosis (less than 1.5 cm in diameter) compared with 41% (7 of 17) by digital examination.

A very recent prostate cancer screening study (Palken et al. 1991), however, revealed very different figures: 5.4% of the cancers were diagnosed by digital rectal examination and only 4.4% by transrectal US (Table 1). This result was attributed to careful digital rectal examination with a high index of suspicion and a very high percentage of biopsies (threefold compared with Lee et al. 1988). The authors conclude that digital rectal examination is considered an effective screening examination, equivalent to transrectal US and preferable because of lower costs.

Table 1. Screening of prostate cancer [28]

−315 self-referred men >50 years old
− 88 biopsies
− 23 prostate cancers:
       14 detected by transrectal US (4.4%)
       17 detected by digital examination (5.4%)
− 7 tumors <1.5 cm:
      4 detected by transrectal US
      5 detected by digital examination
      (2 detected fortuitously: cancer in opposite lobe)

A similar critical comment was given by Carter et al. (1989) that transrectal US may not be a good method to detect clinically unsuspicious prostate cancer, and the false-positive rate would appear to be high.

Torp-Pedersen et al. (1988) calculated the different costs for screening by transrectal US and digital rectal examination based on the results of Lee et al. (1989): Per diagnosed cancer, the costs were US$6520 for transrectal US and US$4108 for digital rectal examination (difference of 37%). However, the costs per early cancer that would have been in an advanced stage if diagnosed without screening were US$22 177 for transrectal US and US$28 528 for digital rectal examination.

Ovaries

The cure rate for stage I epithelial ovarian cancer may be as high as 90% (1990). However, early stage ovarian cancer produces no symptoms, and approximately two-thirds of patients presents with advanced disease at the time of initial diagnosis.

The largest prospective study on transabdominal US screening was carried out by Campbell et al. (1990a,b). This study concerned 5479 self-referred women without symptoms (mean age 52 years and 14594 screenings). Positive results were obtained with 338 screens (2.3%) comprising 326 subjects (5.9%). The authors detected primary ovarian cancers in 5 patients (4 stage Ia, 1 stage Ib; prevalence 0.09%). An additional 4 patients had metastatic ovarian cancer. The authors underlined that it was not possible to differentiate between the US appearance of early malignant and benign tumors. The rate of false-positive results for primary ovarian cancer was 2.3%, the specificity was 97.7%, and the predictive value of a positive result on screening was only 1.5%.

Transvaginal US as a screening method for ovarian cancer (506 asymptomatic patients over 40 years old) was introduced by Higgins et al. (1989). Twelve patients (2.4%) were noted to have abnormal sonograms; 10 patients agreed to undergo surgery. All 10 patients had ovarian tumors with dimensions equal to those predicted by US: 4 serous cystadenomas, 3 endometriomas, 2 cystic teratomas, and 1 adenocarcinoma. Each ovary was measured in 3 planes, and the ovarian volume was calculated using the ellipsoid formula. The upper limit of normal for ovarian volume was $18\,cm^3$ in premenopausal women and $8\,cm^3$ in postmenopausal women.

Van Nagell et al. (1990) screened 1000 women 40 years or older by transvaginal US. Of these, 3.1% had abnormal vaginal sonograms, and 24 of 31 patients underwent exploratory laparatomy. Histologic diagnosis of these tumors included: 1 adenocarcinoma, 8 serous cystadenomas, 6 endometriomas, and 2 cystic teratomas. It must be emphasized that the adenocarcinoma detected by screening measured 11.6 cm in diameter and was palpable on examination.

In 212 postmenopausal women screened by vaginal US, 48 (11.3%) pathological findings were detected (Osmers et al. 1990). Among the histological clarified cases were 2 asymptomatic ovarian cancers. They measured about 5 cm in diameter and were classified as stage Ia.

All these authors (Duda et al. 1990) conclude that further clinical trials are necessary to determine the efficacy of vaginal US as a screening method for ovarian cancer.

Summary

The results of these different studies suggest that US can really contribute to the early detection of cancer. With regard to screening programs, the cost/benefit ratio is rather poor (Miller 1991). For diagnosis and follow-up, US is useful in the early clarification of the clinical situation. Most important for the reliability of the results, however, is the level of knowledge and experience of the examiner.

References

Basset LW, Kimme-Smith C (1991) Breast sonography. AJR 156:449–455
Campbell S, Bhan V, Royston P, Whitehead MI, Collins WP (1990a) Transabdominal ultrasound screening for early ovarian cancer. Br Med J 299:1363–1367
Campbell S, Royston P, Bhan V, Whitehead MI, Collins WP (1990b) Novel screening strategies for early ovarian cancer by transabdominal ultrasonography. Br J Obst Gynaecol 97:304–311
Carter HB, Hamper UM, Sheth S, Sanders RC, Epstein JI, Walsh PC (1989) Evaluation of transrectal ultrasound in the early detection of prostate cancer. J Urol 142:1008–1010
Chodak GW (1989) Screening for prostate cancer. Urol Clin North Am 16:657–661
Cottone M, Turri M, Caltagirone M, Maringhi A, Sciarrino E, Virdone R, Fusco G, Orlando A, Marino L, Pagliaro L (1988) Early detection of hepatocellular carcinoma associated with cirrhosis by ultrasound and alphafetoprotein: a prospective study. Hepatogastroenterology 35:101–103
Csapo Z, Weißmüller J, Sigel A (1987) Sonographie in der Früherkennung von nicht-palpablen Zweit-Hodentumoren: Eine prospektive Studie. Urologe [A] 26:334–338
Damascelli B, Caroroll RLA, Ericson K, Fizzotti G, Gold R, Haynie ThP, van Kaick G, Love L, Stevenson GW, Valcassori L, Salvetti M, Marchiano A, Lutman R (1989) Guidelines on oncologic imaging. Eur J Radiol 9:1–30
Dershaw DD, Scher HI, Smart T (1990) Transrectal sonography for serial evaluation of prostatic malignancy. Urology 36:172–176
Duda V, Rode C, Thein K, Schulz D (1990) Vaginalsonographie: Pilotstudie für den Einsatz als Ovarial-Screening-Verfahren. Geburtshilfe Frauenheilkd 50:388–393
Frank W, Grad O, Jantsch H, Lechner G, Maier A, Pichler W (1989) Sonographie des Gallenblasenkarzinoms, Korrelation mit dem Operationsbefund in 60 Fällen. RÖFO 150:556–561
Hederstrom E, Forsberg L (1987) Ultrasonography carcinoma of the gallbladder. Diagnostic difficulties and pitfalls. Acta Radiol 28:715–718
Hernandez AD, Smith JA Jr (1990) Transrectal ultrasonogroaphy for the early detection and staging of prostate cancer. Urol Clin North 17:745–757
Higgins RV, van Nagell JR, Donaldson ES, Gallion HH, Pavlik EJ, Endicott B, Woods CH (1989) Transvaginal sonography as a screening method for ovarian cancer. Gynaecol Oncol 34:402–406
Hollerweger A, Schuschnigg C, Müller E (1990) Das Nierenzellkarzinom als sonographischer Zufallsbefund. Ultraschall Klin Prax 5:74–77
Kaplan C, Matallana R, Wallack MK (1990) The use of state-of-the-art mammography in the detection of nonpalpable breast carcinoma. Am Surg 56:40–42
Kersjes W, Köster O, Heuer M, Schneider B (1990) Vergleich bildgebender Verfahren in der Diagnostik von Gallenblasen- und Gallengangskarzinomen. ROFO 153:174–180
Kimme-Smith C, Bassett LW, Gold RH (1988) High frequency breast ultrasound. J Ultrasound Med 7:77–81
Kremer H, Dobrinski W, Schreiber MA, Zöllner N (1984) Sonographie des Abdomens als Screeningmethode. Ultraschall 5:272–276
Layer G, Haberkorn U, Lührs H, Bast T, Knopp M, Liebermann D, van Kaick G (1991) Diagnostic ultrasound of Thorotrast induced primary liver tumors. (submitted)
Lee F, Littrup PJ, Torp-Pedersen ST, Mettlin C, McHugh TA, Gray JM, Kumasaka GH, McLeary RD (1988) Prostate cancer: comparison of transrectal US and digital rectal examination for screening. Radiology 168:389–394
Lee F, Torp-Pedersen ST, Siders DB, Littrup PJ, McLeary RD (1989) Transrectal ultrasound in the diagnosis and staging of prostatic carcinoma. Radiology 170:609–615

Mende U, Zöller J, Maier H, Flentje M, Loth M (1991) Ultrasound, and effective imaging method for the early detection of recurrent head and neck tumors. ART91 Symposium, Apr 11–13, Munich

Miller AB (1991) Epidemiological approaches to primary and secondary prevention of cancer. J Cancer Res Clin Oncol 117:177–185

Nesbitt JA, Drago JR, Badalament RA (1989) Transrectal ultrasonography. Urology 34: 120–22

Osmers R, Völksen M, Rath W, Kuhn W (1990) Vaginosonographie als Screeningmethode zur Erkennung von Adnextumoren in der Postmenopause? Onkologie 13:268–270

Omata K, Iguchi K (1986) Clinico-pathological study of thyroid carcinomas detected by mass screening. Gan No Rinsho 32:740–748

Palken M, Cobb OE, Simons CE, Warren BH, Aldape HC (1991) Prostate cancer: comparison of digital rectal examination and transrectal ultrasound for screening. J Urol 145:86–92

Rauschmaier H (1986) Sonographie – die wichtigste Untersuchung zur Früherkennung des Nierenzellkarzinoms. Urologe 25:325–328

Sickles EA, Filly RA, Callen PW (1983) Breast cancer detection with sonography and mammography: comparison using state-of-the-art equipment. AJR 140:843–845

Tanaka S, Kitamura T, Nakanishi K, Okuda S, Yamazake H, Hiyama T, Fujimoto I (1990) Effectiveness of periodic check-up by ultrasonography for the early diagnosis of hepatocellular carcinoma. Cancer 66:2210–2214

Terada Y, Ueki T, Horiuchi D (1989) A study on six cases of renal cell carcinoma detected by renal ultrasound during health screening. Nippon Jinzo Gakkai Shi 31:783–790

Teubner J, van Kaick G, Junkermann H, Pickenhan L, Wesch H, Eggert-Kruse W, Müller A, Tschahargane C, von Fournier D, Kubli F (1985) 5 MHz Realtime-Sonographie der Brustdrüse. Radiologe 25:457–467

Torp-Pedersen ST, Littrup PJ, Lee F, Mettlin C (1988) Early prostate cancer: diagnostic costs of screening transrectal US and digital rectal examination. Radiology 169:351–354

Tremolda F, Benevegnù L, Drago C, Casarin C, Cechetto A, Realdi G, Ruol A (1989) Early detection of hepatocellular carcinoma in patients with cirrhosis by alpha feto protein, ultrasound and fine-needle biopsy. Hepatogastroenterology 36:519–521

Van Kaick G, Wesch H, Lührs H, Liebermann D, Kaul A, Muth H (1989) The German Thorotrast Study – report on 20 years' follow-up. In: Taylor DM, Mays CW, Gerber CB, Thomas RG (eds) Risks from radium and thorotrast, pp 98–104 (BIR report 21) British Institute of Radiology, London

Van Nagell JR, Higgins RV, Donaldson ES, Gallion HH, Powell DE, Pavlik EJ, Woods CH, Thompson EA (1990) Transvaginal sonography as a screening method for ovarian cancer. Cancer 65:573–577

Computed Tomography
and Magnetic Resonance Imaging of the Body
and Musculoskeletal System

P.E. Peters, G. Bongartz, E. Rummeny, K. Wernecke, and W. Wiesmann

Introduction

Early detection of cancer has been defined in the context of this symposium as: (a) the detection of cancer prestages, (b) the diagnosis of small, localized cancers without metastatic spread, and (c) the early detection of recurrent cancers. The first two of these entities do not cause clinical symptoms; thus, our discussion regards the use of computed tomography (CT) and magnetic resonance imaging (MRI) as screening methods. There are certainly many definitions of screening; that given by Miller (1985) is as follows:

"Screening is the presumptive identification of unrecognized disease or defect by the application of tests, examinations, or procedures that can be applied rapidly."

From this definition it is clear that neither CT nor MRI can be seriously considered as screening methods despite the marked progress in shortening scanning times in both techniques.

A screening test is not considered to be diagnostic; a positive finding in screening procedures is generally followed by special diagnostic tests such as CT or MRI. In addition, a screening test should be simple and easy to administer and should entail minimal unpleasant or hazardous side effects (Epstein 1990). Neither technique under discussion fulfills these requirements: they are not simple, they cannot be easily or universally administered, and they do involve unpleasant and even minimally hazardous side effects. With regard specifically to MRI, there are contraindications such as pace makers or implanted ferromagnetic materials, a number of subjects suffer from claustrophobia with it, and the examination is relatively time consuming, very expensive, and not yet widely available. CT is also fairly expensive as a screening procedure and carries a small but definite risk due to the use of ionizing radiation and the frequently required iodinized contrast media.

These methods are therefore not used and not useful for the early detection of cancer in persons without clinical symptoms. A review of the radiologic literature dealing with cancer screening from 1988 to 1990 reveals 56 entries: 47 using mammography in the breast, five using ultrasound in the prostate, two using X-ray and cytology in the lung, one using the guaiac stool test in the colon, and one using VMA in the adrenals. However, none makes use of CT or MRI. The early detection of recurrent disease and metastases following cancer treatment, however, is a very good indication for both methods. The incidental detection of a small neoplasm while performing CT or MRI for unrelated reasons is a very rare occurrence in clinical practice.

Historical Review

This realistic – or perhaps pessimistic – view of the limited usefulness of CT and MRI in the early detection of cancer is the result of controlled studies and clinical experience over many years. The introduction of these methods originally led to many hopes and expectations in the medical community. Tissue characterization by computer analysis of sonographic images, tissue characterisation by measuring the differences in radiation absorption in CT (so-called density measurements in Hounsfield units), and measurement of T1 and T2 relaxation times in MRI do contribute to the diagnosis of a malignant neoplasm, but there is considerable overlap between benign and malignant tissue. Therefore, none of these sophisticated techniques can replace histologic examination of tissue.

In 1971 Damadian observed differences in animal experiments between MRI relaxation times in normal tissue and those in rapidly growing tumor tissue. While his report was not the first application of nuclear magnetic resonance technology to biologic material, it opened a new field of research because of his claim to be able to detect all kinds of cancer noninvasively by this method. In 1972 he designed an apparatus for the detection of cancer and even obtained a United States patent for it. The machine, however, did not work and was never build (Holis 1987).

In 1986 Fossel et al. maintained that water-suppressed proton nuclear magnetic resonance spectroscopy of plasma could detect malignant tumors. This test would be ideally suited as a relatively simple screening procedure for the early detection of cancer; however, other groups have not been able to repeat the results (Okunieff et al. 1990).

Early Detection of Recurrent Disease

In patients with known malignant disease imaging techniques together with physical examinations and laboratory tests are regularly applied in follow-up studies. The philosophy of this type of aftercare is similar to that in screening for the early detection of cancer; one hopes that the early detection of recurrent disease including metastases will have a positive effect on the course of the malignant disease due to early therapeutic consequences. However, there are many factors influencing the prognosis of a malignant tumor once it has recurred or metastasized, and the value of early detection of recurrent disease therefore cannot be assessed in a general way.

As in the initial diagnosis of malignancies, CT and MRI are used primarily as verification modalities, for staging and restaging purposes, and for pre-operative planning. Thus, they are used to solve specific problems rather than

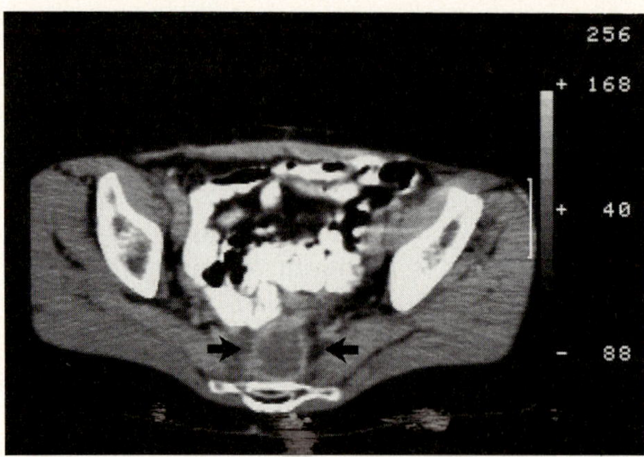

Fig. 1. A 52-year-old patient with severe back pain 2 years after abdominoperineal resection for carcinoma of the rectum. CT of the pelvis following oral and intravenous contrast medium reveals a globoid structure ventral to the sacrum with ring enhancement (*arrows*). Percutaneous biopsy confirmed the presacral cancer recurrence

for routine follow-up examinations. A typical example of this type of specific imaging is the search for recurrent rectal or rectosigmoid carcinoma. CT in this situation is often superior to barium studies and colonoscopy because nearly all recurrent tumors in patients with sphincter-saving resections develop extra-luminally (Freeny et al. 1986). In patients with complete abdominal-perineal resections CT and MRI are the only noninvasive modalities for the evaluation of recurrent tumor (Fig. 1; Thoeni 1989).

Evaluation of Pulmonary Nodules

Solitary pulmonary nodules are a fairly common radiologic finding in asymp-tomatic patients in whom a chest radiograph was performed for other reasons, such as prior to an operation in general anesthesia. In this situation, again, CT is a method not for detection but for further evaluation. The ultimate goal is to select those patients needing surgical removal of the nodule because of a high probability of malignancy. Under the general assumption that the solitary nodule is probably malignant until proven otherwise, a combined analysis of clinical and imaging data is performed. Factors in the patient's history, par-ticularly smoking habits and age, are taken into consideration as well as comparison with previous chest radiographs, if possible. Absence of growth for more than 2 years is considered the best noninvasive proof of benignity (Caskey et al. 1990).

CT is used to ascertain the intraparenchymal position of a suspected nodule and to analyze its size and contours and the presence or absence of calcifications (Fig. 2). It has been shown that specific patterns of calcifications within a pulmonary nodule are associated with benign disease. The technique

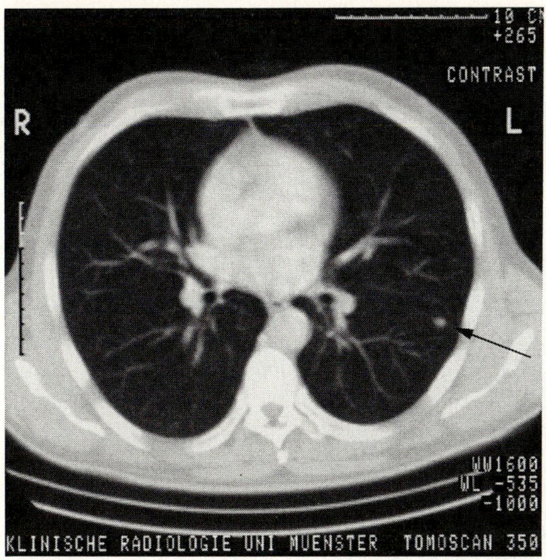

Fig. 2. A 34-year-old man. Incidental finding of a small solitary pulmonary nodule. CT of the chest shows a 0.5-cm well-defined nodule with tiny stippled calcifications (*arrow*; seen better at other window settings). CT diagnosis: probably benign nodule. Unchanged in follow-up examinations

of CT examination with or without special reference phantoms has been extensively discussed in the radiologic literature (Siegelman et al. 1980; Zerhouni et al. 1986; Caskey et al. 1990).

Taking all radiologic criteria such as calcification patterns, fat deposition, and vascular connection into consideration, there remain a significant number of indeterminate nodules. The procedure of choice for these indeterminate pulmonary nodules is transthoracic fine-needle aspiration biopsy (Fig. 3). We prefer CT-guided biopsies using a specially designed biopsy system (Reuther et al. 1990). If the probability of malignancy of a given solitary pulmonary nodule is very high from the history, clinical data, and imaging results, the patient is referred for surgery without prior biopsy.

Conclusion

CT and MRI are indispensable for staging of malignant disease, pretherapeutic planning, and posttherapeutic follow-up examinations. By definition, they are currently not suited as screening tests for the early detection of cancer. Theoretically, MRI offers the possibility of playing a very important role in the early detection of cancer in the future because it is a noninvasive imaging modality that does not use ionizing radiation. Since its introduction into clinical medicine in the early 1980s it has demonstrated a truly breathtaking speed of development. Scanning times, initially in the order of hours, have decreased to less than 1 s, and volume scanning and three-dimensional representation of

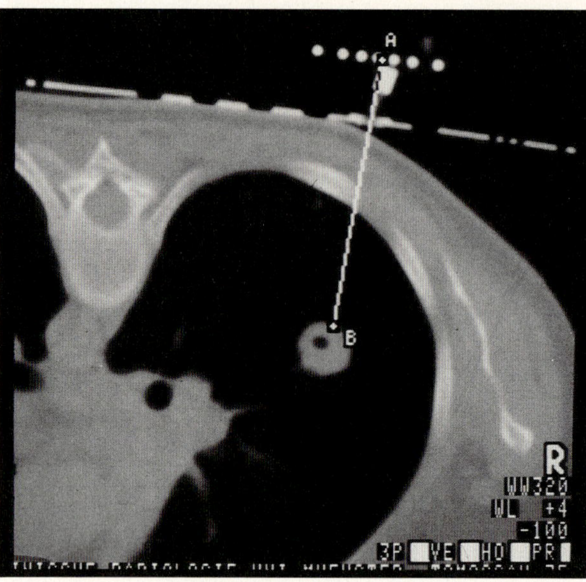

Fig. 3. A 48-year-old woman with known Hodgkin's disease for several years. Newly diagnosed solitary pulmonary nodule. Recurrent disease? Other malignancy? CT-guided fine-needle biopsy ascertained a pulmonary manifestation of Hodgkin's disease

anatomy have become available. Current research is directed to the development of organ-specific paramagnetic contrast media. The preliminary results of this research are very promising.

Finally, there are still very good theoretical reasons why nuclear magnetic resonance spectroscopy, which failed in its first attempt, may be expected to become a valuable tool combined with MRI for the detection of cancer and for the monitoring of response to chemotherapeutic treatment.

References

Caskey CL, Templeton PA, Zerhouni EA (1990) Current evaluation of the solitary pulmonary nodule. Radiol Clin N Am 28:511–520

Damadian R (1971) Tumor detection by nuclear magnetic resonance. Science 171:1151–1153

Epstein DM (1990) The role of radiologic screening in lung cancer. Radiol Clin N Am 28:489–495

Fossel ET, Carr JM, McDonagh J (1986) Detection of malignant tumors. Water-suppressed proton nuclear magnetic resonance spectroscopy of plasma. New Engl J Med 315:1369–1376

Freeny PC, Marks WM, Ryan JA, Boeln JW (1986) Colorectal carcinoma evaluation with CT: preoperative staging and postoperative recurrence. Radiology 158:347

Holis DP (1987) Abusing cancer science. The truth about NMR and cancer. Strawberry Fields Press, Chehalis

Miller AB (1985) Screening for cancer. Academic Press, Orlando

Okunieff P, Zietman A, Kahn J, Singer S et al. (1990) Lack of efficacy of water-suppressed proton nuclear magnetic resonance spectroscopy of plasma for the detection of malignant tumors. New Engl J Med 322:953–958

Reuther G, Wernecke K, Peters PE (1990) Lokalisationstechnik für perkutane Punktionen unter CT-Kontrolle. Radiologe 30:217–220

Siegelman SS, Zerhouni EA, Leo RB et al. (1980) CT of the solitary pulmonary nodule. AJR 135:1–13

Thoeni RF (1989) CT evaluation of carcinomas of the colon and rectum. Radiol Clin N Am 27:731–741

Zerhouni EA, Stitik FP, Siegelman SS et al. (1986) Computed tomography of the pulmonary nodule: a national cooperative study. Radiology 160:318–327

Imaging Techniques: Computed Tomography and Magnetic Resonance Imaging in Neuroradiology

W.J. Huk

Introduction

The early diagnosis of intracranial tumours in statu nascendi is not yet possible. Since many lesions can attain quite a large size without clinical manifestations, diagnosis cannot be made before initial symptoms have become obvious. Prior to the establishment of computed tomography (CT) in the early 1970s, the diagnosis of a brain tumour could only be accomplished when the lesion was large enough to cause indirect morphological signs such as a significant shift of midline structures or displacement of normal vessels, or when pathological vasculature could be demonstrated. CT initiated a diagnostic revolution as brain tissue could, for the first time, be visualised directly. Magnetic resonance imaging (MRI) has further improved the possibility of direct diagnosis.

With the help of these modern imaging techniques the three main goals of diagnostic imaging can almost be achieved (Huk and Heindel 1990):

- Detection of a tumour as early as possible (i.e., at the moment of the initial symptom)
- Exact localisation of the lesion
- Identification of the tumour type

In the following I will try to demonstrate how and to what extent this can be achieved and which limitations still exist.

Detection of a Tumour. Experience has shown that MRI is superior to CT, mainly because of its higher sensitivity and spatial resolution of anatomical detail. Intracranial tumours can be detected earlier with MRI than with CT. For the same reason, a glioma is generally more extensive on MR than on CT images. A neoplasm becomes visible with MRI and CT only when the volume of free intra- and extracellular water has increased sufficiently. This means that there might well be tumour growth beyond the tumour margin outlined in the most sensitive T2-weighted image; this could be demonstrated by Kelly et al. in 1987 with stereotaxic serial biopsies obtained from normal-looking brain tissue surrounding the hyperintense tumour area.

Exact Localisation of a Lesion. MRI is also superior to CT in the evaluation of the spatial relationship of a tumour in order to assess its operability and best suited surgical approach due to its multiplanar facility, the absence of bony artifacts and its superior soft-tissue contrast. This is particularly relevant in the case of small lesions adjacent to bone structures, such as the base of the skull (Baleriaux and Michelozzi 1990, Huk and Heindel 1990) and the spinal canal (Zanella and Friedmann 1990). In addition, knowledge of the anatomical relationship of a tumour helps to identify its matrix and is a valuable contribution to the preoperative differential diagnosis.

Differential Diagnosis of a Tumour. For intracranial tumours, the following parameters should be analysed (Huk and Heindel 1990):

1. Signal contrast with normal brain
2. Tumour structure
3. Tumour margins
4. Presence, absence and extent of perifocal oedema
5. Indirect tumour signs
6. Relation of tumour to blood vessels, richness of tumour blood supply
7. Degree of contrast enhancement

As already mentioned above, the contrast of the majority of neoplasms with neighbouring structures on CT and MR images is based on an increase of the content of free water. The resulting hypodensity on CT and prolongation of relaxation times on MR images may be small, as with some meningiomas and lymphomas, or more distinct, as with gliomas. Shortening of relaxation times of tumour tissue is rarely seen; it can occur only in lesions with a high content of fat, lipid-containing substances or recent haemorrhage. If a tumour appears isointense with the brain, its presence may be indicated by perifocal oedema. When this is also absent, detection must rely on indirect signs or the enhancement of tumour tissue after the intravenous administration of contrast material.

The structure of a tumour may be homogeneous or inhomogeneous. A homogeneous structure is more suggestive of a benign process, such as in meningiomas, low-grade gliomas or cysts, in contrast to the majority of malignant lesions, which appear inhomogeneous. The inhomogeneity may be caused by irregular and patchy, ring- or garlandlike patterns, depending on the composition of the tumour as well as the type and degree of regressive changes. These regressive changes include necrosis, haemorrhage, cyst formation, calcification or a variable combination of all; they can be very helpful in the differential diagnosis.

Haemorrhages generally indicate an increased vascularity, which is more often seen in more malignant tumours of the glioma type and in metastases. However, low-grade gliomas may also be subject to sudden haemorrhage, known as "apoplectic glioma". Thus, in haemorrhages of spontaneous onset or without adequate reason in an atypical location, a neoplasm as the underlying cause has to be excluded. For this purpose, control scans with intravenous contrast enhancement are recommended after the acute haemorrhage has resolved. On MR images, haemosiderin deposits as long-term remnants of previous haemorrhages are a most reliable sign of cavernous haemangiomas, which create an unspecific hyperdensity on CT scans.

Calcifications are usually associated with slowly growing benign lesions, such as oligodendrogliomas, psammomas and craniopharyngiomas. However, they do not rule out higher grades of malignancy. On CT scans they are of increased density. On MRI they are hypointense or isointense, a finding which is nonspecific compared with the typical CT appearance. Thus, CT is necessary if calcifications are to be demonstrated as in craniopharyngiomas.

The signal of the cystic regressive changes depends on the composition of the cystic content. Cysts of benign lesions, like low-grade gliomas, meningiomas, gangliogliomas, etc., generally appear smoother and with more regular margins than the liquefied necrotic cavities of glioblastomas or other malignant tumours. An increased content of protein, blood constituents and lipid-containing substances shortens the relaxation times when compared with CSF or brain tissue, like in craniopharyngiomas or cystic adenomas. Occasionally, fluid levels can be seen due to corpuscular breakdown products of blood. Cystic change is a relatively unspecific finding. In doubtful cases, the walls of a cyst have to be searched thoroughly for a small seam or nodule of tumor tissue which unveils the underlying neoplasm. If pathological tissue cannot be identified, all other causes of cystic lesions have to be included in the differential diagnosis. In rare cases the tumour aetiology of a cyst may become apparent only on control scans performed months or years later.

The tumour margin is another interesting sign in the differential diagnosis of intracranial tumours. Tumours with sharp and regular borders are very likely to be of extra-axial or intraventricular origin, like meningiomas, adenomas, plexus papillomas, etc. Indistinct and ill-defined margins suggest intra-axial lesions or infiltration of neighbouring brain tissue, as in gliomas, invading adenomas, metastases, etc. With intravenous contrast medium the border of these tumours may appear sharper.

The shape of the tumour margin in itself is no reliable parameter for the grade of malignancy.

Vasogenic oedema surrounding a brain tumour is frequently seen in intracerebral tumours. Due to a high content of free water it appears hyperintense on proton density and T2-weighted MR scans, and hypodense on CT scans. The border between tumour and oedema may be clearly defined, or it may be difficult to resolve. In cases with long relaxation times, like low-grade gliomas, the differentiation may even be impossible. Often, however, the tumour tissue is less homogeneous than the perifocal oedema. In many cases, intravenous contrast medium is needed to distinguish tumour and oedema from each other and to delineate small anatomical structures. The vasogenic oedema spreads most easily in the white matter with its comparatively wide interstitial spaces, causing the typical "three finger" pattern corresponding to the distribution of the white matter between the basal ganglia.

Indirect tumour signs are most essential for the detection of space-occupying lesions. They are produced by the deformation and displacement of normal structures in the neighbourhood of the tumour. They often are quite subtle, and the examiner has to analyse the images very carefully, especially in cases where the tumour itself is not clearly visualised. These indirect signs include:

- Compression and deformation of adjacent portions of the ventricles, including the displacement of entire lateral ventricles and midline structures
- Compression of adjacent sulci
- Compression of the basal CSF spaces or filling of these spaces by tumour tissue
- Expansion of the lateral ventricle of the uninvolved hemisphere through constriction of the foramina of Monro or the 3rd ventricle
- Expansion of the prepontine and peripontine cisterns on the involved side by displacement of the brainstem toward the opposite side
- Expansion of the supratentorial portions of the ventricles due to plugging of the aqueduct or 4th ventricle
- Downward displacement of the cerebellar tonsils

To evaluate CSF spaces, T1-weighted sequences are most helpful. When CSF spaces near the skull base or in the spinal canal are to be evaluated, artefacts caused by bone-hardening effects on CT and by pulsatile movements of the CSF on MR images must be considered.

When no mass effect is seen in association with a focal lesion, the differential diagnosis must include all non-neoplastic aetiologies. On the other hand, non-neoplastic lesions such as encephalitis, infarction, MS plaques, heterotopias, etc. may also cause a mass effect.

The blood supply of a tumour and its relationship to large intracranial vessels can, in many cases, be demonstrated by MRI, thus obviating the need for conventional angiography. Examples of this situation are tumours encasing and sometimes compressing the carotid artery and tumour growth within the cavernous and other venous sinuses. Also, the vascularity of a tumour can be defined by the use of flow-sensitive sequences. With intra-axial tumours, however, MRI will not demonstrate the degree of pathological vasculature and its early draining veins, which are quite reliable signs for a higher degree of malignancy in conventional angiography. The same is true for extra-axial tumours, where the feeding vessels arising from the external carotid artery cannot be depicted by MRI to make the diagnosis of a meningioma. Therefore, in doubtful cases evaluation of tumour vascularity with conventional angiography may still be helpful for the differential diagnosis and preoperative establishment of the prognosis.

Enhancement with contrast material is very helpful in detecting a lesion, defining its margins, and analysing its spatial relationship. Enhancement of intracranial tumours beyond the vascular phase signifies the absence or disruption of the blood-brain barrier. It is absent in benign and malignant mesenchymal tumours, such as meningiomas and metastases. Therefore, benign meningiomas cannot be distinguished from those with sarcomatous change. In neuroepithelial brain tumours, however, evidence of disruption of the blood-brain barrier signifies the presence of pathological vessels and thus a higher degree of malignancy. Rare exceptions to this rule are pilocytic astrocytomas, plexus papillomas and other tumours that have fenestrated vessels (Hirano 1983). The same is true for radiation necrosis. In a number of low-grade gliomas, which were non-enhancing on CT, some degree of enhancement could be seen on MRI.

It is important to realise that the limit of contrast enhancement in the early phase after injection corresponds as little to the actual tumour border as does the diffuse spread of the contrast agent in the late phase (Ernest et al. 1986). For the demonstration of contrast enhancement with MRI, T1-weighted images are necessary. On these, the bright tumour contrasts clearly with the dark peritumoural oedema and/or surrounding structures.

With intracerebral lesions, tumours are most sensitively detected by T2-weighted sequences, and the use of contrast medium is only adjunctive to demonstrate a breakdown of the blood-brain barrier and is a helpful sign for the evaluation of the degree of malignancy. With extra-axial tumours, contrast agents substantially increase the reliability of tumour detection.

The different appearances of intracranial lesions described above can be helpful to distinguish a tumour from other intracranial processes and to understand its biological behaviour. In addition, the clinical history can be taken into consideration and is very often essential. A number of cases remain for which the differential diagnosis between a neoplastic and a non-neoplastic lesion cannot be decided. In these cases, the observation of the further development of the lesion with control scans is another important parameter which can be utilised easily with the help of CT and MRI on an outpatient basis. These are reliable tools for non-invasive follow-up studies until the final diagnosis can be established. Nevertheless, there are still patients for whom the diagnosis must be considered very tentative. For these patients, therapeutic decisions without additional pathological proof cannot be made. This can be done with the aid of CT and MRI, which are able to deliver the reliable and exact topographic information needed for stereotaxic biopsies (Huk 1988).

The high standards of modern CT and MRI provide powerful means for the detection of intracranial tumours at the time of the initial clinical symptom. This high sensitivity and reliability were not previously available. The same is true for the detailed description of the shape of a lesion and its relationship to neighbouring structures. The third goal of diagnostic imaging, the identification of the tumour type, however, cannot be achieved, since the specificity of MR findings is in general not much superior to that of CT. An exact diagnosis of intracranial tumours can only be made with varying degrees of confidence from CT and MR images. Histological proof of the diagnosis has to be obtained directly. If this is needed before surgery or before radiotherapy is initiated in inoperable lesions, CT and MRI provide detailed topographic information necessary to pinpoint the site of the most representative biopsy specimen (Huk 1988).

Summary

With CT and MRI the diagnosis of intracranial tumours can now be established at the moment of initial clinical symptoms in the majority of cases. MRI is superior to CT for the detection of a lesion as well as for the evaluation of its anatomical details and its relationship to neighbouring structures. However, since the specificity of MRI is not superior to CT, the diagnosis as to the kind of tumour can only be made with varying degrees of confidence from CT and MR images. If histological proof is needed before therapy, it has to be obtained directly. For stereotaxic biopsies, CT and MRI can provide detailed topographic information necessary to determine the site of the most representative biopsy specimen.

References

Baleriaux D, Michelozzi G (1990) Tumors of the posterior fossa. In: Huk WJ, Gademann G, Friedmann G (eds) MRI of central nervous system diseases. Springer, Berlin Heidelberg New York, pp 277–296

Ernest F IV, Kelly PJ, Scheithauer B, Kall B, Cascino TL, Ehman EL, Forbes G (1986) Pathologic contrast enhancement of cerebral lesions: a comparative study using stereotactic CT, stereotactic MR imaging, and stereotactic biopsy. RSNA '86, Chicago

Hirano A (1983) Praktischer Leitfaden der Neuropathologie. Springer, Berlin Heidelberg New York

Huk WJ (1988) Stereotaxy within the CT scanner: a safe and fast technique for puncture and biopsy. In: Nadjmi M (ed) Imaging of brain metabolism – spine and cord – interventional neuroradiology – free communications. 15th Congress of the European Society of Neuroradiology, Sept 13–17, Würzburg

Huk WJ, Heindel W (1990) Intracranial tumors. In: Huk WJ, Gademann G, Friedmann G (eds) MRI of central nervous system diseases. Springer, Berlin Heidelberg New York, pp 229–276

Kelly PJ, Daumas-Duport C, Kispert DB, Kall BA, Scheithauer BW, Illig JJ (1987) Imaging-based stereotaxic serial biopsies in untreated intracranial glial neoplasms. J Neurosurg 66:865–874

Zanella FE, Friedmann G (1990) Diseases of the vertebral column and spinal cord. In: Huk WJ, Gademann G, Friedmann G (eds) MRI of central nervous system diseases. Springer, Berlin Heidelberg New York, pp 395–425

Positron Emission Tomography (PET) for Tumor Diagnosis and Therapy Management

L.G. STRAUSS

Tumor Perfusion and Metabolism

Colorectal Tumors

PET was used in the follow-up of patients with colorectal malignancies to differentiate recurrent colorectal tumor and scar. The tumor perfusion was evaluated with $[^{15}O]$ water, while $[^{18}F]$ deoxyglucose (FDG) was used for the assessment of tumor metabolism. FDG is transported like glucose but trapped after the phosphorylation step. Therefore, FDG provides information about the regional glucose metabolism. The tracer concentration was quantitatively evaluated by means of a ROI technique and standardized for both injected dose and body volume for each patient. The standardized uptake values (SUV) were evaluated in 27 patients with a recurrent colorectal malignancy and 13 with a nonmalignant mass. The quantitative evaluation of the data demonstrated rapid FDG uptake by the tumor, followed by a slight decrease in uptake values for up to 40 min after FDG administration (Fig. 1). Of the 27 tumors, 25 were correctly identified using the standardized concentration values 1 h after FDG injection, while all 13 benign lesions were correctly classified. Perfusion imaging with $[^{15}O]$ water gave no additional information (Strauss 1989, Strauss and Conti 1991, Strauss et al. 1989a,b, 1990, Haberkorn et al. 1991a).

Lung Tumors

The metabolism of lung tumors was determined by PET using FDG. Furthermore, $[^{15}O]$ water and $[^{13}N]$ glutamate were used with selected patients to evaluate the tumor's perfusion and metabolism. PET studies were performed prior to therapy ($n = 23$) and during chemotherapy ($n = 8$). The change in tumor volume was compared with the change in tumor metabolism during chemotherapy. All tumors showed a significant FDG uptake prior to therapy. Involved lymph nodes were correctly identified in 3 patients. I noted no correlation between the FDG uptake in the tumor and the histology of the lesions. The change in FDG uptake was a more sensitive parameter for therapy response than the change in tumor volume. Furthermore, the FDG uptake prior to therapy was correlated with survival (Strauss and Conti 1991).

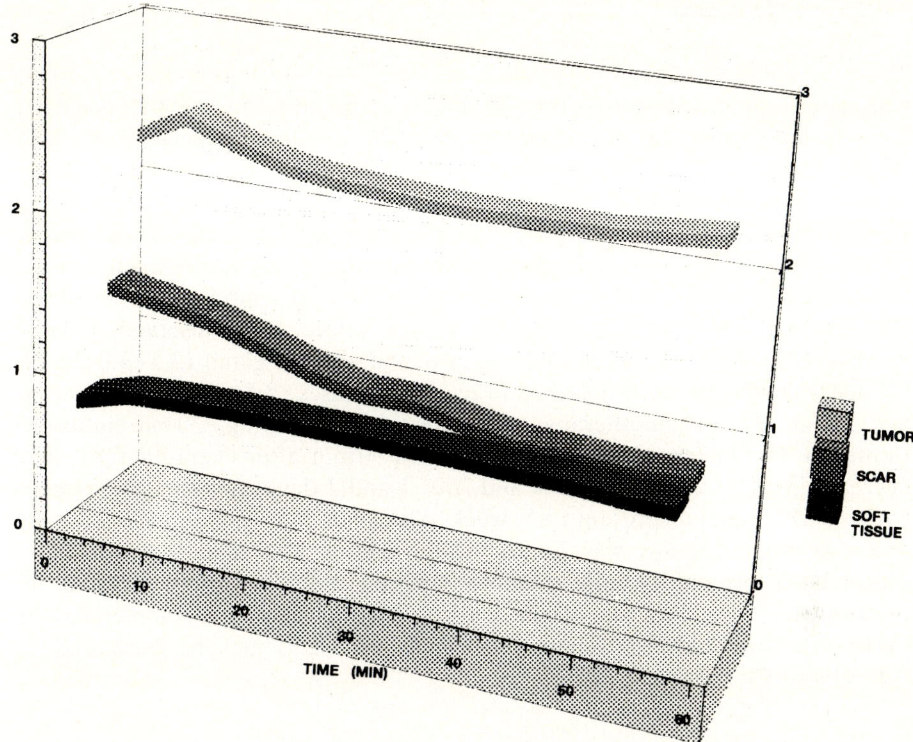

Fig. 1. FDG uptake (in SUV, mean values) up to 60 min after radiotracer injection

Hypopharyngeal Tumors

PET studies were performed in patients with hypopharynx carcinoma in order to evaluate its metabolism and to find the involved lymph nodes prior and after chemotherapy. Furthermore, CT was used to measure the change in tumor volume during chemotherapy. Tumor proliferation was evaluated with biopsy and one-dimensional flow cytometry. All patients ($n = 6$) were given chemotherapy with cisplatin shortly after the first PET study. A second PET examination was performed after the first chemotherapeutic cycle. I noted a high tracer uptake in all malignancies, indicative of high tumor metabolism. Furthermore, a high FDG accumulation was found in involved lymph nodes and bone metastases. The FDG uptake in the lesions decreased in 4 patients and was constant in 2. A correlation was found between the change in tumor volume as measured by CT and the change in FDG uptake. Furthermore, the proliferative index, as determined by one-dimensional flow cytometry, was correlated with the FDG uptake in the malignant lesions (Haberkorn et al. 1991b).

Malignant Melanoma

Different chemotherapeutic protocols are used for the treatment of patients with metastatic melanomas. I used PET here to quantify the metabolic activity in metastases prior to and after therapy. The evaluation included 10 PET studies of 5 patients. CT examinations preceded PET in each patient to determine the target area. PET studies were performed with intravenously injected FDG (370–444 MBq), followed by sequential imaging for 60 min. Standardized uptake values (SUV) were calculated from the iteratively reconstructed cross-sections using a ROI technique. The FDG uptake in lymph node metastases was 2.1–13.1 SUV prior to therapy. Lower values were observed in bone metastases (1.3 SUV) and in metastases of the adrenal gland (2.5–3.0 SUV). Comparable results were obtained in liver metastases (2.5–3.4 SUV). Follow-up studies after chemotherapy with fotemustine (200 mg, 30 min infusion) showed a 3% decrease in tumor metabolism 90 min after chemotherapy. The decrease in FDG uptake was 9% and 26% 1 and 2 days after therapy, respectively, and remained constant for 1 week. The median decrease in FDG uptake following chemotherapy was 27.5%. These results show that PET with FDG can be used to quantify early chemotherapeutic effects on tumor metabolism. Furthermore, the duration of the cytostatic effect can be demonstrated by PET. Therefore, different chemotherapeutic protocols may be compared on the basis of PET studies.

Evaluation of Radiolabeled Fluorouracil for Therapy Management

Primary and Recurrent Colorectal Tumors

I examined 8 patients with colorectal malignancies, who were given intra-arterial chemotherapy (fluorouracil, FU, 750 mg/m^2 for 5 days) and radiation therapy (4 × 2.5 Gy per cycle). A scanning device and/or a two-ring PET were used to evaluate the distribution of intraarterially injected FU and [^{13}N] glutamate. Furthermore, SPECT imaging with ^{99m}Tc-labeled MAA (macro-aggregate) was performed to quantify tumor perfusion and shunting. The median shunting fraction of the tumor was 10.1% of the intraarterially injected activity and exceeded even the median perfusion vlaue (7.5%). The FU accumulation increased with blood flow, until optimal flow values were reached. Increasing the flow further resulted in a decreased FU uptake. A linear correlation existed between glutamate uptake and FU accumulation (Strauss and Conti 1991).

Chemotherapy of Liver Metastases from Colorectal Tumors

Standard Intravenous Fluorouracil Chemotherapy

[^{18}F] FU was used to obtain information about the time-dependent accumulation of the cytostatic agent. Furthermore, [^{15}O] water was used to evaluate the perfusion pattern. Normalized tracer concentrations were determined for metastases, liver parenchyma, and aorta. The data evaluation comprised 52 metastases from 27 patients. The maximum liver activity was noted 28 min (median value) after FU infusion and was three times higher than after 2 h. The ^{18}F activity in the metastases 2 h after FU infusion was 33% the liver activity. A low correlation was noted for FU uptake and perfusion of the lesions. Only 20% of the metastases showed a high tracer uptake. Furthermore, different metastases in the same patient can show different ^{18}F concentrations.

Intraarterial Fluorouracil Chemotherapy

FU has found use for both intravenous and intraarterial chemotherapy. The evaluation comprised 26 double examinations (intravenous and intraarterial studies) in 13 patients with surgically implanted catheters in the gastroduodenal artery. The FU concentration 2 h after tracer application was higher in 10 of 18 metastases using the i.a. approach. I observed a higher systemic toxicity in 33% of the patients. While the accumulation of the perfusion tracer [^{15}O] water was up to 10 times higher in the metastases after intraarterial injection, the FU uptake was not significantly increased by regional application. Therefore, perfusion studies alone cannot be used to estimate the chemotherapy outcome. The results of the ongoing study demonstrate that PET with [^{18}F]-labeled uracil should find preferential use to optimize the regional chemotherapy and to select those patients who will profit from the intraarterial approach.

Fluorouracil Uptake and Tumor Growth

The tumor response to chemotherapy necessitates the accumulation and metabolism of the cytostatic agent in the target area. PET examinations were performed with 12 patients prior to chemotherapy, and the ^{18}F concentrations in the metastases ($n = 18$) were determined. Sequential CT scans were used to calculate the tumor growth rate during chemotherapy. Then, the FU accumulation in the lesions prior to therapy was compared with this. The correlation coefficient for the standardized FU concentration values and the growth rates exceeded 0.8 (Fig. 2). A decrease in tumor volume demands FU concentrations higher than 3.5. The polynomial regression function between FU concentration values and tumor growth rate can be used for therapy planning and optimization (Dimitrakopoulou et al. 1990).

Summary

PET was used in the follow-up of patients with colorectal malignancies to differentiate recurrent colorectal tumor and scar. The tumor perfusion was evaluated with ^{15}O-labeled water, while [^{18}F] deoxyglucose (FDG) was used for the assessment of tumor metabolism. FDG is transported like glucose but

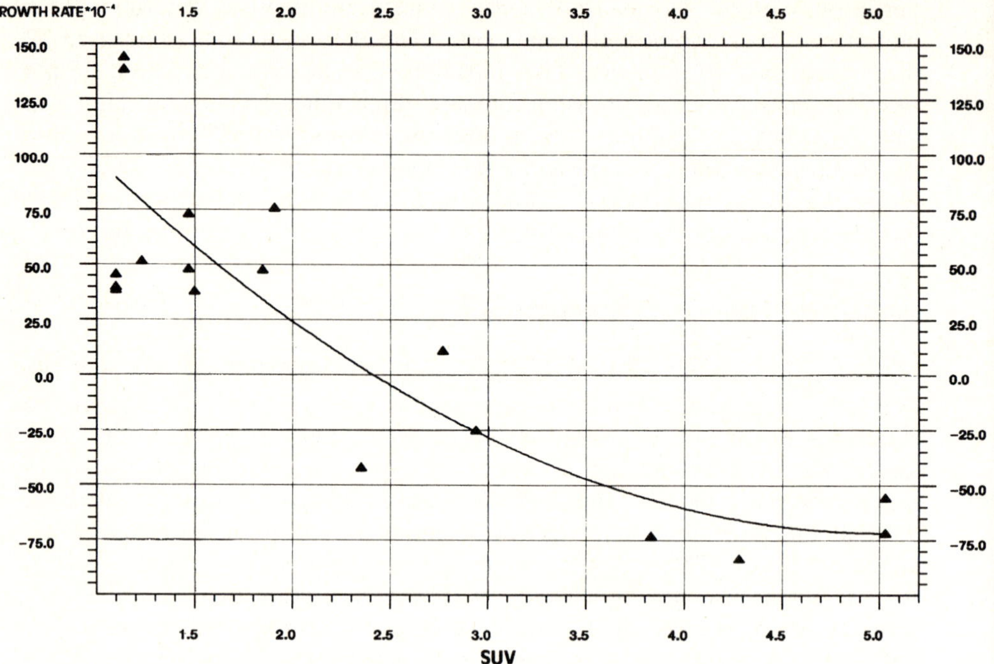

Fig. 2. Correlation between ^{18}F-labeled uracil metabolite concentrations (SUV) prior to therapy and tumor growth after therapy

trapped after the phosphorylation. Therefore, FDG provides information about the regional glucose metabolism. The tracer concentration was quantitatively evaluated by means of a ROI technique and standardized for both injected dose and body volume. The probands included 27 patients with a recurrent colorectal malignancy and 13 with a nonmalignant mass. The quantitative evaluation of the data demonstrated rapid FDG uptake by the tumor, followed by a slight decrease in uptake values for up to 40 min after administration. Of 27 tumors, 25 were correctly identified using the standardized concentration values 1 h after FDG injection, while all 13 benign lesions were correctly classified. Perfusion imaging with ^{15}O-labeled water gave no additional information.

[^{18}F] fluorouracil (FU) was used to obtain information about the time-dependent accumulation of the cytostatic agent. Furthermore, ^{15}O-labeled water was used to evaluate the perfusion pattern. Normalized tracer concentrations were determined for the metastases, liver parenchyma, and aorta. The data evaluation comprised 52 metastases from 27 patients. The maximum liver activity was noted 28 min (median value) after FU infusion and was three times higher than after 2 h. The ^{18}F activity in the metastases 2 h after FU infusion was 33% of the liver activity. A low correlation was noted between the FU uptake and perfusion of the lesions. Only 20% of the metastases showed a high tracer uptake. Furthermore, different metastases in the same patient can show different ^{18}F concentrations.

Tumor response to chemotherapy necessitates the accumulation and metabolism of the cytostatic agent in the target area. PET examinations were perfomed in 12 patients prior to chemotherapy, and the ^{18}F concentrations in the metastases ($n = 18$) were determined. Sequential CT scans were used to calculate the tumor growth rate during chemotherapy. The FU accumulation in the lesions prior to therapy was compared with the growth rate of the lesions. The correlation coefficient for the standardized FU concentration values and the growth rates exceeded 0.8. A decrease in tumor volume demands FU concentrations higher than 3.5. The polynomial regression function between FU concentration values and tumor growth rate can be useful for therapy planning.

References

Dimitrakopoulou A, Strauss LG, Haberkorn U, Knopp M, Schlag P, Helus F, van Kaick G (1990) PET-Untersuchungen mit F-18-Uracil zur Beurteilung des Wachstumsverhaltens von Lebermetastasen. Zentralblatt Radiologie 141:421–422

Haberkorn U, Strauss LG, Dimitrakopoulou A, Engenhart R, Oberdorfer F, Ostertag H, Romahn J, van Kaick G (1991a) PET studies of fluorodeoxyglucose metabolism in patients with recurrent colorectal tumors receiving radiotherapy. J Nucl Med 32:1485–1490

Haberkorn U, Strauss LG, Reisser Ch, Haag D, Dimitrakopoulou A, Ziegler S, Oberdorfer F, Rudat V, van Kaick G (1991b) Glucose uptake, perfusion, and cell proliferation in head and neck tumors: relation of positron emission tomography to flow cytometry. J Nucl Med 32:1548–1555

Strauss LG (1989) Positronenstrahler für die Erforschung des Tumorstoffwechsels. Radiologe 29:318–321

Strauss LG, Conti PS (1991) The applications of PET in clinical oncology. J Nucl Med 32:623–648

Strauss LG, Clorius JH, Schlag P, Lehner B, Kimmig B, Engenhart R, Marin-Grez M, Helus F, Oberdorfer F, Schmidlin P, van Kaick G (1989a) Recurrence of colorectal tumors: PET evaluation. Radiology 170:329–332

Strauss LG, Clorius JH, Kimmig B, Dimitrakopoulou A, Marin-Grez M, Engenhart M, Schraube P (1989b) Imaging positron emitting radionuclides generated during radiation therapy. Europ J Radiol 9:200–202

Strauss LG, Dimitrakopoulou A, Haberkorn U, Knopp M, Helus F, Lorenz WJ (1990) Einsatz der Positronenemissionstomographie (PET) zur onkologischen Diagnostik. Zentralblatt Radiologie 141:255–256

Immunoscintigraphy in the Early Diagnosis
of Tumours of the Abdomen

A. Bischof Delaloye and B. Delaloye

Introduction

Radiolabelled monoclonal antibodies (MoAbs) have been used to detect
various tumours by scintigraphy (Goldenberg et al. 1978; Mach et al. 1980;
Larson 1985; Baldwin and Byers 1985; Delaloye et al. 1986; Chatal 1989;
Nunz and Emrich 1990), but the specific role of antibody imaging in the clinical evaluation of patients still remains to be defined. In the following, the
possible clinical usefulness of immunoscintigraphy in malignant tumours of
the abdomen, especially bladder, ovarian and colorectal carcinoma, will be
analyzed. From this perspective it would be fastidious to enumerate and
describe in detail all the antibodies, radiolabels, labelling and imaging methods
which might be used for immunoscintigraphy. A comprehensive review on the
technical aspects of immunoscintigraphy has been published recently (Britton
et al. 1991).

Primary Tumours

It seems unlikely that immunoscintigraphy will ever be useful for screening
patients with unknown abdominal tumours. When elevated tumour marker
levels indicate possible tumour growth, the presence or absence of tumour can
be reliably defined with other diagnostic procedures. The degree of accuracy of
monoclonal antibody scanning in differentiating benign from malignant ovarian
or colorectal lesions is at present not high enough to decide on the grounds of
immunoscintigraphy in favour of intervention or not.

Except for bladder tumours, where ^{111}In-labelled carcinoembryonic
antigen (CEA)-specific antibodies have been successfully used to evaluate the
tumour stage before resection of the primary tumour (Boeckmann et al. 1990),
immunoscintigraphy will probably not improve preoperative staging of ovarian
and colorectal tumours. In some cases, the detection by immunoscintigraphy of
distant metastases, especially in the liver, might change the clinical management of patients.

Recurrent Tumours and Metastases

Ovarian Cancer

The primary roles of immunoscintigraphy in ovarian cancer are assessing the effects of chemotherapy, demonstrating residual or recurrent disease and distinguishing whether a mass seen on ultrasound (US) or X-ray computed tomography (CT) is due to post-therapy fibrosis or viable tumour and thus reducing the number of second-look laparotomies (Granowska and Britton 1991). Several studies (Epenetos et al. 1986; Granowska et al. 1986; Chatal et al. 1987) have shown a higher sensitivity of immunoscintigraphy (IS) in detecting recurrence after primary surgery of ovarian carcinomas with respect to US and CT. Recently, a French multicenter study (Dutin et al. 1991) tested ^{111}In-labelled MoAbs directed against the CA 125 antigen which is expressed by 90% of serous ovarian cancers. In 47 patients with previously operated ovarian carcinoma, the sensitivity was 0.43 for US, 0.55 for CT and 0.94 for IS. In the same series, specificity was 0.62 for US, 0.71 for CT and 0.67 for IS. The high negative predictive value of IS alone (0.92) and the high positive predictive value of IS combined with CT (0.84) favour the use of IS in the diagnostic approach of suspected recurrent ovarian carcinoma.

Colorectal Cancer

Radical surgery and radiotherapy may cause changes in the anatomical structures of the pelvis so that a presacral mass lesion on CT or US and probably also MRI does not necessarily indicate local recurrence. Thus, it is often very difficult to diagnose tumour recurrence by methods which are based on the detection of morphological changes. Even at laparotomy, the surgeon may sometimes have difficulties distinguishing small tumours from postoperative fibrosis. Inversely, immunoscintigraphy does not show morphological changes, but it demonstrates uptake of antibody in viable tumour tissue and thus allows characterisation of the nature of doubtful nodules. This is also the reason why liver metastases may be detected by immunoscintigraphy before they are large enough to appear as space-occupying lesions on US or CT (Fig. 1).

We have studied prospectively the diagnostic value of IS with ^{123}I-labelled fragments of two MoAbs directed against CEA in 57 patients (Bischof Delaloye 1989a). In patients with a high probability of colorectal cancer, be it primary or recurrent (Fig. 2a), the sensitivity and specificity of immunoscintigraphy was high, 91% and 97%, respectively. However, in 27 patients in whom recurrence was only suspected on the grounds of changes in symptoms and/or slightly raised serum CEA levels, but in whom a complete diagnostic work-up remained inconclusive, only 27 of 38 (71%) tumour deposits could be detected by immunoscintigraphy, and 80 of 90 (87%) tumour-free regions could be described as such (Fig. 2b). In this challenging patient population whose smaller tumours are more likely to respond to therapy, the results seem

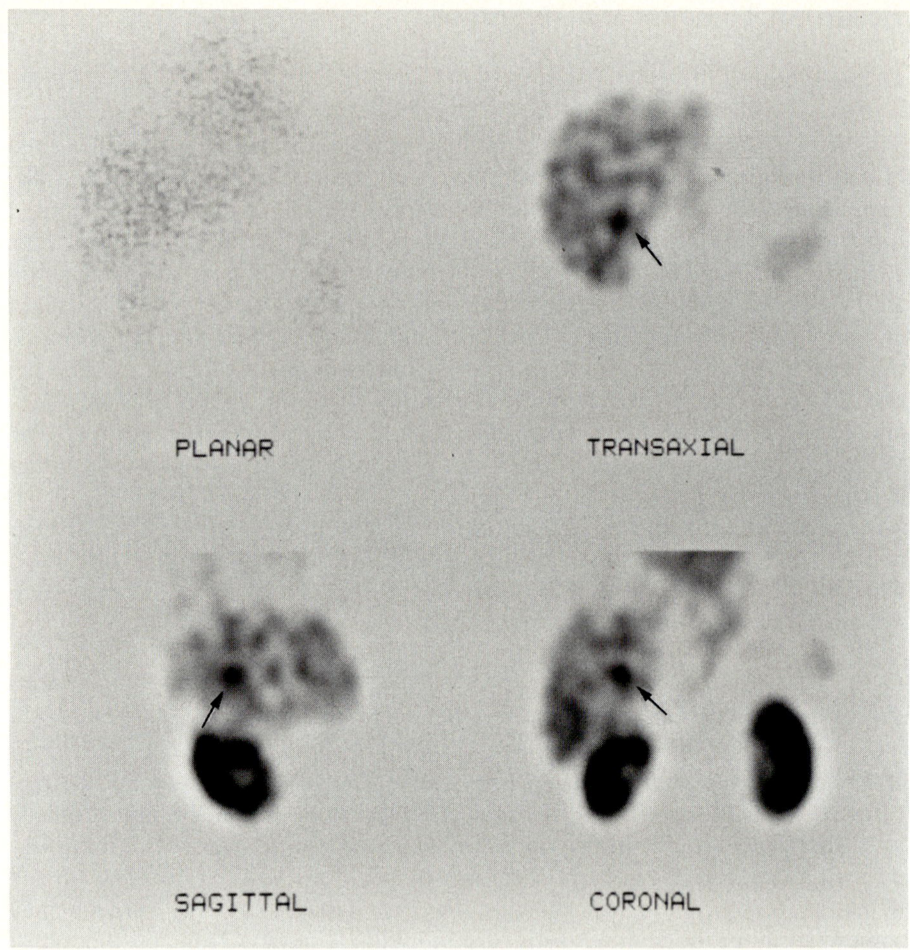

Fig. 1. Uptake of carcinoembryonic antigen-specific antibody in a liver metastasis (*arrows*) 15 months after resection of adenocarcinoma of the sigmoid (Dukes D) on transaxial, sagittal and coronal cross-sectional images of the upper abdomen. The uptake in the metastasis exceeds non-specific uptake in normal liver parenchyma. High non-specific uptake is visible in the kidneys on sagittal and coronal sections

disappointing on first glance, but they compare advantageously with presently available diagnostic modalities. In fact, a simultaneously performed comprehensive diagnostic work-up showed only 14 of the 38 (37%) lesions in these patients. In 6 patients, local recurrence was detected at repeat work-up 1–6 months later; in 8 other patients, the tumour (1 local recurrence and 7 liver metastases) were shown by conventional methods more than 6 months later with respect to immunoscintigraphy, which had been performed only once.

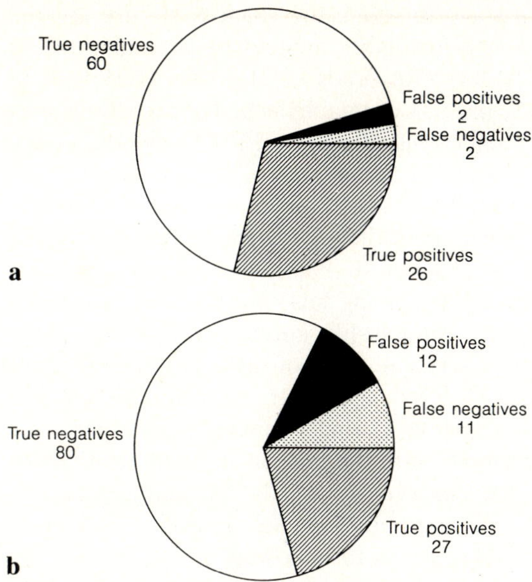

Fig. 2a,b. Results of immunoscintigraphy in patients with suspected relapse after surgery for colorectal carcinoma. In one group of patients (90 sites) the clinical diagnosis of recurrence was probable (**a**), whereas in the other group (130 sites) the clinical and imaging work-up was inconclusive (**b**). Accuracy of immunoscintigraphy was excellent in patients with a high pretest probability but decreased in the indeterminate cases. Even in this latter patient group, immunoscintigraphy allowed the detection of lesions up to 13 months before they were shown by other imaging modalities

Discussion

From the presently available results of prospective studies (Granowska et al. 1986; Bischof Delaloye et al. 1989; Dutin et al. 1991), there is strong evidence that immunoscintigraphy is able to detect tumour relapse earlier than methods which are mainly based on the description of morphological changes. In order to be efficient in terms of patient management, especially when surgical treatment is considered, antibody scans must be interpreted together with US, CT and/or MR images, which are necessary for the exact localization of foci of antibody uptake. On the other hand, immunoscintigraphy allows us to characterise tissues considered as equivocal on anatomic images as tumour or scar, according to the presence or absence of antibody uptake. This combined approach should allow the earlier diagnosis of tumour relapse during the follow-up of patients with ovarian or colorectal carcinomas.

However, in the present point of development Abdomen which most of the monoclonal antibodies used are of murine origin it is not yet possible to perform regular follow-up immunoscintigraphies in order to detect tumour recurrence even before the patients present with new symptoms or a raised level of serum CEA, that is, at a stage in which the chances of cure are the highest. With repeat injections, a non-negligible number of patients develop human antimouse antibodies (HAMA) (Reynolds et al. 1989; Hertel et al. 1990a). In the presence of HAMA, the risk of anaphylactic-type reactions may be slightly increased upon further injections of murine MoAb, but this is not the only drawback. The biokinetics of the injected MoAb may dramatically change in the presence of higher HAMA titers: the radiolabelled MoAb is complexed and trapped in the reticuloendothelial system, especially in the liver, before reaching the tumour (Perkins et al. 1988). Furthermore, HAMA may interfere with tumour marker assays, giving false-positive results (Hertel et al. 1990b). Engineering of chimeric or human-like antibodies (Morrison 1985; Hardman et al. 1989) is expected to overcome some of these problems but not that of development of antibodies directed against the specific binding site of the radiolabelled MoAb which remains murine. Comparing our presently available chimeric CEA-specific antibody with the murine antibody from which it had been derived, we could not observe any really relevant changes in biokinetics and biodistribution as well as tumour uptake (Bischof Delaloye et al. 1989b), but the incidence of HAMA seems to be lower.

We are currently performing a prospective study with chimeric CEA-specific antibodies in patients showing only subtle changes in symptoms and/or serum CEA level in order to evaluate the diagnostic value of the method and the incidence of anti-idiotypic human antimouse antibodies. First results show that the sensitivity and specificity obtained by non-repeated scans are comparable with those published earlier in patients with questionable relapse and studied with murine antibodies (Bischof Delaloye 1989a), which have already been discussed above. Moreover, the present prospective study was undertaken as a feasibility study to evaluate the role of immunoscintigraphy in the possible change of the clinical outcome of such patients in whom relapse could be detected and treated at an earlier stage. In case of promising results, this point will be further evaluated by a randomized, multi-centre trial.

Summary

Immunoscintigraphy is very helpful in the diagnosis of tumour relapse in patients treated surgically for colorectal or ovarian carcinomas at a stage at which other investigations are still negative or equivocal. However, research continues to improve the method so that it can be used in the close follow-up of patients, especially those at high risk of early relapse, in order to reduce further the lapse of time between recurrence and therapy and thus to improve patient survival.

References

Baldwin RW, Byers VS (eds) (1985) Monoclonal antibodies for cancer detection and therapy. Academic, London

Bischof Delaloye A, Delaloye B, Buchegger F, Gilgien W, Studer A, Curchod S, Givel JC, Mosimann F, Pettavel J, Mach JP (1989a) Clinical value of immunoscintigraphy in colorectal carcinoma patients: a prospective study. J Nucl Med 30:1646–1656

Bischof Delaloye A, Delaloye B, Buchegger F, Mach JP, Heusser C, Hardman N (1989b) Chimeric mouse-human anti-CEA antibody of IgG4 isotype used in a pilot immunoscintigraphy study of patients with colorectal carcinomas (Abstr). J Nucl Med 30:809

Bischof Delaloye A, Delaloye B, Buchegger F, Pèlegrin A, Heusser C, Hardman N, Mach JP (1991) Prospective immunoscintigraphy (IS) with chimeric I-123 anti-CEA MAb in patients with raising serum-CEA (Abstr). J Nucl Med 32:941

Boeckmann W, Baum RP, Schuldes H, Kramer W, Hertel A, Baew-Christow T, Hanke P, Jonas D, Hör G (1990) Tumour imaging of bladder carcinomas and their metastases with ^{111}indium-labelled monoclonal anti-CEA antibody BW 431/26. Br J Cancer [Suppl 10] 62:81–84

Britton KE, Granowska M, Mather SJ (1991) Review. Radiolabelled monoclonal antibodies in oncology. I. Technical aspects. Nucl Med Commun 12:65–76

Chatal JF (ed) (1989) Monoclonal antibodies in immunoscintigraphy. CRC, Boca Raton

Chatal JF, Fumoleau P, Saccavini JC, Thedrez P, Curtet C, Bianco-Arco A, Chetanneau A, Peltier P, Kremer M, Guillard Y (1987) Immunoscintigraphy of recurrences of gynecologic carcinomas. J Nucl Med 28:1807–1819

Delaloye B, Bischof Delaloye A, Buchegger F, von Fliedner V, Grob JP, Volant JC, Pettavel J, Mach JP (1986) Detection of colorectal carcinoma by emission computerized tomography after injection of 123-I labelled Fab or F(ab′)$_2$ fragments from monoclonal anti-carcinoembryonic antibodies. J Clin Invest 77:301–311

Dutin JP, Peltier P, Chatal JF, INSERM Clinical Research Network (1991) Bayesian analysis of the utility of In-111 OC 125 immunoscintigraphy (IS) in diagnosing ovarian carcinoma (Abstr). J Nucl Med 32:941

Epenetos AA, Carr D, Johnson P, Bodmer WF, Lavender JP (1986) Antibody guided radiolocalization of tumours in patients with testicular or ovarian cancer using two radioiodinated monoclonal antibodies to placental alkaline phosphatase. Br J Radiol 59:117–125

Goldenberg DM, DeLand FH, Kim EE, Bennet FJ, Primus JR, van Nagell N, Estes P, DeSimone P, Rayburn P (1978) Use of radiolabeled antibodies to carcinoembryonic antigen for the detection and localization of diverse cancers by external photoscanning. N Engl J Med 298:1384–1388

Granowska M, Britton KE (1991) Review. Radiolabelled monoclonal antibodies in oncology. II. Clinical applications in diagnosis. Nucl Med Commun 12:83–98

Granowska M, Britton KE, Shepherd JH, Nimmon CC, Mather S, Ward B, Osborne R, Slevin ML (1986) A prospective study of ^{123}I-labelled monoclonal antibody imaging in ovarian cancer. J Clin Oncol 4:730–736

Hardman N, LeeGill L, de Winter RFJ, Wagner L, Hollis M, Businger F, Ammaturo D, Buchegger F, Mach JP, Heusser C (1989) Generation of a human-mouse chimaeric antibody directed against human carcinoembryonic antigen. Int J Cancer 44:424–433

Hertel A, Baum RP, Auerbach B, Herrmann A, Hör G (1990a) Klinische Relevanz humaner Anti-Maus-Antikörper (HAMA) in der Immunszintigraphie. Nuclearmedizin 29:221–227

Hertel A, Baum RP, Auerbach B, Herrmann A, Hör G (1990b) Effects of human anti-mouse antibodies (HAMA) on tumor marker assays. In: Klapdor R (ed) Recent results in tumor diagnosis and therapy. Zuckschwerdt, Munich, pp 461–463

Larson SM (1985) Radiolabeled monoclonal anti-tumor antibodies in diagnosis and therapy. J Nucl Med 26:538–545

Mach JP, Carrel S, Forni M, Ritschard J, Donath A, Alberto P (1980) Tumor localization of radiolabeled antibodies against carcinoembryonic antigen in patients with carcinoma. N Engl J Med 303:5–10

Morrison SL (1985) Transfectomas provide novel chimeric antibodies. Science 119:1202–1207

Munz DL, Emrich D (eds) (1990) Immunoscintigraphy. Facts and fiction. Elsevier, Amsterdam

Perkins AC, Pimm MV, Powell MC (1988) The implications of patient antibody response for the clinical usefulness of immunoscintigraphy. Nucl Med Commun 9:273–282

Reynolds JC, del Vecchio S, Sakahara J, Lora ME, Carrasquillo JA, Neumann RD, Larson SM (1989) Antimurine antibody response to mouse monoclonal antibodies: clinical findings and implications. Nucl Med Biol 16:121–125

Summary of Discussion: Session 4

G. GADEMANN

The discussion was firstly directed to the clinical value of abdominal screening by ultrasound. Only two systematic approaches can be found in the literature. In one trial including more than 6000 patients, 13 tumors were detected, 10 of which were renal cell carcinomas with a medium size of 5.4 cm. The question of whether the kidney would be a candidate for ultrasound screening revealed the problem of the situation. An estimate of the costs for these 10 renal cell carcinomas reaches DM 30000–50000, excluding all additionally induced examinations like CT for clarifying the findings. In addition, the size of accidentally detected kidney tumors is about 6 cm, which means that there is only a minor difference between screened and accidentally found tumors. Regarding repeated screening in patients with liver scirrhosis, the results of Japanese trials and of the German Thorotrust study recommend a screening interval of 6 months because a high-risk group is selectable. Tumors less than 3 cm in diameter can be visualised by ultrasound – an important point considering the abilities of modern liver surgery. In more superficial organs such as the thyroid or testes, even smaller lesions are detectable with high frequency ultrasound. There the problem arises how to react to these tiny lesions.

P.E. Peters was asked for his opinion about MRI of big breasts. Two German groups in Bonn and Munich deal with MRI of the breast. It requires a lot of time, and in principle, it is not considered to be a screening method. An improvement regarding complicated mammography or questionable findings may be, however, possible. Concerning the indication for MRI in differentiating spinal metastases of breast cancer from degenerative diseases, the ability of MRI is accepted, while its capacity limitation still restricts the indication drastically. The same is true for other bony infiltrations like multiple myeloma for which radionuclear scans are not reliable. The value of abdominal MRI, particularly of the liver, is still debated. CT currently seems to be superior to MRI in the differentiation of liver lesions, but Peters finds the advances in MRI within the past few years significant. By using intraoperative ultrasound as the golden standard, he noted that MRI is now competitive with CT. P.E. Peters was asked whether there is a place for CT in the early detection of lung cancer. He responded that he could not find any publication of screening asymptomatic patients for lung cancer with CT. It certainly cannot be applied to every smoker, but special risk groups could be determined for CT screening. A.B. Miller (Toronto) added that even in new programs of lung, colorectal, and prostate cancer, CT is not considered a primary diagnostic tool. CT and

MRI are always second choice despite a high failure rate of chest X-radiograph diagnosis (30%).

Two questions were posed to W.J. Huk concerning the indication of stereotactic biopsy and intraoperative ultrasound. Biopsy is recommended when the nature of the lesion cannot be found by conventional neuro-radiological diagnostics and if surgery of the lesion is very risky. Intraoperative ultrasound is mainly used for localizing deep-seated small lesions and not for differential diagnosis.

The question of whether the resolution of PET can be improved was answered by G. Strauss. Theoretically, a resolution of 1.6 mm in the plane is possible. It is worse in the Z-direction. The most limiting factor is the movement of organs; thus, PET has a reduced resolution compared with CT or MRI but 4- to 5-fold better than conventional nuclear imaging. Another question concerned the low perfusion of liver metastases of colorectal cancers. The perfusion depends strongly on the size of the lesion. It is relatively high in small lesions and reduced in large lesions; however, perfusion measured with ^{15}O is a quite complicated parameter. It is regarded as tissue perfusion and not from vessels.

The questions and comments on the last topic, immunoscintigraphy presented by A. Bischof-Delaloye, concerned very specific items. It was asked whether imaging can be improved by using technetium as a label or paramagnetic ions in combination with better resolution of MRI. The uptake of less than 0.06% in the tumor certainly limits this method of labelling for MRI. Other substances like Fab and bifunctional molecules were discussed. Conflicting results in using these substances still limit their clinical use.

No diagnostic procedure could really offer an early primary diagnosis. All were more appropriate for the early detection of recurrent tumors. Immunoscintigraphy was able to visualise and localise metastases and recurrences earlier than CT; however, A. Bischof-Delaloye asked herself whether that will change anything for the patients. A.B. Miller commented that he was able to follow the first introduction of CEA many years ago. At that time, he did not have the impression that it would be of any clinical relevance. Now it is widely used. This shows that research on fields that do not look very promising at the beginning should continue. Regarding immunoscintigraphy, research should focus much more on reducing or to avoiding immune reactions with confident antibodies, such as HAMA (human antimouse antibody) which limits repeated drug administration. It was emphasized that radioimmunoscintigraphy is a diagnostic but not a screening technique. There was agreement that this is valid for the other methods discussed. A last rhetorical question was posed by A.B. Miller: Are there any plans to investigate the benefit for the patient of an earlier detection of the recurrence or metastases of a known tumor?

Histo- and Cytopathology

Chairman: H.K. MÜLLER-HERMELINK

Histopathological Diagnosis of Early Cancer and Antecedent Lesions

R.L. Carter

Introduction

Increasing numbers of screening programmes are now being undertaken to identify early cancers and their precursors in a variety of sites (Miller et al. 1990). Morphology in some form is the principal method of detecting such lesions, although other approaches include the use of tumour-associated markers in body fluids (ovarian cancer, neuroblastoma) and serological methods (Epstein–Barr virus antibodies in nasopharyngeal carcinoma). Biopsy techniques have become extremely versatile as a result of advances in endoscopic procedures and in fine localization by stereoscopic methods and computed tomography. The samples obtained from such procedures are often small, and the histopathologist is increasingly required to assess changes which may be subtle and difficult to recognize – quite apart from the related and often contentious issues of descriptive terminology, classification and reproducibility of results. Repeated biopsies may be taken over periods of months or years. The importance of morphology in identifying early cancers and their antecedents is self-evident, but clinicians, pathologists and epidemiologists have to recognize the inherent limitations of histopathology alone and the need for additional, more precise methods. A few selected examples follow which serve to illustrate both the scope and the shortcomings of histopathology in this problematic field.

Invasion

Tumours which infiltrate widely into surrounding tissues are easy to assess, but more restricted invasive growth can be difficult to evaluate. It may be appropriate under such circumstances to measure directly various dimensions of the infiltrating tumour; or the histopathologist can map tumour invasion with reference to local microanatomical landmarks. Thin cutaneous melanomas and microinvasive cancers of the female genital tract serve to illustrate these two approaches.

1. It is now standard practice to evaluate cutaneous melanomas by determining tumour thickness (Breslow) and the level of tumour invasion (Clark), but it is clear that both measurements are subject to considerable intra- and inter-observer variations (EORTC Melanoma Pathologists' Group 1980;

Colloby et al. 1991). Such variations are readily analysed statistically, and the use of kappa statistics is particularly helpful: the calculated kappa values do not depend on a majority diagnosis, and they incorporate a correction for the amount of agreement to be expected purely by chance. Evaluation of thickness and invasive level in thin melanomas is open to several sources of potential variation which may be due to factors in the measuring system, the optics, the observer and, in particular, the biopsy itself. Variations may occur, for example, in normal skin thickness and microanatomical organization; melanomas sometimes show growth patterns which are difficult to measure as in exophytic (polypoid) and ulcerating tumours; and the deepest point of penetration by melanoma cells into the dermis may be obscured by inflammation and fibrosis. The prognostic value of microstaging, particularly for tumour thickness, is not disputed, but it is not infallible.

2. Microinvasive cancers are regarded as tumours of measurable size which show limited local invasion but have minimal potential for metastatic spread. The term is not simply descriptive, and it carries clear clinical and therapeutic implications. These cancers have been extensively studied in the female genital tract. In the cervix, microinvasive carcinomas are generally associated with CIN 3, invasion being either continuous, with protruding "buds" or "pegs", or discontinuous. The continuous protrusions are often better differentiated than the main intraepithelial component, and the surrounding stroma is oedematous and may be infiltrated with lymphocytes. There are two main issues: what defining measurements should be used with respect to depth and lateral extent of the lesions? And what is the relevance of associated features such as spread of neoplastic cells into local "capillary-like" spaces? Both issues remain controversial, but there is sufficient agreement for the category of microinvasive cervical carcinoma to be included within international classifications (Anderson 1987; Burghardt et al. 1991). As far as comparable lesions in the vulva are concerned, analogies with the cervix are difficult to sustain, and it is generally held that a clinically reliable category of microinvasive vulval cancer cannot be formulated at the present time (Buckley et al. 1984; Beilby and Ridley 1987).

More detailed investigation of basement membrane components by electron microscopy and (in particular) immunohistochemistry have not resolved the difficulties of detecting early invasion (D'Ardenne 1989). Some infiltrating tumours retain segments of intact basement membrane on their margins, a feature which varies according to histological type and degree of differentiation. Striking examples are provided by infiltrating squamous cancers in the head and neck (Carter et al. 1985). Conversely, dysplastic and intra-epithelial lesions may show discontinuities in basement membrane staining which vary according to site; any prognostic implications are unclear. Defects in the basement membrane may be associated with non-neoplastic processes such as local inflammation. In everyday practice, immunohistochemical stains for basement membrane components are often more useful in excluding a diagnosis of cancer, for instance, in debatable examples of chronic pancreatitis, sclerosing breast lesions and florid endometrial hyperplasia.

Non-invasive Malignancy: In Situ/Intraepithelial Cancer

The morphological category of in situ malignancy is most clearly exemplified by carcinomas arising from surface epithelia. In situ tumours are demonstrable in certain organs such as the testis, but the existence of in situ malignancy is difficult to sustain in other tissues. Although recognized for many years, there is still no agreed morphological classification of these lesions in several sites, and their natural history remains poorly documented. Even intraepithelial neoplasia in the cervix continues to present problems, despite a vast amount of investigation (Fox and Buckley 1990). Intra- and inter-observer agreement, which is high in assessing CIN 3, falls in the diagnosis of CIN 1 and CIN 2 (Robertson et al. 1989; Ismail et al. 1990). Some authors have advocated a modified classification for CIN, and the discussion continues. It is widely held that CIN evolves according to the sequence CIN 1 → CIN 2 → CIN 3 → invasive carcinoma, but there are several uncertainties (Anderson 1987). How often, for example, does CIN 2 (or even CIN 1) bypass CIN 3 and progress directly to invasive cancer? Very aggressive tumours may develop in women with recent cervical cytology results which are completely negative. The time scale by which CIN, irrespective of grade, evolves to invasive cancer also remains uncertain: lengths of 10–15 years are commonly cited, but results from different studies vary depending on the methods (and consistency) of diagnosis, the number of women observed and the duration of follow-up. There are increasing discrepancies between histopathological appearances and the presence of particular genotypes of human papillomavirus (Griffin et al. 1990). Immunohistochemical methods for detecting oncogenes and/or oncogene products (mainly c-*myc*, h-*ras* and c-*erbB2*) also give divergent results (Hendy-Ibbs et al. 1987; Hughes et al. 1989; Pinion et al. 1991).

Dysplasia

The separation of in situ malignancy from dysplasia is often contentious, and the terminology used is confusing and arbitrary. "Dysplasia" has been discarded for cases in the cervix and is falling into disuse for those in the breast. The term has been retained for cases in the large bowel, but high-grade mucosal dysplasia here is regarded as synonymous with (at least) in situ carcinoma, and the latter term is rarely applied. Borderline neoplastic changes in the large bowel and breast illustrate some of the histopathologist's most tricky problems, and both merit further discussion.

    1. About 3%–5% of patients with long-standing colitis (principally ulcerative colitis) develop colorectal cancers. There is a strong overall association between such cancers and mucosal dysplasia, but anomalies are well recognized (Morson et al. 1990). Dysplasia and cancer, for example, may each be found alone. When they co-exist, they may occur in widely separated regions of the bowel. Increasingly severe dysplasia does not necessarily reflect a correspond-

ing increase in malignant potential. (Low-grade dysplasia, for example, may be associated with cancer in macroscopically raised lesions.) These endoscopic lesions – variously described as plaques, nodules and zones of velvety mucosa – can be difficult to see, and the histopathologist may be confronted by the combined problems of sampling, interpretation and classification.

A detailed scheme for describing and classifying mucosal changes in chronic inflammatory bowel disease was presented by Riddell et al. in 1983, and a slightly simplified version was subsequently proposed by Talbot and Price (1987), who defined 5 categories: dysplasia (high- and low-grade), atypia/ indefinite, active colitis, inactive colitis and normal. The description of atypia/ indefinite is applied to biopsies in which one or a small number of suggestive features are seen, but the overall appearance falls short of that required for low-grade dysplasia. A diagnosis of atypia/indefinite conveys two messages: diagnostic difficulty with the biopsy under consideration and, more generally, the inherent limitations of routine histopathology in recognising mucosal dysplasia. The morphological features of mucosal dysplasia depend on changes in architecture and cytology which are sometimes subtle and difficult to recognise. Features most reliably identified include a villous growth pattern, back-to-back arrangement of glands and deeply staining, heaped-up nuclei which lack normal polarity (Dundas et al. 1987). Considerable degrees of observer variation have been reported (Dundas et al. 1987; Dixon et al. 1988), particularly in the separation of atypia/indefinite from low-grade dysplasia. Wide measures of disagreement have been demonstrated with kappa statistics (Dixon et al. 1988), but it is important to set such findings in perspective. Kappa values are informative but are artificial in that they are based on isolated conclusions drawn from one or more tissue slides divorced from other sources of information such as clinical details, endoscopic appearances and morphological findings in previous biopsies or in additional sections from the current tissues on which such studies are based. The value of regular endoscopy and biopsy in screening high-risk colitis patients for colorectal cancer has been convincingly shown (Lennard-Jones et al. 1983). There is, however, still a lack of an unequivocal marker for identifying dysplastic mucosa. Complementary approaches have been tried such as morphometry (Allen et al. 1987a), histochemistry for sialomucins (Jass et al. 1986), immunohistochemistry for epithelial marker antigens and for *ras* oncogene p21 product (Allen et al. 1985, 1987b) and cell ploidy (Fozard et al. 1986), but none has become established.

2. Studies of observer variation in reporting breast lesions show, entirely predictably, a range of disagreement with respect to ductal and lobular lesions designated by terms such as atypical hyperplasia or epithelial dysplasia (Beck et al. 1985). The importance of these debatable or borderline changes has been accentuated by the increasing use of mammographic screening programmes (Elston and Ellis 1990; Sloane 1991). Such programmes have already stimulated interest in breast pathology and will lead to improvements in histopathological expertise (Royal College of Pathologists Working Group 1990a,b). The patterns of lesions picked up in mammographic screening are already becoming apparent (Sloane 1991). They include increased numbers of in situ

carcinomas, most of which are ductal, and of small (<1 cm) infiltrating cancers, many of which are of the tubular type. *Non-neoplastic* infiltrative lesions which may simulate cancer in the mammogram are increasingly identified such as radial scars, complex sclerosing lesions and sclerosing adenosis. Abnormal patterns of calcification show up in mammograms, mainly due to weddellite (calcium oxalate dihydrate). Sampling of tissues removed after mammography is a time-consuming exercise, particularly when no palpable lesions are found, and standard protocols for examining such material are essential (Royal College of Pathologists Working Group 1990b).

Breast biopsies, irrespective of their source, often show a range of morphological changes. Some of them have implications for the future development of invasive cancer; others do not and may represent "aberrations of normal development and involution" (Hughes et al. 1987). A study by Page and Dupont (1990), based on observations on a large group of women for up to 20 years, proposes four categories of risk with respect to antecedent lesions and the subsequent development of invasive carcinoma:

No risk: adenosis, apocrine changes, duct ectasia, mild hyperplasia of the usual
   type
Risk increased × *2*: moderate and florid hyperplasia of the usual type, sclerosing adenosis, papilloma
Risk increased × *4, 5*: atypical ductal or lobular hyperplasia
Risk increased × *10*: ductal or lobular carcinoma in situ

The importance of atypical ductal hyperplasia as a significant predictive factor for invasive cancer is also emphasised by results from Tavassoli and Norris (1990). Radial scars, despite their sometimes alarming appearances on mammograms and histological sections, apparently do not carry an increased risk for infiltrative cancer (Nielsen et al. 1987). The occurrence of the morphological changes listed here will vary with age: atypical ductal hyperplasia, for example, may persist for several years after the menopause, while atypical lobular hyperplasia tends to decline after this time. All these changes have to be viewed in conjunction with other, non-morphological risk factors. The values quoted for the three "increased risk" groups should (in round figures) be doubled for women with a history of invasive breast cancer in first-degree relatives.

Metaplasia

Metaplasia, a common and non-specific change in both epithelial and stromal tissues, is associated with malignancy in certain contexts. Examples include squamous metaplasia in urothelial and bronchial mucosa and intestinal metaplasia in the stomach, columnar cell-lined segments of the oesophagus, gall bladder and urinary bladder.

Intestinal metaplasia is present in about one-third of unselected gastric biopsies in patients from areas of intermediate risk for gastric cancer; its incidence increases with age (Rothery and Day 1985; Filipe and Jass 1986). It is morphologically heterogeneous and is classified into three types on the basis of light microscopy, ultrastructure, mucin histochemistry and enzymology. Type I, formerly called "complete", is truly metaplastic; types II and III, previously designated as "incomplete", are not. The sulphomucin-secreting type III variant, the least common of the three subgroups, is associated with gastric carcinoma of the intestinal type, but the relationship is unclear. Intestinal metaplasia and gastric cancer commonly co-exist, and tumours may arise within foci of intestinal metaplasia. The metaplastic change is common in gastric biopsies from patients living in high-risk cancer areas, and its incidence declines when people from such areas migrate to low-incidence regions. By contrast, recent studies from intermediate-risk areas have failed to show that type III intestinal metaplasia, unaccompanied by tumour, is a predictor for future gastric cancer over a time scale of >10 years (Ectors and Dixon 1986; Ramesar et al. 1987). These discrepancies remain unsolved, but it is worth stressing the difficulties in comparing results from different studies in this field. Patients need to be matched for age and other risk factors, endoscopy and biopsy protocols should be comparable, the diagnosis of intestinal metaplasia needs to be stringently defined and the duration and completeness of follow-up must be fully documented.

Despite its familiarity, intestinal metaplasia is a poorly understood (and extremely complex) set of tissue changes (Morson et al. 1990). How does intestinal metaplasia arise in the first place? What is its natural history, given that the different types may co-exist and that "mixed" or "transitional" forms can occur? Is intestinal metaplasia an integral part of the tissue changes which make up gastric carcinogenesis, or is it an adaptive, essentially epiphenomenal process?

Chronic Inflammation

Chronic inflammation is a still more common and banal tissue change which presents no diagnostic difficulties. There are, however, certain clinical contexts in which chronic inflammation points to an enhanced risk of developing cancer. An example is provided by the different distribution of chronic oesophagitis, together with mucosal atrophy and dysplasia, in patients from high- and low-risk areas for oesophageal carcinoma in Iran and Northern China (Crespi et al. 1979, 1984; Yang 1980). Chronic oesophagitis and the two associated changes were significantly increased among men and women in high-risk areas, and the separate Chinese studies provided evidence of a progression (chronic oesophagitis → dysplasia → carcinoma) over a 12-year period. The results are not, however, straightforward. The Chinese investigators, for example, based their observations on cytology rather than biopsy. Additional differences between the oesophageal mucosa in patients from high- and low-risk areas may also be relevant: in vitro uptake of tritiated thymidine was found to be higher in mucosa from patients in the high-risk areas, independent of the presence or absence of actual oesophagitis at the time of biopsy (Munoz et al. 1985). Once again, the outstanding problems can be thought of in terms of the natural history of the various lesions. How many, at each stage, persist or regress or advance to a more severe form? What is the time scale? And to what extent are the factors responsible for such changes open to manipulation?

Conclusion

One concluding point merits repetition: the need for additional, non-morphological techniques to supplement conventional histopathology in the recognition of early malignancies and their antecedent changes. There have been striking advances in our knowledge of the development of at least some human tumours at the molecular and genetic levels – notably colorectal cancer – and it seems reasonable to expect that some of the methods of molecular biology can be applied to these problems. An example is provided by the polymerase chain reaction: this technique provides a highly sensitive means of detecting small clones of abnormal lymphoid cells, and methods are now available which can be used with conventionally processed biopsy tissues (McCarthy et al. 1990, 1991).

Summary

Histopathology plays a crucial role in the diagnosis of early cancer and its antecedent lesions, but it must be recognized that morphology has inherent limitations. The histopathological changes may be subtle and difficult to recognise, and there are frequent problems in descriptive nomenclature, classification and reproducibility of results. The examples that are discussed include early invasion and microinvasion with respect to cutaneous melanomas and cancers of the cervix uteri and vulva, cervical intraepithelial neoplasia, dysplasia in the large intestine and breast and intestinal metaplasia in the stomach. The difficulties posed by many of these conditions have not been materially improved by the use of morphometry, electron microscopy, histo-chemistry or immunohisto-chemistry, and there is a clear need for additional, non-morphological approaches. Some of the highly sensitive techniques from molecular biology need to be applied to these problems, and the success of the polymerase chain reaction in demonstrating small clones of abnormal lymphoid cells within lymphoid tissues provides a pointer to possible future developments.

References

Allen DC, Biggart JD, Orchin JC, Foster H (1985) An immunoperoxidase study of epithelial marker antigens in ulcerative colitis with dysplasia and carcinoma. J Clin Pathol 38: 18–29

Allen DC, Hamilton PW, Watt PCH, Biggart JD (1987a) Morphometrical analysis in ulcerative colitis with dysplasia and carcinoma. Histopathology 11:913–926

Allen DC, Foster H, Orchin JC, Biggart JD (1987b) Immunohistochemical staining of colorectal tissues with monoclonal antibodies to *ras* oncogene p21 product and carbohydrate determinant antigen 19–9. J Clin Pathol 40:157–162

Anderson MC (1987) Premalignant and malignant disease of the cervix. In: Fox H (ed) Haines & Taylor obstetrical and gynaecological pathology, vol 1, 3rd edn. Livingstone, Edinburgh, pp 255–301

Beck JS, Members of the Medical Research Council Breast Tumour Pathology Panel (1985) Observer variability in reporting of breast lesions. J Clin Pathol 38:1358–1365

Beilby JOW, Ridley CM (1987) Pathology of the vulva. In: Fox H (ed) Haines & Taylor obstetrical and gynaecological pathology, vol 1, 3rd edn. Livingstone, Edinburgh, pp 64–145

Buckley CH, Butler EB, Fox H (1984) Vulvar intraepithelial neoplasia and microinvasive carcinoma of the vulva. J Clin Pathol 37:1201–1211

Burghardt E, Girardi F, Lahousen M, Pickel H, Tamussino K (1991) Microinvasive carcinoma of the uterine cervix. Cancer 67:1037–1045

Carter RL, Burman JF, Barr L, Gusterson BA (1985) Immuno-histochemical localization of basement membrane type IV collagen in invasive and metastatic squamous carcinomas of the head and neck. J Pathol 147:159–164

Colloby PS, West KP, Fletcher A (1991) Observer variation in the measurement of Breslow depth and Clark's level in thin cutaneous malignant melanoma. J Pathol 163:245–250

Crespi M, Munoz M, Grassi A, Aramesh B, Amiri G, Mojtabi A (1979) Oesophageal lesions in Northern Iran: a premalignant condition? Lancet 1:217–221

Crespi M, Munoz N, Grassi A, Qiong S, Jing WK, Jien LJ (1984) Precursor lesions of oesophageal cancer in a low-risk population in China: comparison with high-risk populations. Int J Cancer 34:599–602

D'Ardenne AJ (1989) Use of basement membrane markers in tumour diagnosis. J Clin Pathol 42:449–457

Dixon MF, Brown LJR, Gilmour HM, Price AB, Smeeton NC, Talbot IC, Williams GT (1988) Observer variation in the assessment of dysplasia in ulcerative colitis. Histopathology 13:385–397

Dundas SAC, Kay R, Beck S, Cotton DWK, Coup AJ, Slater DN, Underwood JCE (1987) Can histopathologists reliably assess dysplasia in chronic inflammatory bowel disease? J Clin Pathol 40:1282–1286

Ectors N, Dixon MF (1986) The prognostic value of sulphomucin positive intestinal metaplasia in the development of gastric cancer. Histopathology 10:1271–1277

Elston CW, Ellis IO (1990) Pathology and breast screening. Histopathology 16:109–118

EORTC Melanoma Pathologists' Group (1980) Difficulties encountered in the application of Clark classification and the Breslow thickness measurement in cutaneous malignant melanoma. Int J Cancer 26:159–163

Filipe MI, Jass JR (eds) (1986) Gastric carcinoma. Livingstone, Edinburgh

Fox H, Buckley CH (1990) Current problems in the pathology of intra-epithelial lesions of the uterine cervix. Histopathology 17:1–6

Fozard JB, Quirke P, Dixon MF, Giles GR, Bird CC (1986) DNA aneuploidy in ulcerative colitis. Gut 27:1414–1423

Griffin NR, Bevan IS, Lewis FA, Wells M, Young LS (1990) Demonstration of multiple HPV types in normal cervix and in cervical squamous cell carcinoma using the polymerase chain reaction on paraffin wax embedded material. J Clin Pathol 43:52–56

Hendy-Ibbs P, Cox H, Evan GI, Watson JV (1987) Flow cytometric quantitation of DNA and c-*myc* oncoprotein in archival biopsies of uterine cervix neoplasia. Br J Cancer 55:275–282

Hughes LE, Mansel RE, Webster DJT (1987) Aberrations of normal development and involution (ANDI): a new perspective on pathogenesis and nomenclature of benign breast disease. Lancet 2:1316–1319

Hughes RG, Neill WA, Norval M (1989) Papillomavirus and c-*myc* antigen expression in normal and neoplastic cervical epithelium. J Clin Pathol 42:46–51

Ismail SM, Colclough AB, Dinnen JS, Eakins D, Evans DMD, Gradwell E, O'Sullivan JP, Summerell JM, Newcombe R (1990) Reporting cervical intra-epithelial neoplasia (CIN): intra- and interpathologist variation and factors associated with disagreement. Histopathology 16:371–376

Jass JR, England J, Miller K (1986) Value of mucin histochemistry in follow up surveillance of patients with long standing ulcerative colitis. J Clin Pathol 39:393–398

Lennard-Jones JE, Morson BC, Ritchie JK, Williams CB (1983) Cancer surveillance in ulcerative colitis. Lancet 2:149–152

McCarthy KP, Sloane JP, Wiedemann LM (1990) A rapid method for distinguishing clonal from polyclonal B-cell populations in surgical biopsies. J Clin Pathol 43:429–432

McCarthy KP, Sloane JP, Kabarowski JHS, Matutes E, Wiedemann LM (1991) The rapid detection of clonal T-cell proliferations in patients with lymphoid disorders. Am J Pathol 138:821–828

Miller AB, Chamberlain J, Day NE, Hakama M, Prorok PC (1990) Report on a workshop of the UICC Project on Evaluation of Screening for Cancer. Int J Cancer 46:761–769

Morson BC, Dawson IMP, Day DW, Jass JR, Price AB, Williams GT (1990) Morson and Dawson's gastrointestinal pathology, 3rd edn. Blackwell, Oxford

Munoz N, Lipkin M, Crespi M, Wahrendorf J, Grassi A, Shih-Hsien L (1985) Proliferative abnormalities of the oesophageal epithelium of Chinese populations at high and low risk for oesophageal cancer. Int J Cancer 36:187–189

Nielsen M, Christensen L, Andersen J (1987) Radial scars in women with breast cancer. Cancer 59:1019–1025

Page DL, Dupont WD (1990) Anatomic markers of human premalignancy and risk of breast cancer. Cancer 66:1326–1335

Pinion SB, Kennedy JH, Miller RW, MacLean AB (1991) Oncogene expression in cervical intraepithelial neoplasia and invasive cancer of cervix. Lancet 337:819–820

Ramesar KCRB, Sanders DSA, Hopwood D (1987) Limited value of type III intestinal metaplasia in predicting risk of gastric carcinoma. J Clin Pathol 40:1287–1290

Riddell RH, Goldman H, Ransohoff DF, Appelman HD, Fenoglio CM, Haggitt RC, Ahren C, Correa P, Hamilton SR, Morson BC, Sommers SC, Yardley JH (1983) Dysplasia in inflammatory bowel disease. Hum Pathol 14:931–968

Robertson AJ, Anderson JM, Beck JS, Burnett RA, Howatson SR, Lee FD, Lessells AM, McLaren KM, Moss SM, Simpson JG, Smith GD, Tavadia HB, Walker F (1989) Observer variability in histopathological reporting of cervical biopsy specimens. J Clin Pathol 42:231–238

Rothery GA, Day DW (1985) Intestinal metaplasia in endoscopic biopsy specimens of gastric mucosa. J Clin Pathol 38:613–621

Royal College of Pathologists Working Group (1990a) NHS Breast Screening Programme: guidelines for pathologists. Screening Publications, London

Royal College of Pathologists Working Group (1990b) NHS Breast Screening Programme: pathology reporting in breast cancer screening. Screening Publications, London

Sloane JP (1991) Changing role of the pathologist. Br Med Bull 47:433–454

Talbot I, Price AB (1987) Biopsy pathology in colorectal disease. Chapman and Hall, London

Tavassoli FA, Norris HJ (1990) A comparison of the results of long-term follow-up for atypical intraductal hyperplasia and intraductal hyperplasia of the breast. Cancer 65:518–529

Yang CS (1980) Research on esophageal cancer in China: a review. Cancer Res 40:2633–2644

Cytodiagnosis of Precancerous States and Early Human Cancer

L.G. Koss

Introduction

Cytologic techniques have been instrumental in the detection and diagnosis of precancerous lesions and early stages of human cancer and have contributed in a major way to the current knowledge of these lesions (summary in Koss 1992). The success in these endeavors is best illustrated by cervix cancer detection programs that contributed to a statistically significant drop in the rate of invasive cancer of the cervix in societies where such programs were appropriately executed (summary in Koss 1989). Besides the uterine cervix, the targets of these techniques have included other organs of the female genital tract such as the endometrium (Koss et al. 1984), several organs of the gastrointestinal tract, mainly the esophagus (Shu 1985) and stomach (Takeda 1984), organs of the lower urinary tract, mainly the urinary bladder (Koss et al. 1985), and the larynx and the lung (Fontana 1986). Other incidental applications of these techniques to the diagnosis of precancerous lesions have also been described.

The concept upon which these diagnostic efforts have been based is the recognition that microscopically visible cell abnormalities occur in the precancerous state and that these abnormalities can be recognized in cytologic samples obtained from the target organs. These abnormalities pertain mainly to the nuclei of affected cells, with a resulting change in the nucleocytoplasmic ratio (Koss 1992).

Uterine Cervix and Endometrium

In reference to the uterine cervix, the cervical smear has now been used for some 50 years in many countries. It has been well documented that cellular abnormalities, such as abnormal cell forms and nuclear enlargement and hyperchromasia, may be related with histologically documented precancerous states of various levels of atypia. It is of note that, in competent hands, not only the histologic type of these abnormalities but also their anatomic location can be determined. For example, within the uterine cervix, lesions of the squamous epithelium of the portio and of the endocervical canal can be accurately identified. Further, the participation of the human papillomavirus (HPV) in these precancerous events can be recognized by specific cell abnormalities known as koilocytosis (Koss and Durfee 1956).

One of the biologic puzzles that so far has remained unsolved and which urgently requires additional research is the natural history of the precancerous lesions of the cervix. It can be safely assumed that only about one-third of these lesions has the potential for becoming invasive cancers. Thus, about two-thirds are unnecessarily treated out of ignorance of their destiny rather than because they constitute a direct danger to the patient. So far, no reliable criteria allowing the differentiation between the dangerous and not dangerous lesions have been developed.

A somewhat similar situation occurs in the endometrium where, by direct sampling, it could be documented that approximately 8 per 1000 of post-menopausal women have occult endometrial carcinomas (Koss et al. 1984). There is some evidence, although not nearly as reliable as for the uterine cervix, that at least some of these occult carcinomas would not have progressed during the lifetime of the patient to a clinically obvious cancer. This evidence is based on a review of autopsy material of elderly women dying of other causes in whom clinically unsuspected endometrial carcinomas were discovered (Horwitz et al. 1981).

Esophagus and Stomach

Within the past 20 years, a major effect toward the cytologic detection of precancerous stages of carcinoma of the esophagus has been conducted in China. The techniques used by the Chinese investigators were based on balloon sampling of the esophageal epithelium in high-risk areas. The results strongly suggest that precancerous events in the esophagus can be identified by cytologic sampling and that these detection efforts may lead to a substantial reduction in the rate of invasive esophageal carcinoma in the target population (Shu 1984). There is evidence that surgical resection of carcinoma in situ and related precancerous events in the esophagus has significantly improved the survival of patients with this dreaded disease, when compared with cohorts of patients with fully invasive carcinoma (Li et al. 1989). There is also some evidence, although perhaps anecdotal, that not all of the precancerous events recognized by cytologic techniques will necessarily progress to invasive cancer. Thus, Shu reported that at least some patients with "dysplasia" may revert to normal and show no progression to invasive cancer (Shu 1985).

The efforts at cytologic detection of gastric cancer were initiated by Schade in patients with pernicious anemia (Schade 1956). With the use of simple cytologic lavage techniques, Schade was able to diagnose carcinoma in situ and related lesions of the stomach in several patients. This work found a keen following among Japanese investigators aware of the nearly epidemic occurrence of gastric cancer in·Japan (Takeda et al. 1981). The initial success with early cancer detection in Japan was based on cytologic sampling, although this technique has been now largely replaced by gastric endoscopy or biopsies. The evidence from Japan strongly suggests that detection of precancerous states and early gastric cancer, regardless of histologic or cytologic type, has a very beneficial effect on the survival of patients (Kasugai and Kobayashi 1974).

Urinary Bladder and Ureter

Carcinoma in situ and related abnormalities of the urinary bladder, and to some lesser extent of the renal pelves and ureters, have been shown to be important precancerous lesions. The use of cytologic techniques based on the microscopic examination of the sediment of voided urine has led to the recognition of a flat carcinoma in situ of the urinary bladder, a lesion that is more aggressive than similar abnormalities in other organs. There is evidence from several sources that, if untreated, carcinoma in situ of the bladder will progress to invasive cancer in at least 70% of patients within 5 years (summary in Koss 1975, 1985). There is also persuasive evidence that carcinoma in situ appears to be the most common source of origin of invasive bladder cancer (Brawn 1982, Kaye and Lange 1982). Anecdotal, similar cases from the renal pelves and ureters, recognized by cytologic techniques, have also been described (Koss 1992). In this target area, cytology has not only contributed to the identification of precancerous events but also to the recognition that tumors of the urothelium display two pathways of behavior, the papillary and the nonpapillary, with different DNA ploidy values and very different clinical behavior patterns (Koss 1988). The nonpapillary lesions are clearly the more dangerous of the two, and their recognition as of today is based mainly on cytologic techniques (Koss et al. 1985).

Respiratory Tract

Within the respiratory tract, there are numerous documented cases of carcinoma in situ of the bronchus, identified by cytologic techniques in sputum (Fontana et al. 1975). With the changing smoking patterns, the classic, flat epidermoid carcinoma in situ has become less frequent and has been, to a large extent, replaced by adenocarcinomas which are not successfully diagnosed in early stages by cytologic techniques. Further, there is some question as to whether the massive public health services and laboratory measures leading to the diagnosis of bronchogenic carcinoma in situ are justified because of their enormous cost (Fontana 1986). There is also evidence that carcinoma in situ of the larynx can be identified either in a sputum sample or by direct swabbing of the larynx (Koss 1992).

Comment

The recurrent theme in all of these efforts is the unpredictable behavior of precancerous events, as shown best for the uterine cervix, but possibly also occurring in other organs and organ systems. Precancerous events may either revert to normal, remain the same, or progress to more aggressive forms of intraepithelial neoplasia or directly to invasive carcinoma. It is of special interest in this regard that the so-called progression of the precancerous lesions in the uterine cervix is not based on a transformation of one type of epithelial abnormality into another but rather on the occurrence of new neoplastic events in the adjacent epithelium. There are no good explanations for this sequence of events at this time.

It can be stated without any ambiguity whatsoever that were it not for the introduction of cytologic techniques on a large scale, much of our current knowledge of precancerous events in humans would have remained anecdotal and based on incidental biopsies or on postmortem examinations of patients dying of other causes. There are, at this time, many mysteries pertaining to the events leading to precancerous lesions. With regard to lesions of the squamous epithelium, be it in the cervix, larynx, bronchus, or esophagus, the role of HPV needs to be elucidated further. Whether this infection, now known to be very widespread, is in fact the trigger or merely the follower of these neoplastic events remains to be elucidated. A further clue to the onset of the neoplastic events may be in the realm of molecular biology. Studies of oncogene product expression suggest that overexpression of the Ha-*ras* gene occurs in precancerous gastric lesions at a higher level than in invasive gastric cancer (Czerniak et al. 1989). Inactivation of some of the inhibitory genes, such as the Rb gene, may also underlie some of the changes. Single nucleotide mutations have been observed in the Ha-*ras* gene in bladder tumors (Czerniak et al. 1990). At this point in time, no single pathway of these changes has been defined, and the possibility that a synchronous, multigene abnormality must take place for these events to occur has to be entertained.

References

Brawn PN (1982) The origin of invasive carcinoma of the bladder. Cancer 50:515–519

Czerniak B, Herz F, Gorczyca W, Koss LG (1989) Expression of *ras* oncogene protein in early gastric carcinoma and adjacent gastric epithelia. Cancer 64:1467–1473

Czerniak B, Deitch D, Simmons H, Etkind P, Herz F, Koss LG (1990) Ha-*ras* gene codon 12 mutation and DNA ploidy in urinary bladder carcinoma. Br J Cancer 62:762–763

Fontana RS (1986) Screening for lung cancer: recent experience in the United States. In: Hansen HH (ed) Lung cancer: basic and clinical aspects. Nijhoff, Boston, pp 91–111

Fontana RS, Sanderson DR, Woolner LB, Miller WE, Bernatz PE, Payne WS, Taylor WF (1975) The Mayo lung project for early detection and localization of bronchogenic carcinoma: a status report. Chest 67:511–522

Horwitz RI, Feinstein AR, Horowitz SM, Robboy SJ (1981) Necropsy diagnosis of endometrial cancer and detection-bias in case/control studies. Lancet 2:66–68

Kasugai T, Kobayashi S (1974) Evaluation of biopsy and cytology in the diagnosis of gastric cancer. Am J Gastroenterol 62:199–203

Kaye KW, Lange PH (1982) Mode of presentation of invasive bladder cancer: reassessment of the problem. J Urol 128:31–33

Koss LG (1975, 1985) Tumors of the urinary bladder. Armed Forces Institute of Pathology, Washington (Atlas of tumor pathology, fasc 11, 2nd ser and Suppl)

Koss LG (1988) Precursor lesions of invasive bladder cancer. Eur Urol 14 [Suppl 1]:4–6

Koss LG (1989) The Papanicolaou test for cervical cancer detection. A triumph and a tragedy. JAMA 261:737–743

Koss LG (1992) Diagnostic cytology and its histopathologic bases, 4th edn. Lippincott, Philadelphia

Koss LG, Durfee GR (1956) Unusual patterns of squamous epithelium of uterine cervix; cytologic and pathologic study of koilocytotic atypia. Ann NY Acad Sci 63:1245–1261

Koss LG, Schreiber K, Oberlander SG, Moussouris HF, Lesser M (1984) Detection of endometrial carcinoma and hyperplasia in asymptomatic women. Obstet Gynecol 64: 1–11

Koss LG, Deitch D, Ramanathan R, Sherman AB (1985) Diagnostic value of cytology of voided urine. Acta Cytol 29:810–816

Li J-Y, Ershow AG, Chen Z-J, Wacholder S, Li G-Y, Guo W, Li B, Blot WJ (1989) A case-control study of cancer of the esophagus and gastric cardia in Linxian. Int J Cancer 43:755–761

Schade ROK (1956) Cytological diagnosis of gastric carcinoma. Gastroenterologia 85: 190–194

Shu Y-J (1984) Detection of esophageal carcinoma by the balloon technique in the People's Republic of China. In: Koss LG, Coleman DV (eds) Advances in clinical cytology, vol 2. Masson, New York, pp 67–102

Shu Y-J (1985) Cytopathology of esophageal cancer. Masson, New York

Takeda M (1984) Gastric cytology: recent developments. In: Koss LG, Coleman DV (eds) Advances in clinical cytology vol 2. Masson, New York, pp 49–65

Takeda M, Gomi K, Lewis PL, Tamura K, Ohoki S, Fujimoto Y, Kikyo S (1981) Two histologic types of early gastric carcinoma and their cytologic presentation. Acta Cytol 25:229–236

Differentiation Markers in the Early Detection of Cancer

R. MOLL, R. BAUMANN, and C. HAGE

Introduction

Our current understanding of carcinogenesis indicates that it is a multistage process involving various genetic alterations (e.g., mutations of proto-oncogenes, allelic losses). This suggests the possible existence of markers that may be specific indicators of malignant transformation and early neoplastic stages at the tissue level (see the contributions of H. Höfler and D. Lohmann and P. Bannasch et al. in the present volume). Our paper is concerned with the question of whether differentiation markers, i.e., the standard type of histological markers, are useful in the diagnosis of early stages of cancer.

Most histological differentiation or cell-type markers (so-called tumor markers) are characterized by the fact that their expression remains relatively constant and stable throughout tumorigenesis, this being an essential prerequisite for any potential tumor marker. Thus, most of these substances are used to determine the origin and classification of tumors in diagnostically problematic cases, such as very poorly differentiated tumors or metastases whose primary tumor is unknown. Since standard differentiation markers such as prostate-specific antigen (PSA), thyreoglobulin, and most intermediate filament (IF) proteins are expressed in both certain normal tissues and their corresponding tumors, these cannot be used as markers for neoplasia. In addition, although carcinoembryonic antigen (CEA), as an oncofetal antigen, is serologically fairly specific for malignancy (albeit principally for advanced stages), it is unable to make an immunohistochemical distinction between normal colonic mucosa, colonic adenomas, and adenocarcinomas; therefore, it is also unsuitable for use as a marker of malignancy at the histological level.

Intermediate Filaments and Cytokeratins as Differentiation Markers

The IFs, which are almost ubiquitous cytoskeletal filaments with diameters of about 10 nm, comprise a particularly complex yet important system of differentiation markers. On the basis of their protein subunits, it is possible to distinguish several IF classes, whose expression is both differentiation-dependent and, in general, very stable during malignant transformation and tumor progression (for review, see Nagle 1988). Thus, cytokeratin (CK) filaments are markers of epithelial tumors in general, vimentin filaments are typical features of mesenchymal tumors, desmin filaments are markers of muscle tumors, glial filaments occur in certain glial tumors, and neurofilaments are found in neural tumors.

Among these IF classes, the epithelial CKs are especially striking due to their remarkable molecular complexity. Up to now, 20 different CK polypeptides (1–20) have been identified in the various (soft) human epithelia, and the expression of these is also – among the various epithelia – differentiation- and cell-type-dependent (Moll et al. 1982, 1990; Sun et al. 1984; Moll 1987). The larger CKs (1–6 and 9–17) are typically expressed in stratified epithelia, while the smaller ones (7, 8, 18–20) mainly occur in simple epithelia. Within these broad epithelial categories, even finer specificities can be observed. For example, whereas CKs 8 and 18 are expressed in all simple epithelia, the newly identified CK 20 is restricted to intestinal and gastric mucosa (Moll et al. 1990).

In many instances, these cell-type-specific expression patterns of CK polypeptides observed in normal epithelia are maintained in the corresponding carcinomas. For example, both normal intestinal epithelium and colonic adenocarcinomas (including poorly differentiated tumors) are characterized by the co-expression pattern of CKs 8, 18, 19 and 20 (Moll et al. 1990). Far-reaching similarities between the normal epithelium and malignant tumor tissue have also been found for the liver (CKs 8 and 18 being the CKs typical of normal hepatocytes and well-differentiated hepatocellular carcinomas), exocrine pancreas, and urothelium. The last of these exhibits a particularly complex CK pattern that includes the stratified epithelium CK 13, whose expression is retained in the majority of transitional cell carcinomas; however, this CK may be present at reduced levels or even entirely absent in poorly differentiated tumors (Moll et al. 1988).

In the examples listed above, the stable and persistent nature of CK expression makes it feasible to use them as cell-type markers in the differential diagnosis of metastases but precludes their application in the diagnosis of early stages of neoplasia. The partial or complete absence of certain CKs in poorly differentiated tumors (e.g., CK 13 in bladder tumors; a similar decrease in or complete lack of expression also occurs in the case of other differentiation markers) is probably of no practical value with respect to the early detection of cancer.

Modulations in the Expression of Intermediate Filaments (Particularly Cytokeratins) During Tumorigenesis

In some instances, however, differences in the IF and, especially, CK polypeptide patterns have been observed in normal epithelia and their corresponding carcinomas; thus, in the following, we discuss whether such changes might serve as a basis for these proteins being used as markers of the early stages of certain types of carcinoma.

Renal Cell Carcinomas

In the kidney, a remarkable, apparently consistent alteration distinguishes normal proximal tubular cells from their corresponding tumors, i.e., renal cell carcinomas: While the former only express CKs, the latter (except for the rare chromophobe type) are characterized by the constant co-expression of CKs and vimentin (Pitz et al. 1987). Unfortunately, this does not necessarily indicate a transformation-specific onset of vimentin expression, since vimentin is also switched on in proximal tubular cells in the event of chronic damage (Gröne et al. 1987). Therefore, the onset of vimentin expression in proximal tubular cells must be regarded as a nonspecific occurrence influenced by various cellular alterations, so that it cannot usefully be applied as an early tumor marker.

Early Neoplastic Changes in Oropharyngeal and Laryngeal Stratified Squamous Epithelium

Along with the predominant CKs of stratified epithelia, normal oral mucosa usually also expresses CK 19, although this CK is restricted to the basal cell layer. Recently, Lindberg and Rheinwald (1989) have shown that, in dysplastic oral epithelium and in carcinoma in situ, this restriction ceases to apply, with CK 19 also being expressed in suprabasal epithelial layers. These investigators concluded that suprabasal CK 19 staining is correlated with premalignant changes in the oral epithelium. In fact, earlier biochemical studies have revealed an increase in CK 19 levels in squamous cell carcinomas as compared with normal stratified squamous epithelium (Moll et al. 1982). However, it should be borne in mind that nonspecific inflammatory processes also appear to be capable of inducing suprabasal CK 19 expression, as previously shown for the gingival epithelium (Bosch et al. 1989). Therefore, although it may be of some diagnostic value, it is highly questionable whether suprabasal CK 19 expression has an exclusively malignancy- or premalignancy-specific character.

In laryngeal squamous epithelium, dysplasia has been shown to be accompanied by the novel expression of certain simple epithelial CKs (Hellquist and Olofsson 1988). Using three CK antibodies, Vigneswaran et al. (1989) found differences between oral leukoplakias exhibiting and lacking epithelial dysplasia; however, these findings were not constant enough to be considered diagnostically decisive. In other studies, in contrast to the normal tissue, reduced levels or the absence of (suprabasal) CK 13 expression was found in premalignant and malignant lesions of the oropharyngeal stratified squamous epithelium (Moll et al. 1982; Wild and Mischke 1986; Klijanienko et al. 1989), indicating a failure to achieve terminal differentiation. Whether these observations are sufficiently specific to be of diagnostic relevance remains to be demonstrated.

Metaplastic, Preneoplastic, and Neoplastic Lesions of the Uterine Cervical Epithelium

The exact histopathological classification of premalignant and early malignant lesions of the cervix uteri is of great clinical importance. Several studies have focussed on the potential diagnostic value of the immunohistochemical staining for CK 8 produced by applying the monoclonal antibody, CAM 5.2, to trypsinized paraffin sections. Positive staining has been found in invasive cervical (squamous cell) carcinomas and, to a lesser extent, in CIN III lesions, but not in normal ectocervical squamous epithelium and mildly dysplastic lesions (Bobrow et al. 1986; Angus et al. 1988; Raju 1988). However, Wells et al. (1986) obtained generally negative results in most of their cases. In a recent study, the majority of both the in situ and invasive cervical carcinomas investigated was found to be positive for CK 8, and most of these were classified as being of the small cell (reserve cell) type (Dallenbach-Hellweg and Lang 1991). Using frozen sections, Smedts et al. (1990) demonstrated the presence of CK 8 expression in most of their cases of CIN III lesions.

However, it should be borne in mind that, in contrast to the situation in the oropharyngeal epithelium, carcinogenesis in the uterine cervix is topographically generally localized around the squamocolumnar border and is

Table 1. Cytokeratin immunohistochemistry (paraffin material) of normal, metaplastic, and neoplastic cervical epithelium

		CK 8 (CAM 5.2)			CK 19 (K_s 19.1)			CK 13 (K_s 13.1)[a]		
		−	+	++	−	+	++	−	+	++
Normal ectocervical epithelium	($n = 16$)	14	2[b]	0	5	11[b]	0	0	0	16
Ectocervicitis	($n = 3$)	3	0	0	2	1[b]	0	0	0	3
Reserve cell hyperplasia	($n = 7$)	2	2	3	0	0	7	6	1	0
Squamous metaplasia										
Immature[c]	($n = 10$)	3	4	3	0	1	9	2	5	3
Mature	($n = 9$)	4	5[d]	0	1	2[d]	6[d]	0	2	7
CIN II	($n = 4$)	2	2[d,e]	0	2	2[d]	0	0	0	4
CIN III, carcinoma in situ	($n = 6$)	3	2[f]	1	0	1	5	1	0	5
Invasive squamous cell carcinoma	($n = 3$)	0	2[e]	1	1	0	2	1	1	1

−, negative; +, <30% of cells positive; ++, 30%−100% of cells positive.
[a] This antibody binds weakly also to CKs 14 and 16. Basal cells were consistently negative with this antibody.
[b] Only basal cells positive.
[c] Superficial residual columnar cells were positive for CK 8 (strongly) and CK 19 and negative for CK 13.
[d] Predominantly lower cell layers positive.
[e] In one case, very few cells were positive.
[f] Very few cells were positive.

therefore intimately linked with processes of squamous metaplasia. In cases of cervical squamous metaplasia, the initial alteration is the appearance of sub-columnar reserve cells. These exhibit both primitive squamous properties, as reflected by their expression of certain stratified epithelial CKs (5, 17), as well as certain simple epithelial features, as evidenced by the expression of CKs 8 and 19; this combination clearly demonstrates their bipotent character (Weikel et al. 1987). CKs 5 and 17 are further prominent components of the cervical squamous metaplastic epithelium (Moll et al. 1983). Since the majority of cervical carcinomas develop via endocervical reserve cell hyperplasia and squamous metaplasia rather than arising from the exocervical squamous epi-thelium, the significance of the expression of CK 8 in CIN III and cervical carcinomas and its alleged transformation specificity needs to be reconsidered.

Therefore, we investigated immunohistochemically a limited series of paraffin-embedded cervical specimens, both normal and with various lesions, with particular emphasis on squamous metaplasia. Paraffin-embedded tissue blocks from 32 patients (24–75 years old, mean age 45.5 years) were used. After trypsination, sections were stained, using the avidin-biotin complex (ABC) peroxidase method, with antibodies CAM 5.2 against CK 8 (Becton-Dickinson, Neckargemünd, FRG), $K_S19.1$ against CK 19 (Progen, Heidelberg, FRG; see Moll et al. 1988), and $K_S13.1$ that reacts mainly with CK 13 (Progen; Moll et al. 1988). The results are summarized in Table 1.

While normal ectocervical epithelium was, in most cases, completely negative for CK 8, this CK was found to be focally distributed in some CIN II and CIN III lesions (Fig. 1a). Invasive squamous cell carcinomas were generally positive for CK 8 but exhibited wide variations with respect to the proportion of positive tumor cells (Fig. 1b). These results are essentially in agreement with those of previous studies (Bobrow et al. 1986; Angus et al. 1988). However, we also found significant positive CK 8 staining in reserve cells (albeit irregularly) and reserve cell hyperplasia (Table 1). Moreover, CK 8 was also detected in immature squamous metaplasia (most cases; Fig. 1c) and even, although less frequently and extensively, in mature squamous metaplasia. While the earlier investigations of paraffin-embedded material (for references, see above) failed to detect CK 8 in squamous metaplasia, the present results are well in line with those obtained by Smedts et al. (1990) using frozen material. The positive reaction for CK 19 was generally more extensive than that for CK 8 (Table 1; cf. Gigi-Leitner et al. 1986; Raju 1990). The stratified epithelial CK 13 was often detected even in immature squamous metaplasia (Fig. 1d) but was more extensively expressed in more mature forms of squamous epithelia as well as in CIN lesions (Table 1).

It is generally accepted that the majority of cervical neoplasias originate from the proliferation of reserve cells (cf. Dallenbach-Hellweg and Lang 1991). Thus, in CK-8-positive CIN III cases, the expression of CK 8 may simply have been retained from the precursor lesions, reserve cell hyperplasia or squamous metaplasia; in other cases, though, the expression of CK 8 may in fact be a new development occurring during malignant transformation and tumor pro-gression. At any rate, owing to the frequent presence of CK 8 positivity

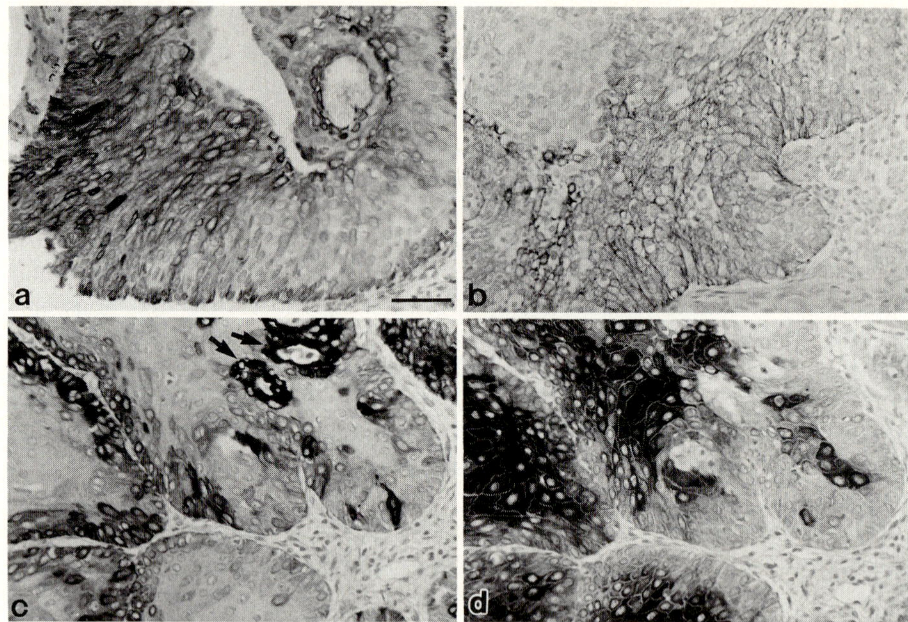

Fig. 1a–d. Immunohistochemical detection of cytokeratins in metaplastic, preneoplastic, and neoplastic lesions of the uterine cervix (trypsinized paraffin sections; ABC-peroxidase reaction). **a** A case of CIN III (severe dysplasia) heterogeneously positive for CK 8 (antibody CAM 5.2). **b** Invasive squamous cell carcinoma of cervix showing delicate staining of many tumor cells for CK 8 (CAM 5.2). **c, d** Immature squamous metaplasia involving near-surface cervical glands, exhibiting significant staining of lower cell layers for CK 8 (**c**, CAM 5.2) and suprabasal staining for CK 13 (**d**, K_S13.1), the latter being molecular evidence of the process of squamous maturation. Note the strongly positive CK 8 reaction of residual cervical columnar cells (**c**, *arrows*). *Bar* in **a**, 50 μm

in squamous metaplastic epithelium, this CK cannot be regarded as a good indicator of malignant transformation or invasive potential. In summary, when making a histodiagnosis of early neoplastic lesions of the cervix, CK 8 staining may provide some accessory information, but the diagnosis of malignancy per se should not be primarily based on this reaction. Furthermore, in the potentially difficult differential diagnosis of metaplastic lesions and CIN, CK staining patterns would not appear to be a useful diagnostic aid.

Squamous Metaplasia of the Bronchial Epithelium

Another important tumor whose development involves squamous metaplasia is squamous cell carcinoma of the bronchus. Both morphologically and in terms of CK patterns, the situation at this site is quite well comparable, albeit not identical, to that in the endocervix, except that, in the bronchus, basal cells are constantly present. In the bronchus, stratified epithelial CKs are expressed both in normal basal cells and in squamous metaplasia. Preliminary data suggest that the additional expression of simple-epithelial CKs in squamous metaplastic lesions may be due to dysplasia and/or immaturity (Rustad et al., unpublished data).

Cytokeratins in the Diagnosis of Early Stages of Breast Cancer

For certain histodiagnostic problems arising in the case of breast carcinoma, the application of CKs as differentiation markers may usefully complement other procedures in the following instances:

1. In intraductal carcinoma, the intact myoepithelial layer may be immuno-histochemically demonstrated using CKs 14 or 17 as myoepithelial markers (e.g., Jarasch et al. 1988).
2. Similarly, the disruption or absence of the myoepithelial layer may be demonstrated in ductal carcinomas at an early stage of invasion.
3. CKs may be helpful in the differential diagnosis of sclerosing adenosis (CK-14/17-positive proliferating myoepithelial cells) as opposed to invasive ductal carcinoma (CK-7/8/18/19-positive; Jarasch et al. 1988).
4. In the early stages of invasive lobular carcinomas, the invasive tumor cells, which are often single and scattered so that they are morphologically inconspicuous can easily be identified by their staining for CK 8/18/19.
5. Simple epithelial CKs are good markers for intraepidermal tumor cells in Paget's disease of the nipple, a condition which may present as an early symptom of an underlying breast carcinoma.

Conclusions

In conclusion, differentiation markers are not of primary diagnostic importance in the early detection of cancer. In the case of IFs, there are some instances in which changes in their expression, reflecting changes in cellular differentiation, may proceed in tandem with malignant changes. However, since these altera-tions in IF expression are not *directly* correlated with the molecular biological processes of carcinogenesis, caution is required in the diagnostic application of IF markers for such purposes, and such results should always be interpreted in the context of findings obtained concerning other parameters.

Summary

Most established histological tumor markers are differentiation markers whose main application is to assist in the classification of malignant tumors with respect to type and origin. However, their stable and constant expression during malignant transformation precludes their employment for the histo-logical detection of early neoplastic changes. This is also generally true for the intermediate filaments (IFs), including the epithelial cytokeratins (CKs), all of which are important differentiation markers. However, there are some cases of IF and CK expression being different in normal epithelia and their corresponding carcinomas. For example, (nonchromophobe) renal cell carcinomas, unlike proximal tubular cells, express not only CKs but also vimentin, although this additional IF expression is clearly not transformation-specific. Changes in the distribution of CK 19 in the event of dysplasia have been described for oral squamous epithelium, but inflammation would also appear to be able to induce similar alterations. With regard to normal and neoplastic squamous epithelium of the uterine cervix, several investigators have suggested that the expression of CK 8 (as detected by antibody CAM 5.2) is a marker for malignant transformation or invasiveness. We immunohistochemically stained various cervical specimens using antibodies against CKs 8 (CAM 5.2), 19, and 13. CK 8 was found to be focally distributed in some CIN II and CIN III lesions as well as in invasive cervical carcinomas. Most interestingly, this CK was also often found in reserve cell hyperplasia and squamous metaplasia, so that it is not truly specific for malignancy. In the mammary gland, CKs may be of assistance in the histological identification of myoepithelial cells and the recognition of (early) carcinoma invasiveness. In conclusion, since the changes in IF expression outlined here are not directly correlated with processes of carcinogenesis, caution is required in the application of IF markers for the diagnosis of early stages of cancer, and such results should always be interpreted in the context of findings obtained concerning other parameters.

References

Angus B, Kiberu B, Purvis J, Wilkinson K, Horne CHW (1988) Cytokeratins in cervical dysplasia and neoplasia: a comparative study of immunohistochemical staining using monoclonal antibodies NCL-5D5, CAM 5.2, and PKK1. J Pathol 155:71–75

Bobrow LG, Makin CA, Law S, Bodmer WF (1986) Expression of low molecular weight cytokeratin proteins in cervical neoplasia. J Pathol 148:135–140

Bosch FX, Ouhayoun J-P, Bader BL, Collin C, Grund C, Lee I, Franke WW (1989) Extensive changes in cytokeratin expression patterns in pathologically affected human gingiva. Virchows Arch [B] 58:59–77

Dallenbach-Hellweg G, Lang G (1991) Immunohistochemical studies on uterine tumors. I. Invasive squamous cell carcinomas of the cervix and their precursors. Pathol Res Pract 187:36–43

Gigi-Leitner O, Geiger B, Levy R, Czernobilsky B (1986) Cytokeratin expression in squamous metaplasia of the human uterine cervix. Differentiation 31:191–205

Gröne HJ, Weber K, Gröne E, Helmchen U, Osborn M (1987) Coexpression of keratin and vimentin in damaged and regenerating tubular epithelia of the kidney. Am J Pathol 129:1–8

Hellquist HB, Olofsson J (1988) Expression of low molecular weight cytokeratin proteins in laryngeal dysplasia. APMIS 96:971–978

Jarasch E-D, Nagle RB, Kaufmann M, Maurer C, Böcker WJ (1988) Differential diagnosis of benign epithelial proliferations and carcinomas of the breast using antibodies to cytokeratins. Hum Pathol 19:276–289

Klijanienko J, Micheau C, Carlu C, Caillaud JM (1989) Significance of keratin 13 and 6 expression in normal, dysplastic and malignant squamous epithelium of pyriform fossa. Virchows Arch [A] 416:121–124

Lindberg K, Rheinwald JG (1989) Suprabasal 40 kd keratin (K 19) expression as an immunohistologic marker of premalignancy in oral epithelium. Am J Pathol 134:89–98

Moll R (1987) Epithelial tumor markers: cytokeratins and tissue polypeptide antigen (TPA). Curr Top Pathol 77:71–101

Moll R, Franke WW, Schiller DL, Geiger B, Krepler R (1982) The catalog of human cytokeratins: patterns of expression in normal epithelia, tumors and cultured cells. Cell 31:11–24

Moll R, Levy R, Czernobilsky B, Hohlweg-Majert P, Dallenbach-Hellweg G, Franke WW (1983) Cytokeratins of normal epithelia and some neoplasms of the female genital tract. Lab Invest 49:599–610

Moll R, Achtstätter T, Becht E, Balcarova-Ständer J, Ittensohn M, Franke WW (1988) Cytokeratins in normal and malignant transitional epithelium: maintenance of expression of urothelial differentiation features in transitional cell carcinomas and bladder carcinoma cell culture lines. Am J Pathol 132:123–144

Moll R, Schiller DL, Franke WW (1990) Identification of protein IT of the intestinal cytoskeleton as a novel type I cytokeratin with unusual properties and expression patterns. J Cell Biol 111:567–580

Nagle RB (1988) Intermediate filaments: a review of the basic biology. Am J Surg Pathol 12 [Suppl 1]:4–16

Pitz S, Moll R, Störkel S, Thoenes W (1987) Expression of intermediate filament proteins in subtypes of renal cell carcinomas and in renal oncocytomas. Lab Invest 56:642–653

Raju GC (1988) Expression of the cytokeratin marker CAM 5.2 in cervical neoplasia. Histopathology 12:437–443

Raju GC (1990) The expression of cytokeratin 19 in cervical neoplasia. Histopathology 16:297–300

Smedts F, Ramaekers F, Robben H, Pruszczynski M, van Muijen G, Lane B, Leigh I, Vooijs P (1990) Changing patterns of keratin expression during progression of cervical intraepithelial neoplasia. Am J Pathol 136:657–668

Sun T-T, Eichner R, Schermer A, Cooper D, Nelson WG, Weiss RA (1984) Classification, expression and possible mechanisms of evolution of mammalian epithelial keratins: an unifying model. In: Levine A, Topp W, Vande Woude G, Watson JD (eds) The cancer cell, vol 1. The transformed phenotype. Cold Spring Harbor Laboratory, Cold Spring Harbor, pp 169–176

Vigneswaran N, Peters K-P, Hornstein OP, Haneke E (1989) Comparison of cytokeratin, filaggrin and involucrin profiles in oral leukoplakias and squamous carcinomas. J Oral Pathol Med 18:377–390

Weikel W, Wagner R, Moll R (1987) Characterization of subcolumnar reserve cells and other epithelia of human uterine cervix: demonstration of diverse cytokeratin polypeptides in reserve cells. Virchows Arch [B] 54:98–110

Wells M, Brown LJR, Jackson P (1986) Low molecular weight cytokeratin proteins in cervical neoplasia. J Pathol 150:69–71

Wild GA, Mischke D (1986) Variation and frequency of cytokeratin polypeptide patterns in human squamous non-keratinizing epithelium. Exp Cell Res 162:114–126

Molecular Genetic Approaches to Early Cancer Detection

H. Höfler and D. Lohmann

Introduction

Today, most cancer diagnoses are made by pathologists on the basis of classic histological features of histomorphological alterations of tissue or single cells. Recent insights into the molecular biology of cancer, particularly the discovery of oncogenes and – probably more importantly – tumor suppressor genes, imply new concepts for the detection of premalignant changes and early cancer. For most tumors, a multistage model of tumor development is proposed, in which one or several steps of genetic alterations most likely precede the first morphological changes of the premalignant or early tumor cell, respectively. The ultimate challenge for the pathologist remains the detection of changes associated with high risk of malignant cell transformation before the occurrence of phenotypic changes. The methods necessary accomplish this goal should be applicable in "routine diagnosis."

Prerequisites to achieve these goals include an advanced knowledge of the basic mechanisms of carcinogenesis and tumor progression and the development of methods to detect these alterations in tissue sections and to compare "genetic" alterations with the classic morphological criteria of neoplastic transformation and clinical parameters of prognosis. Generally, this "genetic" approach of (pre)cancer characterization had at least partially been made possible by the development of techniques which allow the detection of minimal alterations at the DNA (and RNA) level in tissue sections and single cell preparations.

Oncogenes in Early Cancer Diagnosis

(Proto)oncogenes (c-*onc*) are involved in the control of mitosis and differentiation and play an important role in embryonic development and tissue repair. Most authors believe that the activation of c-*onc* represents a crucial event in cell transformation and for the expression of the malignant phenotype (Egan et al. 1987). Activation of c-*onc* is in most cases caused by mutational events, including transduction, insertional mutagenesis, gene amplification, or point mutations (for review, see Marks 1987; Höfler 1991). Such activated oncogenes have gained tumorigenic potential and are thought to be actively involved in tumor initiation and maintenance.

Diagnosis-related alterations of c-*onc* in human tumors can be devided into two subgroups: (1) tumor type-specific alterations which may contribute to tumor classification and (2) non-tumor type-specific alterations. Among the former, rearrangement of oncogenes in non-Hodgkin's lymphomas, such as the translocation t(8;14) of the c-*myc* gene in Burkitt's lymphomas and the translocation of bcl-1 t(11;14) and bcl-2 t(14;18) are of well-known diagnostic significance (Taub et al. 1982). Furthermore, the specific c-*abl* translocation in chronic myeloid leukemias is already well established, particularly for the detection of early stages of disease or minimal residual disease. Finally, certain alterations of the *ret*/PTC genes are only found in thyroid papillary carcinomas.

To the group of non-tumor type-specific alterations of c-*onc* belong the point mutations of the *ras* genes. Forrester et al. (1987) and Bos et al. (1987) reported point mutations of the 12th codon of the Ki-*ras* gene in 39% of primary colorectal carcinomas, but without any correlation to sex, age, tumor localization, histological grade, and stage.

Similarly, Ki-*ras* mutations are reported in an even higher percentage (up to 96%!) in exocrine pancreatic carcinomas. The relatively high incidence of point mutations in colorectal and pancreatic carcinomas, however, could not be confirmed by other groups more recently. Nevertheless, the detection of point mutations involving the hot spots of the *ras* genes (codons 12, 13, 61) in a given tissue or body fluid sample (blood, urine, etc.) is highly suspicious of the existence of malignancy or a premalignant stage.

The detection of altered oncogene expression in a heterogeneous tissue, blood, or other body fluid is feasible by several methods, particularly Southern blot analysis, in situ hybridization, and polymerase chain reaction (PCR) of microdissected – even formalin-fixed – tissue in combination with other techniques (see below and Höfler 1991 for review).

Tumor Suppressor Genes in Early Cancer Diagnosis

As already mentioned above, most neoplasias are thought to result of multiple events involving the activation of multiple genes (Knudson 1985; Friend et al. 1988). Some of these genes may interact with the activity of growth-regulating (onco)genes, perhaps via *trans*-acting mechanisms, by restraining cell growth and by preventing clonal cell proliferation. These genes have been called "anti-oncogenes" because they were originally considered to interact with oncogenes. However, tumor-suppressor gene is a more appropriate term, since it includes the possibility of their interaction with genes other than oncogenes. The best characterized representative of these tumor-suppressing genes is the retinoblastoma (RB-1) gene, which not only seems to be involved in the prevention of retinoblastoma but was also found to play a role in the development of osteosarcomas, soft-tissue sarcomas, melanomas, breast carcinomas, bladder carcinomas, etc. RB-1 gene inactivation is thought to represent an early step in tumorigenesis, whereas the loss of p53 gene function seems to occur in later stages of carcinogenesis and tumor progression. Other

Table 1. Specific loss of suppressor gene loci in tumors

Gene	Locus	Tumor
RB1	13q14	Retinoblastoma, osteosarcoma, etc.
p53	17q12	Breast, colon, and lung carcinoma, osteosarcoma, etc.
WT1	11p13	Wilms' tumor (also 11p15.5)
DCC	18Q21	Colon carcinoma
NM23	17q11	Breast carcinoma
NF1	17q11.2	Neurofibromatosis type 1
NF2	22	Neurofibromatosis type 2
FAP	5q21	Familial adenomatous polyposis colon carcinoma
MEN	10,11	Tumors of endocrine tissues

suppressor loci are implicated in liver, lung, kidney, and breast carcinoma and neuroblastoma (compare Table 1).

The characterization of alterations of tumor suppressor genes may contribute to tumor diagnosis, classification, and most importantly to evaluating the risk of tumor susceptibility (genetic counselling!).

Methods for Detection of Tumor Suppressor Genes

All known tumor suppressor genes reside on autosomal chromosomes and therefore exist in two homologous copies. As a consequence, the functional loss of a tumor suppressor requires two mutations (hits) to inactivate both alleles. Functional inactivation can be caused by a variety of genetic alterations. Different methods of detection have to be employed to cover the whole spectrum of mutations known to occur at tumor suppressor loci. More problems with regard to sensitivity exist for the detection of suppressor gene alterations because of their recessive mode of action. Several approaches for the detection of genetic alterations and altered gene expression will be discussed here.

The most evident example of an inactivating mutation is the *loss of one chromosome or chromosome arm* that harbours the suppressor locus. Small interstitial deletions also lead to the complete loss of the loci involved. These gross alterations can be identified by karyotype analysis of metaphase spreads as long as chromosome staining techniques show the loss of a chromosome band. If appropriate hybridization probes for the chromosomal region of interest are available, the resolution of morphological analysis can be extended by the use of chromosomal in situ hybridization. With the help of this technique loss of genetic material can be detected far beyond the scope of banding techniques. Furthermore, it can be applied to the study of interphase nuclei and thereby allows the investigation of material that precludes tissue culture. With the rapidly growing repertoire of probes, chromosomal in situ hybridization will play an increasingly important role not only for the detection of gene loss at tumor suppressor loci, but also for the visualization of gene translocations and amplifications.

Loss of genetic material can also be revealed by the use of *polymorphic markers*. A great number of genetic loci are known to harbor different alleles. The reduction of constitutional heterozygosity for a given locus to hemi- or homozygosity in tumor cells indicates the loss of this locus. The majority of allelic polymorphisms have been described for variant restriction enzyme digestion patterns. The classic approach for the detection of these restriction fragment length polymorphisms (RFLPs) is Southern hybridization. Recently, the possibility of in vitro enzymatic amplification of distinct sequences by the PCR has extended the spectrum of investigation. Amplification of regions that span polymorphic restriction sites followed by digestion of the PCR products and electrophoretic analysis obviates the need for laborious hybridization techniques. Moreover, polymorphisms that are due to a variable number of repeated sequence units may easily be identified by electrophoretic analysis alone.

All methods described so far are directed to the detection of genetic alterations that involve the physical loss of an allele. In fact, in most cases the loss of one allele can be revealed by one of these techniques. However, the remaining allele is often inactivated due to comparatively small mutations. In order to identify these alterations exact knowledge of the genomic organization and sequence of the suppressor gene under investigation is necessary. The RB-1 gene and the p53 gene both fulfil these prerequisites, and a variety of inactivating mutations has been detected in diverse human malignancies.

These mutations comprise deletions or insertions that lead to gross structural rearrangements of the gene. The appropriate method to detect alterations of this kind is Southern analysis. For a detailed evaluation multiple hybridization probes and restriction enzyme digestions are often indispensable. Even then only 15%–30% of all RB-1 gene mutations in retinoblastoma are detectable (Gallie et al. 1990; Kloss et al. 1991). Mutations of the p53 gene even more seldom lead to an altered hybridization pattern in most tumor types.

Gene function may also be impaired by small deletions and insertions or even point mutations. Whereas known point mutations (e.g., for the *ras* genes) can be detected by the use of allele-specific oligonucleotides, mismatch PCR, or RFLPs, for the detection of unknown mutations more laborious techniques including RNAse cleavage or denaturing gradient gel analysis have to be applied. The ultimate way to detect mutations of this kind is DNA sequencing. To this end a part of the sequence to be investigated is amplified by PCR first. After purification, the synthesized DNA serves as a template for sequencing. Numerous amplification and sequencing rounds have to be performed to cover the entire sequence that may harbor the inactivating mutation. The bulk of alterations that have been found in the p53 gene are missense mutations (Levine et al. 1991). These are localized in four regions of the gene (hot spots) corresponding to evolutionary conserved domains in the protein. This fact notably reduces the expenditure of investigation. In contrast to p53 all the mutations found in the RB-1 gene so far show no preferential localization that would indicate a mutation hot spot. Therefore, for RB-1 it is necessary to screen all of the 27 exons and adjacent intronic sequences. Since this is quite laborious, efforts have been made to develop screening methods for the detection of small genetic alterations. Among other methods high-resolution electrophoresis of amplified DNA on polyacrylamide gels enables the detection of small length alterations within the region surveyed by the amplification primers. When combining this type of analysis with coamplification of multiple regions of the gene in one single reaction (multiplex-PCR), a rapid screening for small length alterations even in large genes such as RB-1 becomes feasible (Lohmann et al. 1992).

Beside the often very small amount of tumor tissue and the need for specific tissue processing (e.g., shock freezing), the heterogeneity of tumor tissue is a limiting factor for the sensitivity of all methods. Tumor tissue always contains a varying proportion of non-tumorous cells. Tumor stroma with often high numbers of lymphoid cells contributes genetic material that is not expected to share the tumor-specific mutations. When investigating the activation of dominant oncogenes, gene amplification or overexpression often overrides the dilutional effect of contaminant tissues. In contrast, loss-of-function type alterations as displayed by recessive oncogenes (tumor suppressor genes) are hardly detected against a high background of unaffected genome. Methods to diminish the problem of tissue heterogeneity include microdissection of tissue sections and highly laborious cloning techniques followed by PCR analysis and direct sequencing.

Summary

1. Currently, individual steps involved in malignant transformation can be detected in routinely processed tissue samples by molecular methods.
2. Risk of tumor susceptibility can be evaluated for certain tumors by the detection of constitutional alterations of tumor suppressor genes (genetic counselling!).
3. Detection of alterations of oncogenes may contribute to early tumor diagnosis, detection of minimal residual disease, and tumor classfication.

The "modern" pathologist will have to know the most recent concepts of tumorigenesis and should understand the techniques to detect "premicroscopic," genetic changes in the tissue but must not forget the classic histomorphological features of early cancer. It can be anticipated that pathologists will be increasingly involved in genetic counselling.

References

Bos JL, Fearon ER, Hamilton StR, Verlaan-de Vries M, van Boom JH, van der Erb AJ, Vogelstein B (1987) Prevalence of *ras* gene mutations in human colorectal cancers. Nature 327:293–297
Egan SE, Wright JA, Jarolim L, Anagihara K, Bassin RH, Greenberg AH (1987) Transformation by oncogenes encoding protein kinases induces the metastatic phenotype. Science 238:202–205

Forrester K, Almoguera C, Han K, Grizzle WE, Perucho M (1987) Detection of high incidence of K-*ras* oncogenes during human colon tumorigenesis. Nature 327:298–303

Friend SH, Dryja TP, Weinberg RA (1988) Oncogenes and tumor-suppressing genes. N Engl J Med 318(10):618–622

Gallie BL, Squire JA, Goddard A, Dunn JM, Canton M, Hinton D, Zhu XP et al. (1990) Mechanism of oncogenesis in retinoblastoma. Lab Invest 62:394–408

Höfler H (1991) Oncogene and receptor expression. Curr Top Pathol 83:435–453

Kloss K, Währisch P, Greger V, Messmer E, Fritze H, Höpping W, Passarge E et al. (1991) Characterization of deletions at the retinoblastoma locus in patients with bilateral retinoblastoma. Am J Med Genet 39:196–200

Knudson AG (1985) Hereditary cancer, oncogenes, and antioncogenes. Canc Res 45:1437–1443

Levine AJ, Momand J, Finlay CA (1991) The p53 tumor suppressor gene. Nature 351:453–456

Lohmann D, Horsthemke B, Gillesen-Kaesbach G, Stefani FH, Höfler H (1992) Detection of small RB-1 gene deletions by multiplex PCR and high-resolution gel electrophoresis. Human Genetics (in press)

Marks F (1987) What's new in oncogenes and growth factors? Pathol Res Pract 182:831–848

Taub R, Kirsh I, Morton C (1982) Translocation of the c-*myc* gene into the immunoglobulin heavy chain locus in human Burkitt's lymphoma and murine plasmacytoma cells. Proc Natl Acad Sci USA 79:7837–7841

Preneoplastic Lesions as Early Indicators of Neoplastic Development

P. BANNASCH, U.R. JAHN, and H. ZERBAN

Introduction

In human pathology, the terms "preneoplasia" and "precancer" have traditionally been used as synonyms indicating a pathological condition carrying increased risk for the development of malignant neoplasia (cancer). In addition to definite proliferative lesions such as nodular hyperplasia, papilloma, or carcinoma in situ, dysplastic lesions have been considered potential prestages of cancer and have, hence, been widely involved in the early diagnosis of neoplasia (Carter 1984, and this volume; Koss 1979, and this volume). However, investigations in several animal models and some studies in man revealed that characteristic changes in the biochemical and morphological phenotype of focal cell populations, which initially deviate only slightly from the normal differentiated state, precede the appearance of both benign and malignant neoplasms in a number of tissues by weeks and months or even years (Bannasch 1986; Sirica 1989). This holds especially true for epithelial tissues endowed with a low cell turnover under normal conditions, such as the hepatic parenchyma (Bannasch et al. 1989a; Symposium 1989), exocrine pancreatic parenchyma (Longnecker and Millar 1990; Woutersen et al. 1991), and renal tubular system (Bannasch and Zerban 1990; Dietrich and Swenberg 1991), but it also relates to some epithelial tissues with a high cell turnover like the colonic mucosa (Mayer et al. 1987; Barrow et al. 1990) and bronchial mucosa (Gusterson 1984) (Table 1). Based on these findings, preneoplasia may be defined as phenotypically altered cell populations which have no obvious neoplastic nature but indicate an increased risk for the development of benign or malignant neoplasia in the respective tissue (Bannasch 1986).

Table 1. Preneoplasia in various epithelial tissues

Hepatic parenchyma	Foci of altered hepatocytes
Bile ductular epithelia	Cholangiofibrosis
Exocrine pancreatic parenchyma	Foci of altered acinar cells
Pancreatic duct system	Ductal proliferations
Renal tubular system	Foci of altered renal cells
Colonic mucosa	Foci of altered epithelia
Bronchial mucosa	Goblet cell hyperplasia, squamous cell metaplasia

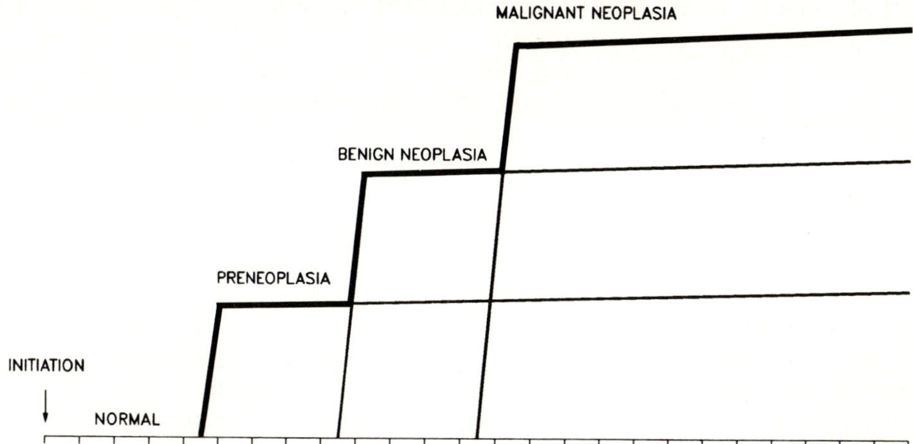

Fig. 1. Schematic presentation of the relationship between preneoplasia, benign neoplasia, and malignant neoplasia

Stages of Neoplastic Development

Observations from different models of neoplastic development indicate that preneoplasia and benign neoplasia represent, as a rule, subsequent stages in a biological continuum leading from the normal state to malignant neoplasia (Fig. 1). However, some findings suggest that carcinomas may also arise directly from preneoplastic lesions without passing a benign intermediate stage. Another exception to the rule is that specific types of epithelial neoplasms such as renal oncocytoma are usually benign end-stages which do not progress to malignant neoplasia. There is no doubt that focal preneoplastic lesions frequently persist over long lag periods without giving rise to overt neoplasia, but this should not detract from their significance as early indicators of a neoplastic response. This property is being increasingly utilized for the identification of carcinogenic agents in laboratory animals (Bannasch 1986; Symposium 1989; Dietrich and Swenberg 1991; Woutersen et al. 1991), but it should also be of advantage for the early detection and secondary prevention of neoplasia in man.

Phenotypic Patterns of Preneoplasia

The phenotypic patterns of preneoplasia appear to be as varied as those of neoplasia, each histologically and cytologically defined tumor type presenting its own histo- and cytogenesis (Bannasch 1984). In contrast to dysplastic and neoplastic cell populations which are conventionally mainly defined by nuclear alterations, the phenotypic cellular changes associated with preneoplasia pertain predominantly to the cytoplasm and may be classified into four main categories (Bannasch 1988):

1. Alterations in the expression of enzymes, particularly enzymes of the carbohydrate and drug metabolism
2. Changes in the content of metabolites, especially an excessive storage of macromolecules such as glycogen, glycosaminoglycans, ribonucleoproteins, or lipids
3. Alterations in the organization of organelles, such as mitochondria, peroxisomes, or endoplasmic reticulum
4. Increased cell proliferation and nuclear alterations

At first glance, these alterations may appear extremely heterogeneous. In different tissues or even in subpopulations of the same tissue, the phenotype of the preneoplastic lesions may indeed vary considerably, but it may also show striking similarities. Many of the cytoplasmic alterations observed in preneoplastic lesions suggest early aberrations in energy metabolism during neoplastic development.

In order to exemplify this concept, we shall present some types of early focal lesions induced in the liver and kidney of rats by various carcinogenic agents. Among the first phenotypic cellular changes appearing during hepato-carcinogenesis in different species are alterations in the expression of enzymes of carbohydrate metabolism, such as a decrease in the activities of glucose-6-phosphatase and glycogen phosphorylase and an increase in the activity of glucose-6-phosphate dehydrogenase, the key enzyme of the pentose phosphate pathway (Hacker et al. 1982). These enzyme histochemical findings have been confirmed and extended by the results of immunohistochemical (Moore et al. 1986; Seelmann-Eggebert et al. 1987), microbiochemical (Klimek et al. 1984; Fischer et al. 1987), and molecular genetic approaches which have been discussed in detail elsewhere (Bannasch et al. 1991). In this context, it is interesting to note that the early reduction in the activity of glycogen phosphorylase is not due to a loss of the enzyme protein but to a posttranscriptional modification of its expression (Seelmann-Eggebert et al. 1987), whereas the increased activity of glucose-6-phosphate dehydrogenase apparently results from a marked overexpression of the coding gene as demonstrated by in situ hybridization to antisense messenger RNA (Bannasch et al. 1992).

Serial cryostat and paraffin sections revealed that the enzymatic alterations appearing early during hepatocarcinogenesis are regularly associated with an excessive storage of glycogen (glycogenosis). The accumulation of glycogen leads to cellular enlargement and a clearing of the cytoplasm as seen in conventional H&E-stained tissue sections, since the glycogen is eluted during tissue preparation (Bannasch 1968). Foci consisting of clear cells can readily be identified and are now widely used as early indicators of neoplastic development possibly induced in laboratory animals by test compounds (Bannasch 1986; Goldsworthy et al. 1986; Symposium 1989; Bannasch and Zerban 1992).

An early lesion resembling focal hepatic glycogenosis is the tubular glycogenosis induced in rat kidney by chemical carcinogens (Bannasch et al. 1978a; Nogueira et al. 1989; Dietrich and Swenberg 1991). This lesion is a precursor of the rat renal clear cell tumor, which largely corresponds to the predominant type of renal cell carcinoma in man. The abnormality of an excessive storage of glycogen in preneoplastic and neoplastic lesions is much more evident in the kidney than in the liver since the normal renal parenchyma is nearly free of glycogen. In addition to the tubular glycogenosis, there are at least two other types of preneoplastic tubular lesions in rat kidney, which, however, do not exhibit a pronounced storage of glycogen (Bannasch and Zerban 1990; Dietrich and Swenberg 1991). One type is composed of oncocytes which are overcrowded with a dense population of atypical mitochondria as seen under the electron microscope (Bannasch et al. 1978b; Krech et al. 1981; Nogueira and Bannasch 1988). In the past few years, similar tubular lesions have been observed in the human kidney (Zerban et al. 1987; Ortmann et al. 1988; Störkel et al. 1988). In both man and laboratory animals, the oncocytic tubules arise from the collecting duct system and may slowly progress to renal oncocytomas, which in contrast to renal clear cell tumors have a favorable prognosis. This example shows that critical prognostic implications may already be evident from phenotypic cellular changes at very early stages of neoplastic development.

It is essential to realize, however, that the cellular phenotype of putative preneoplastic lesions is by no means stable under all conditions. This has mainly been demonstrated for hepatocarcinogenesis induced in rodents by various chemicals (Bannasch 1986; Moore and Kitagawa 1986; Goldsworthy et al. 1986; Farber and Sarma 1987).

Reversion- and Progression-Linked Phenotypic Instability in Hepatic Preneoplasia

Two basically different types of phenotypic instability have been distinguished in foci of altered hepatocytes, namely a reversion-linked and a progression-linked form (Bannasch et al. 1985b). The reversion-linked phenotypic instability has particularly been found under extreme experimental conditions such as the repeated administration of high sublethal doses of hepatocarcinogens or the widely applied Solt/Farber procedure. These schedules do not only result in a very large number of phenotypically altered hepatic foci but also in pronounced, unspecific toxic liver lesions including necrotic cellular changes (Moore and Kitagawa 1986; Farber and Sarma 1987). However, when the toxic compounds are withdrawn, a high percentage of the phenotypically altered foci disappear, although complete reversibility of all foci has never been observed. In addition, some observations suggested that phenotypically reverted foci may reappear later on (Watanabe and Williams 1978; Tatematsu et al. 1983). The reason for the reversion-linked phenotypic instability is poorly understood, but cessation of regenerative stimuli elicited by the toxic necrosis may play an important role (Bannasch and Zerban 1992).

In order to avoid any interference with unspecific toxic effects and reversion-linked phenotypic instability of putative preneoplastic hepatic foci, we studied the behavior of the persisting lesions in stop experiments from the time of withdrawal of the carcinogen up to the appearance of hepatocellular adenomas and carcinomas in several series using *N*-nitrosomorpholine (NNM) in different dosing schedules. Cytomorphological, cytochemical, microbiochemical, and stereological approaches invariably revealed that there is a progression-linked phenotypic instability of hepatic preneoplasia (Bannasch 1968; for recent reviews, see Bannasch et al. 1989a; Bannasch 1990). The predominant sequence of cellular changes leads from the preneoplastic clear (and acidophilic) glycogenotic cells via mixed cell populations to neoplastic cells poor in glycogen but rich in ribosomes, which prevail in hepatocellular carcinomas. These cytomorphological changes are associated with a metabolic shift from the glycogenotic state to alternative metabolic pathways, such as glycolysis and the pentose phosphate pathway (Bannasch et al. 1984, 1991; Mayer et al. 1989). At the same time, there is an ever increasing proliferative activity as demonstrated by the incorportion of [^{3}H]-thymidine which is the greater the more glycogen-poor, basophilic cells appear in mixed cell foci, hepatocellular adenomas, and carcinomas (Zerban et al. 1989). Baba et al. (1989) have shown that the increase in glucose-6-phosphate dehydrogenase activity is closely related to the increase in cell proliferation. The results of several stereological studies indicated that there is always an early peak of clear and acidophilic glycogen storage foci, followed by an increase in mixed cell foci, and the occurrence of adenomas and carcinomas (Moore et al. 1982; Enzmann and Bannasch 1987; Weber 1989). Although this sequence appears to be well established in various species including primates, recent findings in rodents suggest that alternative lineages of altered hepatocytes may lead to hepatic tumors under certain conditions (Bannasch et al. 1985a; Weber et al. 1988; Harada et al. 1989; Kraupp-Grasl et al. 1990). In any case, there are now numerous arguments in favor of the preneoplastic nature of persistent foci of altered hepatocytes (Bannasch et al. 1989a): They show many similarities in their morphological and biochemical phenotype to hepatic tumors; they emerge prior to the appearance of hepatic tumors induced by chemicals in various species, by radiation in rats, and by the woodchuck hepatitis virus in woodchucks; they persist in stop experiments with chemical carcinogens; they show a cell proliferation rate which is significantly higher than in the normal liver parenchyma but lower than in adenomas and carcinomas; morphological transitions to adenomas and carcinomas are frequent; and there is a close statistical correlation to the incidence of hepatocellular neoplasms.

Human Hepatic Preneoplasia

Various types of foci of altered hepatocytes have been fortuitously observed in the human liver (Balász 1976; Cain and Kraus 1977; Shapiro et al. 1977; Altmann 1978; Heine 1981; Mori et al. 1982; Fischer et al. 1986; Schaff et al. 1986; Karhunen and Pentillä 1987), but their relationship to hepatic neoplasms has not been studied systematically. In the past 2 years we started a more extensive investigation in explanted livers which we received from our col-

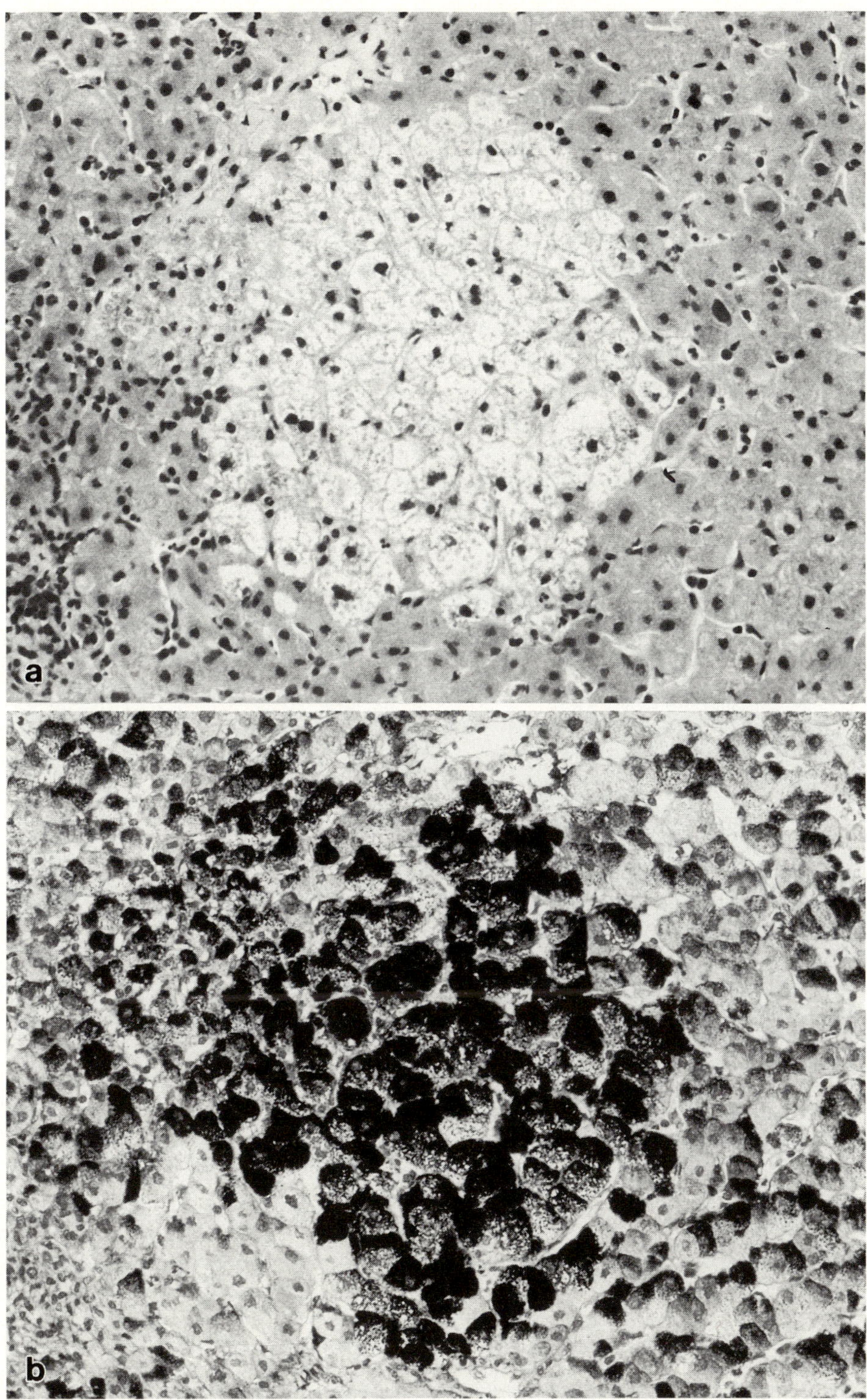

Fig. 2a,b. Focal hepatic glycogenosis in male patient with a hepatocellular carcinoma. **a** Clear cell appearance of glycogen storage focus after staining with H&E. **b** Serial section to **a** exhibiting excessive storage of glycogen as demonstrated by the periodic acid–Schiff reaction. Both images ×565 leagues in the Surgical Departments of the Universities of Heidelberg and Hannover. We found focal lesions storing glycogen in excess (Fig. 2) and exhibiting various enzymatic changes, particularly a decrease in the activities of glycogen phosphorylase and glucose-6-phosphatase, in both non-cirrhotic and cirrhotic livers (Figs. 3, 4). From 32 livers which have been evaluated in detail up to the present (Table 2), 10 contained hepatocellular carcinomas, whereas 14 showed a posthepatitic and 8 an alcoholic liver cirrhosis. Foci of altered hepatocytes comparable to preneoplastic hepatic foci in rodents were observed in 8 out of 10 livers bearing hepatocellular carcinomas and in 15 out of 22 cirrhotic livers, which are generally considered to represent a preneoplastic condition. In spite of the relatively low number of cases studied, along with earlier relevant findings these results suggest that the sequence of cellular changes leading to hepatocellular tumors is, in principle, identical in laboratory animals and man as proposed years ago (Bannasch and Klinge 1971).

There is a second line of evidence supporting this conclusion. It has been known for some time that patients suffering from inborn hepatic glycogen storage disease type 1, which is due to a genetically fixed defect in glucose-6-

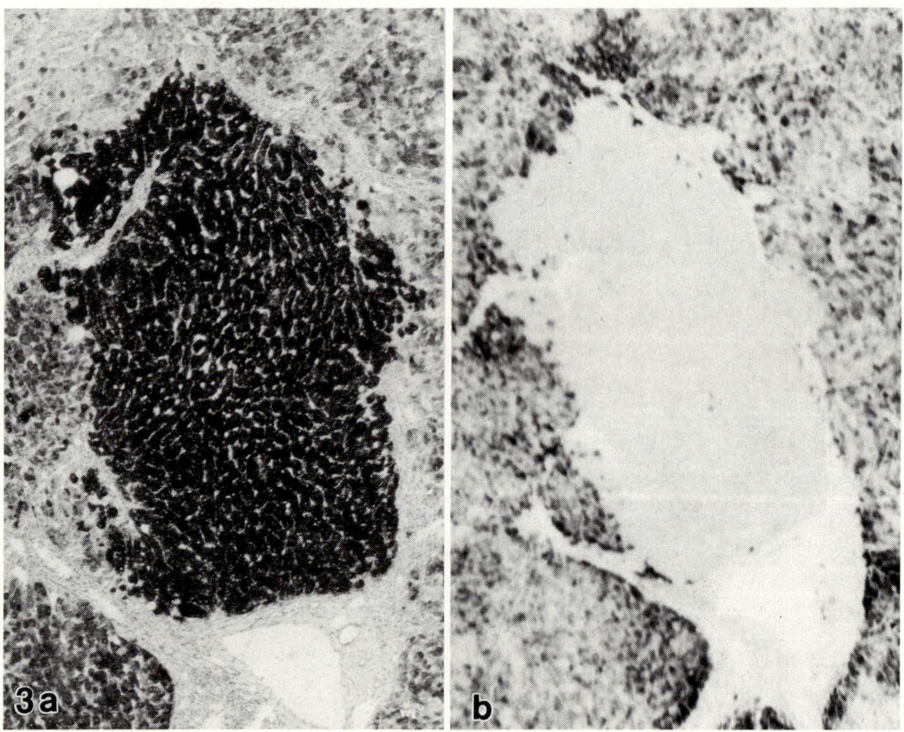

Fig. 3a,b. Focal hepatic glycogenosis in male patient with a hepatocellular carcinoma. **a** Hepatic focus storing glycogen in excess as demonstrated by the periodic acid–Schiff reaction. **b** Serial section to **a** exhibiting decreased activity of glycogen phosphorylase as demonstrated by iodine staining of newly formed glycogen. Both images ×30

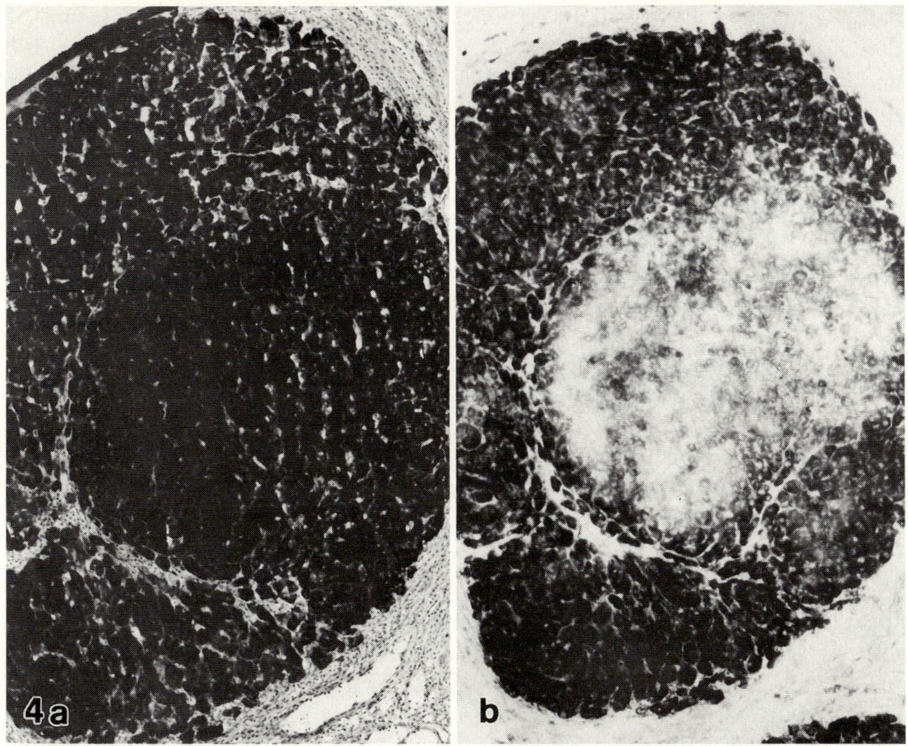

Fig. 4a,b. Focal hepatic glycogenosis in cirrhotic human liver. **a** Excessive storage of glycogen as demonstrated by the periodic acid–Schiff reaction. **b** Serial section to **a** exhibiting focally decreased activity of glycogen phosphorylase as demonstrated by iodine staining of newly formed glycogen. Both images ×45

Table 2. Preneoplastic hepatic lesions in cirrhotic and tumor-bearing human livers

Pathological condition	No. of patients	Livers with preneoplastic lesions
Posthepatitic liver cirrhosis	14	9 (64%)
Alcoholic liver cirrhosis	8	6 (75%)
Hepatocellular carcinoma	10	8 (80%)

phosphatase, have an exceedingly high risk of developing multiple hepatic tumors. We have recently collected all data published on the combination of this inborn storage disease and liver cell tumors and found 67 patients with this syndrome (Brözel 1989). Whereas the tumors were relatively rare in young children, the risk of developing adenomas and carcinomas exceeded 90% when the patients passed through adolescence. In some patients the clinical course of the disease suggested an adenoma-carcinoma sequence as observed in the majority of experimental models of hepatocarcinogenesis. These findings favor the concept that the molecular changes underlying hepatocellular glycogenosis emerging early during hepatocarcinogenesis might trigger a sustained cascade of adaptive metabolic events eventually leading to neoplastic transformation of the hepatocytes (Bannasch et al. 1984).

Relevance of Preneoplastic Lesions for Early Detection

In laboratory animals, there is increasing evidence of the usefulness of preneoplastic lesions, especially preneoplastic hepatic foci, as early indicators of a neoplastic response (Bannasch and Zerban 1992). However, stereological studies have indicated that the number of preneoplastic hepatic foci by far exceeds the number of neoplasms appearing after long lag periods. Using glycogen retention after starvation as a marker for foci of altered hepatocytes induced in rat liver by an initiation-promotion protocol, Kaufmann et al. (1985, 1987) estimated that only one carcinoma developed for every 1000 to 10 000 focal lesions that were observed either prior to or concurrent with the appearance of neoplasms. Although this discrepancy is difficult to understand from a mechanistic point of view, the large number of preneoplastic lesions implies a great advantage for the detection of early stages of neoplastic development.

Depending on the dose and duration of the carcinogenic treatment the lag period between the first appearance of glycogenotic hepatic foci and hepatic neoplasms may vary widely. In NNM-treated rats, Weber (1989) observed lag periods for the occurrence of adenomas of between 15 and more than 50 weeks. There is at present no additional marker which would permit us to predict precisely from the appearance of preneoplastic hepatic foci at which time point hepatic adenomas or carcinomas will develop. However, for many experimental situations the assumption of a lag period of 6–12 months, corresponding to about 15%–30% of the average life span of the rat, appears to be reasonable. It is interesting to note that in relation to the average life span these figures are very close to the 15–30 years which pass in the majority of children suffering from inborn hepatic glycogenosis type I until multiple hepatocellular tumors occur.

The main shortcoming for utilization of this long lag period in the progression of preneoplastic hepatic lesions for the early detection of neoplastic development in man is the small size of the lesions and their location in an organ which is not easily accessible. Thus, the majority of preneoplastic hepatic glycogen storage foci are smaller than a liver lobule which has an average diameter of 1–2 mm in both rodents and man. This small size precludes a non-invasive identification by all imaging procedures available. However, the enzymatic alterations observed in foci of altered hepatocytes might help to diagnose such lesions in fine-needle biopsies. The further elucidation of the metabolic aberrations associated with neoplastic cell conversion in the liver and other tissues should eventually provide a rational basis for the chemoprevention of neoplasia.

Summary

Definite proliferative lesions such as nodular hyperplasia, papilloma, or carcinoma in situ have been considered prestages of malignant neoplasms (cancer) and have, hence, been widely employed in the early diagnosis of neoplasia. "Preneoplasia" and "precancer" were used as synonyms for a long time. However, investigations in several animal models and some studies in man revealed that characteristic changes in the biochemical and morphological phenotype of focal cell populations precede the appearance of both benign and malignant neoplasms in a number of tissues by weeks and months or even years. Consequently, preneoplasia has been defined as phenotypically altered cell populations which have no obvious neoplastic nature but indicate a high probability of progression to benign or malignant neoplasms.

Focal preneoplastic lesions according to the definition given have been discovered in various tissues, such as liver parenchyma, renal tubular system, exocrine pancreas, and colonic mucosa. The phenotypic patterns of preneoplasia appear to be as varied as those of neoplasia, each histologically and cytologically defined tumor type presenting its own histo- and cytogenesis. The changes characterizing preneoplastic lesions include many cytoplasmic alterations and may be classed into four main categories: (1) alterations in the expression of enzymes, (2) changes in the content of metabolites, especially an excessive storage of macromolecules (e.g., glycogen, glycosaminoglycans, lipids), (3) alterations in the organization of organelles (e.g., mitochondria, peroxisomes, endoplasmic reticulum), (4) increased cell proliferation and nuclear alterations. Many of the cytoplasmic alterations observed suggest early aberrations in energy metabolism during neoplastic development.

Hepatic preneoplasia has been studied extensively in several species including primates. Stereological studies have indicated that the number of preneoplastic hepatic lesions by far exceeds the number of neoplasms appearing after long lag periods. This discrepancy is difficult to understand from a mechanistic point of view, but the large number of preneoplastic lesions implies a great advantage for the detection of early stages of neoplastic development.

Acknowledgements. We gratefully acknowledge the supply of surgical specimens by Dr. G. Otto (Department of Surgery, University of Heidelberg) and Professor R. Pichlmayr (Department of Surgery, Medical School, University of Hannover). We would also like to thank Gabriele Becker for preparing the photomicrographs and Brigitte Pétillon for typing the manuscript.

References

Altmann HW (1978) Pathology of human liver tumors. In: Remmer H, Bolt H, Bannasch P, Popper H (eds) Primary liver tumors. MTP Press, Lancaster, pp 53–71

Baba M, Yamamoto R, Iishi H, Tatsuta M, Wada A (1989) Role of glucose-6-phosphate dehydrogenase on enhanced proliferation of pre-neoplastic and neoplastic cells in rat liver induced by N-nitrosomorpholine. Int J Cancer 43:892–895

Balázs M (1976) Licht- und elektronenmikroskopische Untersuchungen in einem Fall von primärem Leberkarzinom im Säuglingsalter. Zentralbl Allg Pathol 120:3–13

Bannasch P (1968) The cytoplasm of hepatocytes during carcinogenesis. Electron and light microscopic investigations of the nitrosomorpholine-intoxicated rat liver. Recent Results Cancer Res 19:1–100

Bannasch P (1984) Sequential cellular changes during chemical carcinogenesis. J Cancer Res Clin Oncol 108:11–22

Bannasch P (1986) Preneoplastic lesions as end points in carcinogenicity testing. I. Hepatic preneoplasia. II. Preneoplasia in various non-hepatic tissues. Carcinogenesis 7:689–695, 849–852

Bannasch P (1988) Phenotypic cellular changes as indicators of stages during neoplastic development. In: Iversen OH (ed) Theories of carcinogenesis. Hemisphere, Washington, pp 231–249

Bannasch P (1990) Pathobiology of chemical hepatocarcinogenesis: recent progress and perspectives. I. Cytomorphological changes and cell proliferation. II. Metabolic and molecular changes. J Gastroenterol Hepatol 5:149–159, 310–320

Bannasch P, Klinge O (1971) Hepatozelluläre Glykogenose und Hepatombildung beim Menschen. Virchows Arch [A] 352:157–164

Bannasch P, Zerban H (1990) Animal models and renal carcinogenesis. In: Eble JN (ed) Contemporary issues in surgical pathology. Tumors and tumor-like conditions of the kidneys and ureters. Livingstone, Edinburgh, pp 1–34

Bannasch P, Zerban H (1992) Predictive value of hepatic preneoplastic lesions as indicators of carcinogenic response. IARC Sci Publ (in press)

Bannasch P, Krech R, Zerban H (1978a) Morphogenese und Mikromorphologie epithelialer Nierentumoren bei Nitrosomorpholin-vergifteten Ratten. II. Tubuläre Glykogenose und die Genese von klar- oder acidophilzelligen Tumoren. Z Krebsforsch 92:63–86

Bannasch P, Krech R, Zerban H (1978b) Morphogenese und Mikromorphologie epithelialer Nierentumoren bei Nitrosomorpholin-vergifteten Ratten. III. Onkocytentubuli und Onkocytome. Z Krebsforsch 92:87–104

Bannasch P, Hacker HJ, Klimek F, Mayer D (1984) Hepatocellular glycogenosis and related pattern of enzymatic changes during hepatocarcinogenesis. Adv Enzyme Regul 22: 97–121

Bannasch P, Benner U, Enzmann H, Hacker HJ (1985a) Tigroid cell foci and neoplastic nodules in the liver of rats treated with a single dose of aflatoxin B_1. Carcinogenesis 6:1641–1648

Bannasch P, Moore MA, Hacker HJ, Klimek F, Mayer D, Enzmann H, Zerban H (1985b) Potential significance of phenotypic instability in focal and nodular liver lesions induced by hepatocarcinogens. In: Brunner H, Thaler H (eds) Hepatology: a Festschrift for Hans Popper. Raven, New York, pp 191–209

Bannasch P, Enzmann H, Hacker HJ, Weber E, Zerban H (1989a) Comparative pathobiology of hepatic preneoplasia. In: Bannasch P, Keppler D, Weber G (eds) Liver cell carcinoma. Kluwer, Dordrecht, pp 53–73

Bannasch P, Enzmann H, Klimek F, Weber E, Zerban H (1989b) Significance of sequential cellular changes inside and outside foci of altered hepatocytes during hepatocarcinogenesis. Toxicol Pathol 17:617–629

Bannasch P, Hacker HJ, Klimek F, Mayer D, Stumpf H, Zerban H (1991) Cytochemical, microbiochemical and molecular genetic analysis of chemical carcinogenesis. Prog Histochem Cytochem 23:45–60

Barrow BJ, O'Riordan MA, Stellato TA, Calkins BM, Pretlow TP (1990) Enzyme-altered foci in colons of carcinogen-treated rats. Cancer Res 50:1911–1916

Brözel U (1989) Hepatozelluläre Tumoren bei angeborener Glykogenspeicherkrankheit. Thesis, University of Heidelberg

Cain H, Kraus B (1977) Entwicklungsstörungen der Leber und Leberkarzinom im Säuglings- und Kindesalter. Dtsch Med Wochenschr 102:505–509

Carter RL (ed) (1984) Precancerous states. Oxford University Press, London

Dietrich DR, Swenberg JA (1991) Preneoplastic lesions in rodent kidney induced spontaneously or by non-genotoxic carcinogens. Mutat Res 248:239–260

Enzmann H, Bannasch P (1987) Potential significance of phenotypic heterogeneity of focal lesions at different stages in hepatocarcinogenesis. Carcinogenesis 8:1607–1612

Farber E, Sarma DSR (1987) Hepatocarcinogenesis: a dynamic cellular perspective. Lab Invest 56:4–22

Fischer G, Hartmann H, Droese M, Schauer A, Bock KW (1986) Histochemical and immunohistochemical detection of putative preneoplastic liver foci in women after long-term use of oral contraceptives. Virchows Arch [B] 50:321–337

Fischer G, Ruschenburg J, Eigenbrodt E, Katz N (1987) Decrease in glucokinase and glucose-6-phosphatase and increase in hexokinase in putative preneoplastic lesions of rat liver. J Cancer Res Clin Oncol 113:430–436

Goldsworthy TL, Hanigan HM, Pitot HC (1986) Models of hepatocarcinogenesis in the rat – contrasts and comparisons. CRC Crit Rev Toxicol 17:61–89

Gusterson BA (1984) Precancerous changes in the lungs and the potential of cells to have modulated phenotypes. In: Carter RL (ed) Precancerous states. Oxford University Press, London, pp 161–184

Hacker HJ, Moore MA, Mayer D, Bannasch P (1982) Correlative histochemistry of some enzymes of carbohydrate metabolism in preneoplastic and neoplastic lesions in the rat liver. Carcinogenesis 3:1265–1272

Harada T, Maronpot RR, Morris RW, Boorman GA (1989) Observations on altered hepatocellular foci in National Toxicology Program two-year carcinogenicity studies in rats. Toxicol Pathol 17:690–708

Heine WD (1981) Experimentelle und menschliche hepatozelluläre Lebertumoren und ihre Vorstufen – histologische, enzymhistochemische und zellkinetische Charakteristika. In: Zelder O, Röher HD, Fischer M, Bode JC (eds) Experimentelle und klinische Hepatologie. Schattauer, Stuttgart, pp 13–24

Karhunen PJ, Pentillä A (1987) Preneoplastic lesions of human liver. Hepato-gastroenterology 34:10–15

Kaufmann WK, MacKenzie SA, Kaufman DG (1985) Quantitative relationship between hepatocytic neoplasms and islands of cellular alteration during hepatocarcinogenesis in the male F344 rat. Am J Pathol 119:171–174

Kaufmann WK, Rahija RJ, MacKenzie SA, Kaufman DG (1987) Cell cycle-dependent initiation of hepatocarcinogenesis in rats by (±) 7r, 8t-dihydroxy-9t, 10t-epoxy-7,8,9,10-tetrahydrobenzo(a)pyrene. Cancer Res 47:3771–3775

Klimek F, Mayer D, Bannasch P (1984) Biochemical microanalysis of glycogen content and glucose-6-phosphate dehydrogenase activity in focal lesions of the rat liver induced by N-nitrosomorpholine. Carcinogenesis 5:265–268

Koss LG (1979) Diagnostic cytology and its histopathologic bases, 3rd edn. Lippincott, Philadelphia

Kraupp-Grasl B, Huber W, Putz B, Gerbracht U, Schulte-Hermann R (1990) Tumor promotion by the peroxisome proliferator nafenopin involving a specific subtype of altered foci in rat liver. Cancer Res 50:3701–3708

Krech R, Zerban H, Bannasch P (1981) Mitochondrial anomalies in renal oncocytes induced in rat by N-nitrosomorpholine. Eur J Cell Biol 25:331–339

Longnecker DS, Millar PM (1990) Tumours of the pancreas. IARC Sci Publ 99:199–240

Mayer D, Trocheris V, Hacker HJ, Viallard V, Murat JC, Bannasch P (1987) Sequential histochemical and morphometric studies on preneoplastic and neoplastic lesions induced in rat colon by 1,2-dimethylhydrazine. Carcinogenesis 8:155–161

Mayer D, Klimek F, Hacker HJ, Seelmann-Eggebert G, Bannasch P (1989) Carbohydrate metabolism in hepatic preneoplasia. In: Bannasch P, Keppler D, Weber G (eds) Liver cell carcinoma. Kluwer, Dordrecht, pp 321–337

Moore MA, Kitagawa T (1986) Hepatocarcinogenesis in the rat; the effect of the promoters and carcinogens in vivo and in vitro. Int Rev Cytol 101:125–173

Moore MA, Mayer D, Bannasch P (1982) The dose-dependence and sequential appearance of putative preneoplastic populations induced in the rat liver by stop experiments with *N*-nitrosomorpholine. Carcinogenesis 3:1429–1436

Moore MA, Nakamura T, Shirai T, Ito N (1986) Immunohistochemical demonstration of increased glucose-6-phosphate dehydrogenase in preneoplastic and neoplastic lesions induced by propylnitrosamine in F344 rats and Syrian hamsters. Jpn J Cancer Res 77:131–138

Mori H, Tanaka T, Sugie S, Takahashi M, Williams GM (1982) DNA content of liver cell nuclei of *N*-2-fluorenylacetamide-induced altered foci and neoplasms in rats and human hyperplastic foci. JNCI 69:1277–1282

Nogueira E, Bannasch P (1988) Cellular origin of rat renal oncocytoma. Lab Invest 59:337–343

Nogueira E, Klimek F, Weber E, Bannasch P (1989) Origin of rat renal clear cell tumors from the collecting duct. Virchows Arch [3] 57:275–283

Ortmann M, Vierbuchen M, Koller G, Fischer R (1988) Renal oncocytoma. I. Cytochrome C oxidase in normal and neoplastic renal tissue as detected by immunohistochemistry – a valuable aid to distinguish oncocytomas from renal cell carcinomas. Virchows Arch [B] 56:165–173

Schaff Z, Lapis K, Henson DE (1986) Liver. In: Henson DE, Albores-Saavedra J (eds) The pathology of incipient neoplasia. Saunders, Philadelphia, pp 167–202

Seelmann-Eggebert G, Mayer D, Mecke D, Bannasch P (1987) Expression and regulation of glycogen phosphorylase in preneoplastic and neoplastic hepatic lesions in rats. Virchows Arch [B] 53:44–51

Shapiro P, Ikeda RM, Ruebner BH, Coonors MH, Halsted CC, Abildgaard CF (1977) Multiple hepatic tumors and peliosis hepatis in Fanconi's anemia treated with androgens. Am J Dis Child 131:1104–1106

Sirica AE (1989) Preneoplasia and precancerous lesions. In: Sirica AE (ed) The pathobiology of neoplasia. Plenum, New York, pp 199–215

Störkel S, Pannen B, Thoenes W, Steart PV, Wagner S, Drenckhahn D (1988) Intercalated cells as a probable source for the development of renal oncocytoma. Virchows Arch [B] 56:185–189

Symposium (1989) Significance of foci of cellular alteration in the rat liver. Toxicol Pathol 17:557–735

Tatematsu M, Nagamine Y, Farber E (1983) Redifferentiation as a basis for remodeling of carcinogen-induced hepatocyte nodules to normal appearing liver. Cancer Res 433:5049–5058

Watanabe K, Williams GM (1978) Enhancement of rat hepatocellular-altered foci by the liver tumor promoter phenobarbital: evidence that foci are precursors of neoplasms and that the promoter acts on carcinogen-induced lesions. JNCI 61:1311–1314

Weber E (1989) Dosisabhängigkeit der Sequenz zellulärer Veränderungen bei der *N*-Nitrosomorpholin-induzierten Hepatokarzinogenese in der Ratte. Thesis, University of Darmstadt

Weber E, Moore MA, Bannasch P (1988) Enzyme histochemical and morphological phenotype of amphophilic foci and amphophilic/tigroid cell adenomas in rat liver after combined treatment with dehydroepiandrosterone and *N*-nitrosomorpholine. Carcinogenesis 9:1049–1054

Woutersen RA, van Garderen-Hoetmer A, Lamers CBHW, Scherer E (1991) Early indicators of exocrine pancreas carcinogenesis produced by non-genotoxic agents. Mutat Res 248:291–302

Zerban H, Nogueira E, Riedasch G, Bannasch P (1987) Renal oncocytoma: origin from the collecting duct. Virchows Arch [B] 52:375–387

Zerban H, Rabes HM, Bannasch P (1989) Sequential changes in growth kinetics and cellular phenotype during hepatocarcinogenesis. J Cancer Res Clin Oncol 115:329–334

Summary of Discussion: Session 5

P. MÖLLER

The pertinent problem of early detection of neoplasia as the best way towards curative treatment has many aspects. Neoplasia or the tendency to develop a tumor during a lifetime can be inborn, even inherited. Therefore, molecular genetic probes detecting, e.g., (recessive) tumor genes and homozygosity or acquired loss of heterozygosity concerning a critical allele may be the earliest indicator for an elevated oncogenic potential. This aspect was part of the contribution of H. Höfler (Munich) dealing with molecular genetic approaches to the problem. For example, structural alterations of the retinoblastoma gene are known to initiate retinoblastoma. Mutations within the p53 tumor suppressor gene are presently thought to be involved in initiating events of many solid tumors and even leukemias. Methods are available or are being developed to detect specifically and sensitively these genomic changes in a preneoplastic stage. P. Bannasch (Heidelberg) stressed the fact that functional defects of cells induced by carcinogenic agents can clearly procede the apparent neoplastic transformation. Functional carcinogen-induced damage within the cytoplasmic compartment may through mechanisms like altered enzyme expression, disturbed organization of organelles, etc. (per se eventually leading to increased cell turnover) secondly induce genetic alterations. As examples of this line of evidence, he presented and discussed chemical hepatic and renal carcinogenesis. Once a preneoplastic or neoplastic lesion has developed somewhere in an organism, the next problem is the early detection of the initially minimal tumor burden. This aspect is the realm of preventive medical care and mass screening. However, early detection through screening is scientifically possible for only a limited number of cancers and ethically feasible for only a few. Preventional mass screening is – apart from its efficacy which is positively influenced by scientific progress – primarily a subject of health politics, which, in turn, is largely influenced by socioeconomic parameters only very vaguely linked to the problem itself. L. Koss (New York) as basic cytologist and one of the pioneers in preventive cancer care gave an impressive lecture on the influence of both politics and scientific progress on the development in cyto-diagnosis of precancerous states and early human cancer, paradigmatically focussing on urinary bladder carcinoma. As R. Moll (Mainz) pointed out, the role of immunohistochemical and immunocytochemical characterization of cells via determination of intermediate filament patterns is still subordinated to other, largely classic, micromorphological parameters. Immunomorphology clearly has its place in diagnostic pathology but is most powerful in detecting single tumor cells in a non-neoplastic context and, secondly, in the histogenetical assignment of morphologically undifferentiated malignant cells. Last but not least (and therefore it was dealt as the first topic of this session), although the borderline questions in diagnostic pathology are mostly situated at the interface of established knowledge and hypothesis, and although they are in certain aspects identical with the limits of our methodological repertoire, a good number of them, however, are semantical ones. What does "early" mean in the context of cancer? The contribution by R.L. Carter (Sutton) analyzed the connotative field of terms like metaplasia, dysplasia, borderline, early cancer, early invasion pointing at "hot spots" in routine histopathology.

In several aspects, the limits of a scientist in this field can be best described by the words of E.A. Clark (Seattle), who once characterized our knowledge on B-lymphocyte activation with the phrase: "We don't see the bullet – we just see the smoking gun."

SESSION 6

Cytogenetics and Molecular Genetics

Chairman: F. VOGEL

Chromosome Aberrations in Human Neoplasia

N. Mandahl

Introduction

It is established beyond doubt that most neoplasms, benign and malignant, have karyotypic changes detectable with cytogenetic techniques. To date more than 14 000 human neoplasms with karyotypic abnormalities, analyzed by means of chromosome banding, have been reported (Mitelman 1991). The chromosome aberrations are of three different kinds: (1) primary changes, which are essential in establishing the tumor and may occur already as solitary cytogenetic changes in the earliest disease phase; (2) secondary changes developing only after the neoplasm is established but which nonetheless may be important in tumor progression; and (3) cytogenetic noise, which is the background level of inconsequential changes. Primary and often also secondary aberrations are nonrandom. The more than 100 primary abnormalities identified correlate strictly with particular neoplastic disorders and even with histopathological subgroups within a given tumor type (Mitelman et al. 1990), providing convincing evidence for the fundamental role of chromosomal rearrangements in the carcinogenic process. This is further supported by the coincident localization of neoplasia-associated chromosomal breakpoints and the two functionally different classes of directly cancer-relevant genes, the dominant oncogenes and the recessive, tumor-suppressing antioncogenes (Mitelman and Heim 1988).

It is important to stress that the cytogenetic information presently available is in many respects incomplete. The data are heavily biased in favor of hematologic neoplasms; of the total database 68% involves hematologic disorders, 11% lymphomas, and 21% solid tumors, which is highly disproportionate to the relative contribution of these disorders to human cancer morbidity and mortality. This discrepancy is largely due to the technical difficulties encountered in solid tumor cytogenetics. Moreover, the karyotypic changes are typically much more complex in solid tumors, which makes it difficult to identify which aberrations are primary and secondary and which represent cytogenetic noise. Obviously, in most types of solid tumors, many more samples will have to be studied. The preferential involvement of different chromosomes or chromosome segments in different neoplasms also make these aberrations clinically useful as diagnostic and prognostic parameters in hematologic disorders where substantial data are available (Heim 1990, Heim and Mitelman 1987, Sandberg 1990). In this respect, cytogenetic analysis in solid tumors is still less useful. Improved techniques, utilizing short-term tissue culturing and refined culture media, now seem to change this situation.

Nomenclature

The standardized nomenclature of human chromosome classification is outlined in ISCN (1985). The symbol "p" designates the short arm and "q" the long arm of a chromosome. Transverse banding of chromosomes may be induced by a variety of staining methods. Each chromosome is seen as consisting of a continuous series of dark and light bands. These are allocated to certain defined regions along the chromosome arms, and the regions are delimited by specific landmarks (the centromere, the two chromosome ends, and some prominent bands). Regions and bands are numbered consecutively from the centromere outward along each chromosome arm. To describe a particular band, four items are required: the chromosome number, the arm symbol, the region number, and the band number within that region. Thus, 12q15 indicates chromosome 12, long arm, region 1, band 5.

Plus (+) and minus (−) signs are placed before the appropriate symbol to indicate additional or missing whole chromosomes (numerical aberrations). Structurally abnormal chromosomes are defined by their breakpoints. Translocations, transfer of material within or between chromosomes, are specified by the symbol "t", and t(11;22)(q24;q12) means exchange between chromosomes 11 and 22. The breakpoints are in bands 11q24 and 22q12. The symbol "del" denotes deletion (loss of part of a chromosome), "inv" inversion (rotation of a chromosome segment 180°), and "i" isochromosome (homologous arms, p or q, that are mirror images of one another).

Chromosome Aberrations in Human Neoplasms

Before turning to the clinical applicability of cytogenetic analysis in human neoplasms, a brief summary of consistent and specific karyotypic changes will be presented. The aberrations of, in particular, hematologic disorders and also solid tumors have been reviewed extensively (Heim and Mitelman 1987, 1991, Mitelman and Heim 1990, Rowley 1988, Sandberg 1990, Sandberg et al. 1988) and will only be superficially described here.

Acute Nonlymphocytic Leukemia

Clonal chromosome abnormalities are found in two-thirds of all cases at diagnosis. Several of the about 50 primary karyotypic abnormalities identified are associated with particular acute nonlymphocytic leukemia (ANLL) subtypes as defined by the French-American-British (FAB) classification and are of clinical importance. Some of the best characterized primary, structural aberrations are:

inv(3)(q21q26), AML with abnormal megakaryocytes and thrombocytosis; t(6;9)(p23;q34), M2 and M4 with basophilia; t(8;16)(p11;p13), M5 with phagocytosis; t(8;21)(q22;q22), M2 with Auer rods and eosinophilia; t(9;11)(p21–22;q23), M5 (mostly M5a); t(15;17)(q22;q11–12), M3; and inv(16)(p13q22), M4 with eosinophilia. None of the numerical changes (the most common are +4, −5, −7, +8, +21, and −Y) is restricted to any particular FAB subgroup.

Myelodysplastic Syndromes

Several hematopoietic dysfunction states that carry an increased risk for the ultimate development of ANLL are included. Karyotypic changes are found in one-third to half of the cases. The fact that chromosome changes may be found in myelodysplastic syndromes (MDS) strongly supports the presently held view that these syndromes do in fact represent truly neoplastic disorders. About 80% of karyotypically abnormal MDS patients has one of the following changes: t(1;3)(p36;q21), t(1;7)(p11;q11), inv(3)(q21q26), del(5q), t(6;9)(p23;q34), −7, +8, t/del(11q), t/del(12p), del(13q), i(17q), del(20q), and −Y.

Chronic Myeloid Leukemia

About 90% of patients with clinically typical chronic myeloid leukemia (CML) has the Philadelphia chromosome, which originates through the reciprocal translocation t(9;22)(q34;q11). Additional, nonrandom aberrations are acquired at the time of blastic crisis; 80% of the cases has at least one of four changes: +8, i(17q), +19, and an extra copy of the Philadelphia chromosome.

Acute Lymphocytic Leukemia

About two-thirds of patients with acute lymphocytic leukemia (ALL) have clonal chromosome aberrations in their bone marrow cells at diagnosis. About 40 consistently occurring rearrangements are known. The most prominent aberrations associated with particular immunological and morphological ALL subtypes are: t(1;19)(q23;p13), pre-B ALL, L1; t(4;11)(q21;q23), early B-precursor ALL, L1, L2; del(6q), various lymphoid malignancies; t(9;22)(q34;q11), pre-B or early B-precursor ALL, L1, L2; t/del(9p), T-ALL, L1, L2; t/del(12p), common ALL, L1; abnormalities of 14q11, T-ALL, L1, L2; and t(8;14)(q24;q32), t(8;22)(q24;q11), and t(2;8)(p12;q24), B-ALL, L3, and in particular in Burkitt's lymphoma.

Lymphoma

The characteristic aberrations of Burkitt's lymphoma are described above. In non-Burkitt's, non-Hodgkin's lymphoma the characteristic aberrations are less consistently associated with histopathological subtype than the changes in Burkitt's lymphoma. The best candidates for primary rearrangements are: t(2;5)(p23;q35), +3, del(6p), del(6q), t(11;14)(q13;q32), and t(14;18)(q32; q21).

Solid Tumors

Benign Epithelial, Mesenchymal, and Neurogenic Tumors

Four tumor types have been studied in sufficient number to permit reasonably well-founded conclusions: pleomorphic adenoma, lipoma, uterine leiomyoma, and meningioma.

Pleomorphic Adenoma. Three cytogenetic subgroups, characterized by aberrations involving 3p21, 8q12, and 12q13–15, may be distinguished. Often, but not always, 3p21 and 8q12 recombine in a t(3;8).

Lipoma. Different cytogenetic subgroups may be distinguished: reciprocal, apparently balanced translocations between 12q13–15 and various other chromosomes, t(3;12)(q27–28;q13–15) and less frequently t(2;12)(q35; q13–15) are recurrent aberrations; supernumerary ring chromosomes, particularly in atypical lipomas; t/del(13q); and aberrations other than those mentioned above.

Uterine Leiomyoma. The reciprocal translocation t(12;14)(q14–15;q23–24) has been found as the sole aberration in a substantial proportion of tumors with an abnormal karyotype. Other cytogenetic subtypes include del(7q) (q21q31) and trisomy 12.

Meningioma. The vast majority of cases are characterized by the loss of one chromosome 22. Occasionally, del(22q) may be found.

Malignant Mesenchymal Tumors

Apart from hematologic disorders, the largest number of consistent and specific karyotypic changes have been identified in the group of malignant mesenchymal tumors. These include the highly specific aberrations: t(12; 16)(q13;p11) in myxoid liposarcoma; t(X;18)(p11;q11) in synovial sarcoma; t(2;13)(q35–37;q14) in rhabdomyosarcoma, primarily of the alveolar type; t(9;22)(q22;q12) in extraskeletal myxoid chondrosarcoma (only identified in three of four tumors analyzed); and the aberration t(11;22)(q24;q12), which is found in Ewing's sarcoma, neuroepithelioma, and the Askin tumor. Nonrandom, secondary aberrations (+8 and an unbalanced 1;16 translocation) have also been identified in Ewing's sarcoma and myxoid liposarcoma (+8).

Malignant Epithelial Tumors

Few cases of most types of malignant epithelial tumors have been investigated cytogenetically. Many of these have highly complex karyotypic changes. Hence, it is in general difficult to distinguish between primary and secondary aberrations in these tumors. However, although more data are needed, a number of consistent cytogenetic abnormalities have been revealed.

The majority of small cell lung carcinomas, the only one of the four histologic subtypes investigated to any extent, has deletion of the short arm of chromosome 3, with loss of 3p14–23 as the least common denominator. Also, in carcinoma of the kidney, rearrangements of 3p with breakpoints mapping to 3p11–21 and often giving rise to loss of 3p material are frequent. In Wilms' tumor, half of all cases has rearrangements of chromosome 1 and one-fourth has deletions or translocations of 11p13. Chromosome 1 abnormalities appear to be the most common changes in carcinoma of the ovary; the breakpoints have mostly been mapped to 1p36. A 19p+ marker chromosome has been reported in a subset of ovarian seropapillary cystadenocarcinomas. Other commonly involved chromosomes are 3, 6, 11, and 14. Carcinomas of the large bowel have most frequently structural changes of chromosomes 1 and 17, and +7 and +12. In carcinomas of the bladder, the most common anomalies are structural changes of chromosomes 1 and 11, i(5p), +7, and −9.

Malignant Neurogenic Tumors

The most frequent findings in malignant glioma are double minutes (dmin), rearrangements of 1p, 7q, 9q, 19q, +7, −10, and −22. The predominant abnormality in neuroblastoma involves aberrations of the terminal portion of the short arm of chromosome 1. Half of all retinoblastomas has changes of chromosome 1, one-third has i(6p), and only one-fifth has changes involving chromosome 13.

Germ Cell Tumors

An isochromosome for the short arm of chromosome 12 has consistently been found in various histologic types of germ cell tumors of the testis.

Clinical Implications of Cytogenetic Findings

The finding of clonal, acquired chromosome aberrations gives, according to the generally accepted opinion, the information that a neoplastic process is present. The finding of a normal karyotype is inconclusive. The presence of clonal chromosome abnormalities in samples taken from an effusion of unknown cause reveal the neoplastic nature of origin in situations where cytology or other diagnostic methods may fail to detect a cancer. Due to the specificity of some consistent rearrangements, they may be diagnostically useful. However, in several cases it will be impossible to determine the type of neoplasm just on the basis of karyotypic findings. Given additional information, the detection of, for example, t(9;22)(q34;q11) in a myeloproliferative disorder or t(15;17)(q22;q11) in AML, the specificity of these aberrations makes possible the diagnosis of CML and AML M3. The karyotypic findings may also give information of prognostic value.

Another important diagnostic role for cytogenetic analyses in hematological neoplasms is in the monitoring of remission and relapse. During induction treatment, normalization of the bone marrow karyotype occurs if complete remission is achieved; persisting cytogenetic changes mean that the patient is not yet disease-free. When therapy is discontinued, another cytogenetic analysis may be performed to be sure that no aberrant clone is present. The recurrence of the chromosome aberrations found at diagnosis demonstrate relapse. At times, cytogenetic analysis may be more sensitive than morphological bone marrow examination in detecting leukemic relapse and in the early diagnosis of secondary leukemia. The acquisition of additional chromosome aberrations may occur occasionally and indicate progression. Cytogenetic monitoring may also be applied after bone marrow transplantation, but since the data are still insufficient the interpretations should be made with caution.

In solid tumors, cytogenetic analysis is clinically less important, in part because of lack of sufficient data and in part because of the extreme complexity of the karyotypic changes. There is a great hope that the diagnostic impact of cytogenetic analysis will increase with the growing number of tumors investigated. Indications that cytogenetic analysis may also be helpful in prognostication in solid tumors have emerged in recent years (reviewed in Heim and Mitelman 1991). The cytogenetic findings should be interpreted together with histopathologic information. Cytogenetic analysis may be diagnostically useful particularly in mesenchymal tumors. In small, round cell tumors in children, a difficult differential diagnostic situation, cytogenetics may help to discriminate between Ewing's sarcoma/neuroepithelioma [t(11;22)], neuroblastoma [del(1p) and amplification shown as homogeneously staining regions or dmin], rhabdomyosarcoma [t(2;13)], and malignant lymphoma (various other aberrations). Fast, preoperative diagnosis by cytology and cytogenetics on samples obtained through fine-needle aspiration has been successful in smaller series of cases of Ewing's sarcoma and osteosarcoma. Thereby, open biopsy before operation can be avoided.

The generally held view that clonal acquired chromosome aberrations indicate a neoplastic process may be challenged by some recent findings (Limon et al. 1990, Lindström et al. 1991, Salk 1982, Scappaticci et al. 1989). Trisomy 7 has frequently been found in the cytogenetic analysis of tumors from the brain, lung, kidney, and intestines, sometimes as the sole anomaly. In at least malignant glioma and renal cell carcinoma, it has been revealed that +7 is rarely present in the clones that carry structural chromosome changes, i.e., those cells certainly representing the neoplasm. Moreover, trisomy 7 has been found also in nonneoplastic tissue from patients with carcinoma of the lung, kidney, large bowel, and malignant brain tumor, as well as in tissue from kidney and liver from patients without a neoplasm. An extra chromosome 7 has also been found in cultures from Dupuytren's contracture and placenta. Besides these simple numerical changes, clonal structural aberrations have been detected in patients with certain inherited disorders predisposing to cancer: ataxia telangiectasia, Werner's syndrome, porokeratosis of Mibelli, and Gorlin's syndrome. Similar findings have been reported from a few cases of tissue from the upper aerodigestive tract and sun-exposed skin. The significance of these findings is at present not clear.

Summary

Benign as well as malignant neoplasms are characterized by nonrandom chromosome aberrations. Of the more than 14 000 karyotypically abnormal neoplasms reported, only one-fifth is solid tumors, and four-fifths is hematologic disorders and lymphomas. The most common aberrations in various groups of neoplasms are briefly reviewed. The consistency and specificity of the chromosome changes make them useful as diagnostic and prognostic parameters, particularly in hematologic disorders. Cytogenetic analysis is also useful in the monitoring of remission and relapse and may at times be more sensitive than morphological examination. The finding of clonal, acquired chromosome aberrations is generally accepted as a sign of a neoplastic process, although recent findings of clonal changes in nonneoplastic tissue may challenge this opinion.

References

Heim S (1990) Cytogenetics in the investigation of haematological disorders. Baillières Clin Haematol 3:921–948

Heim S, Mitelman F (1987) Cancer cytogenetics. Liss, New York

Heim S, Mitelman F (1991) Cytogenetics of solid tumours. Recent Adv Histopathol (in press)

ISCN (1985) An international system for human cytogenetic nomenclature. Birth Defects 21(1)

Limon J, Mrózek K, Heim S, Elfving P, Nedoszytko B, Babinska M, Mandahl N, Lundgren R, Mitelman F (1990) On the significance of trisomy 7 and sex chromosome loss in renal cell carcinoma. Cancer Genet Cytogenet 49:259–263

Lindström E, Salford LG, Heim S, Mandahl N, Strömblad S, Brun A, Mitelman F (1991) Trisomy 7 and sex chromosome loss need not be representative of tumor parenchyma cells in malignant glioma. Genes Chromosomes Cancer (in press)

Mitelman F (1991) Catalog of chromosome aberrations in cancer, 4th edn. Wiley-Liss, New York

Mitelman F, Heim S (1988) Consistent involvement of only 71 of the 329 chromosomal bands of the human genome in primary neoplasia-associated rearrangements. Cancer Res 48:7115–7119

Mitelman F, Heim S (1990) Chromosome abnormalities in cancer. Cancer Detect Prev 14: 527–537

Mitelman F, Kaneko Y, Trent JM (1990) Report of the committee on chromosome changes in neoplasia. Cytogenet Cell Genet 55:358–386

Rowley JD (1988) Chromosome abnormalities in leukemia. J Clin Oncol 6:194–202

Salk D (1982) Werner's syndrome: a review of recent research with an analysis of connective tissue metabolism, growth control of cultured cells, and chromosomal aberrations. Hum Genet 62:1–5

Sandberg AA, Turc-Carel C, Gemmill RM (1988) Chromosomes in solid tumors and beyond. Cancer Res 48:1049–1059

Sandberg AA (1990) The chromosomes in human cancer and leukemia, 2nd edn. Elsevier, New York

Scappaticci S, Lambiase S, Orecchia G, Fraccaro M (1989) Clonal chromosome abnormalities with preferential involvement of chromosome 3 in patients with porokeratosis of Mibelli. Cancer Genet Cytogenet 43:89–94

Amplified *N-myc* Gene
as a Genetic Marker for the Prognosis
of Human Neuroblastoma

M. Schwab

Introduction

Cytogenetic analyses have brought to light the frequency of DNA amplification
in tumor cells and have provided a starting point to define the contribution for
tumorigenesis that comes from an increase of the dosage of cellular oncogenes
by amplification. Chromosomal abnormalities associated with DNA amplification are mainly of two types: double minutes (DMs), originally discovered
in direct preparations of human neuroblastoma cells (Cox et al. 1965) and
homogeneously staining chromosomal regions (HSRs), again detected in
neuroblastoma cells (Biedler and Spengler 1976). In metaphase spreads, DMs
appear as small, spherical, usually paired, chromosome-like structures that lack
a centromere and may contain circular DNA in chromatin form. HSRs stain
with intermediate intensity throughout their length rather than with the normal
pattern of alternating dark and light bands in trypsin-Giemsa-stained preparations. Both kinds of abnormalities contain amplified DNA and are found in
metaphases of freshly isolated cancer cells, but not of normal cells (Barker
1982). Exact data about the frequency of DMs and HSRs in tumor cells in vivo
are difficult to obtain since the abnormalities are easily missed in routine
cytogenetic analysis. DMs and HSRs have been described in most types of in
vitro cultured malignant cells.

Initial growth in cell culture apparently selects for tumor cells that contain
either DMs or HSRs. Moreover, in culture the DMs are frequently lost,
concomitant with the appearance of clonal population of cells that have developed a HSR, suggesting that the two cytogenetic abnormalities are alternative
forms of gene amplification. It has been assumed that HSRs can break down
to form DMs and that DMs can integrate into chromosomes to generate
HSRs (Cowell 1982). However, this hypothesis lacks experimental evidence.
Amplified genes may also occupy abnormally banding regions (ABRs) and C
bandless chromosomes (CMs) (Levan and Levan 1982; Alitalo et al. 1984;
Schwab et al. 1985a).

Experimental work on drug-resistant cells has shown that in the absence of
a selection pressure, the DMs and the amplified genes contained within are
lost, whereas amplified DNA in the form of HSRs is retained in the cells
(for a review, see Schimke 1984). This is explained by the fact that DMs are
segregated unevenly in mitosis and are frequently lost from the nucleus due to
their lack of centromeres (Levan and Levan 1982). HSR chromosomes carry

centromeres and are therefore divided equally between daughter cells at mitosis. If DMs and HSRs contain amplified genes that encode drug-resistant or growth-stimulating protein products, it would follow that the more stable chromosomal form, the HSR, confers a greater selective growth advantage for cells.

The same gene can be amplified either chromosomally or extra-chromosomally within a cell population, but the intrachromosomal and extra-chromosomal forms do not usually co-exist within the same cell. However, a few exceptions to this rule have been described (Gudkov and Kopnin 1987). Although DMs and HSRs have been described predominantly in tumor cells selected for resistance to cytotoxic drugs, it is also clear that they can be present in cancer before the start of therapy.

Cytogenetic manifestations for DNA amplification in settings unrelated to drug resistance have been encountered as yet exclusively in tumor cells. They do not seem to be restricted to vertebrate cells but have been found in malignant cells of insects as well (Mukhergee and Krawczum 1983). Among solid human tumors, DMs and HSRs can be seen in virtually any type, at least in some cases, and detection is usually a matter of patience. The chance to detect DMs or HSRs is increased when tumor cells are established in culture and when cells carrying amplification are selected for. In no instance has amplification been found as a tissue culture artifact. Detection of DMs and HSRs in direct preparations of solid tumors is often difficult. This may be due either to the general difficulty of obtaining good karyotypes from solid tumors or to the heterogeneity of tumor cells. It is well established that tumor cell populations are heterogeneous for many characteristics, and it is possible that amplification varies among members. For instance, growth in peripheral regions of the tumor could be subjected to selective forces different from those that operate in a more central environment. Failure to detect amplified DNA in a particular type of tumor by analyzing DNA with known gene probes does not exclude the presence of amplified DNA. We should be open to the possibility that the human genome contains genes involved in growth control in addition to the 50 or so that have been identified and designated "cellular oncogenes." Identifying and defining amplified DNA in tumor cells could be a strategy for the isolation of additional cellular genes involved in growth control and possibly in tumorigenesis.

The first instance of oncogene amplification concerned the cellular oncogene *MYC* and was originally observed in the human cell line HL-60 (Collins and Groudine 1982; Dalla-Favera et al. 1982). This was thought to represent an exceptional situation, however. A more systematic study ensued when tumor cells that carried cytogenetic manifestations for amplified DNA, DMs, CMs, or HSRs, were surveyed for amplified cellular oncogenes. The tumor cells containing DMs, CMs, or HSRs also consistently revealed amplified cellular oncogenes. The list of amplified oncogenes includes among others *ABL*, *KRAS1*, *KRAS2*, *MYC*, *N-myc*, *L-myc*, *NRAS*, *MYB*, *EGFR*, *ERBB2*, *GLI* and *HST*, with copy numbers ranging from 5 to 700.

N-myc Amplification in Neuroblastomas

N-myc was the first amplified oncogene that turned out to be of clinical significance due to its association with aggressively growing tumor phenotypes (for a review see Schwab 1985, 1986). *N-myc* was originally identified when human neuroblastoma cells showing DMs or HSRs were analyzed with various oncogene probes (Schwab et al. 1983; Kohl et al. 1983). These surveys quickly established that, with few exceptions, cultured neuroblastoma cell lines carry the gene *N-myc* in amplified form. At the same time, neuroblastoma tumors were also found to carry amplified *N-myc* (Schwab et al. 1983). The initial surveys suggested that *N-myc* amplification was specific for neuroblastoma. It turned out later that *N-myc* amplification can be seen in small cell lung cancer, retinoblastoma, malignant gliomas, and peripheral neuroectodermal tumors (PNETs), although at a much lower incidence. As a common feature, all these tumors have neural qualities. Until now, however, *N-myc* has been the only gene found amplified in neuroblastomas.

The oncogenic potential of enhanced expression of *N-myc* as the consequence of amplification has been addressed in various experimental systems. Enhanced expression resulting after introduction of *N-myc* expression vector can assist mutationally activated HRAS in tumorigenic conversion of primary rat embryo cells (Schwab et al. 1985b), converts established cells of the rat (Small et al. 1987) and of humans (Schweigerer et al. 1990) to tumorigenicity, and rescues primary rat embryo cells (Schwab and Bishop 1988) and neural precursor cells (Bernard et al. 1989) from senescence. Furthermore, *N-myc* has frequently been found activated by proviral insertion in MuLV-induced T-cell lymphomas (van Lohuizen et al. 1989) and is involved in tumorigenesis in transgenic mice (Dildrop et al. 1989; Rosenbaum et al. 1989). These results clearly attest to the capacity of high *N-myc* expression to modulate the growth of cells, and it appears reasonable, therefore, to suggest that enhanced expression consequent to amplification contributes to tumorigenesis. The available evidence suggests that the nucleotide sequence of *N-myc* in neuroblastoma cells is unaltered compared with that of normal cells (Ibson and Rabbits 1988). Consistent with this result, the biological activities of *N-myc* derived from normal or from neuroblastoma cells have not been found to differ (Schwab et al. 1985; Schwab and Bishop 1988).

Structural Arrangement of Amplified *N-myc*

A direct determination of the size and the structure of the amplified DNA in human neuroblastoma cells has been done by pulsed field gel electrophoresis, which is capable of fractionating DNA fragments in the size range from 100 to several thousand kbp. The analysis was facilitated by the finding that the 5'-region of *N-myc* is a CpG island and has recognition sequences for several rare cutting enzymes (Amler and Schwab 1989). This situation made it possible to

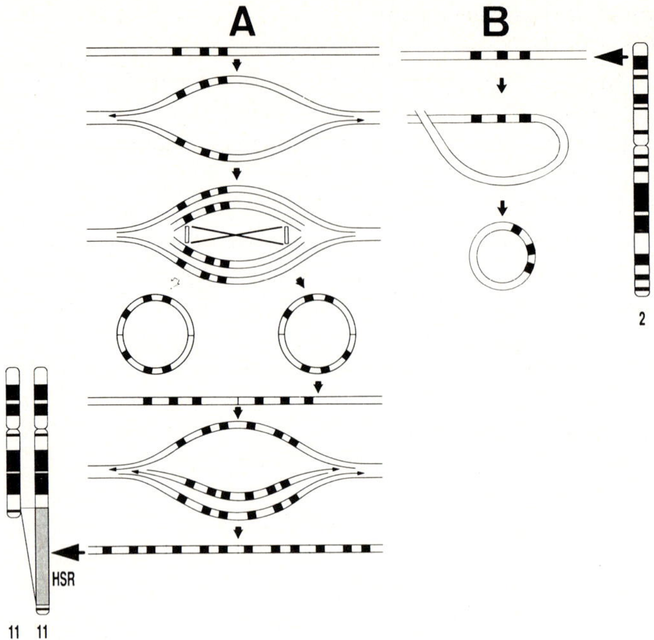

Fig. 1A,B. Models illustrating amplification of *N-myc* in neuroblastoma cells. Amplification starts when DNA becomes extrareplicated (**A**) or when DNA becomes excised following loop formation (**B**). The extrachromosomal DNA is integrated into a chromosome, where it may undergo in situ amplification to yield tandem DNA amplicons that can be cytogenetically demonstrated as an homogenously staining chromosomal region (*HSR*)

map the DNA encompassing *N-myc* over a distance of more than 1000 kbp. By employing suitable *N-myc* probes derived from the 5′- and 3′-region of recognition sites for rare cutting restriction endonucleases with *N-myc*, the amplified DNA was found in most cases arranged in precise head-to-tail units. These units varied in length among different neuroblastomas and ranged from about 100 to 800 kbp in size (Amler and Schwab 1989). The precise and ordered head-to-tail arrangement is stable over long periods of time and does not change upon establishment of tumor cells in culture or during passages of tumor cells through athymic mice.

There are principally two mechanisms that might be involved in the initiation of amplification. Amplification may start with the unscheduled replication of DNA encompassing *N-myc* which maps to chromosome 2p23–24 (Schwab et al. 1984) (Fig. 1A). Alternatively, amplification may start with loop formation and excision of the DNA (Fig. 1B). In either event, extrachromosomal DNA molecules appear to result that integrate into a distant chromosomal region and undergo in situ amplification (for a detailed discussion, see Schwab 1990). The amplified *N-myc* copies in neuroblastoma cell lines map in most instances to HSRs that are localized on different chromosomes in cells derived from different tumors.

Table 1. Risk groups in neuroblastoma and *N-myc* amplification (criteria according to the pilot protocol of the German Neuroblastoma Study Group NB90P)

Risk group (% survival)	Tumor
A (90%–100%)	Tumor localized, almost completely resectable
	Stage 1; microscopic residual tumor acceptable
	Stage 2; minimal macroscopic residual tumor acceptable; <10%
	Patients with amplification positive tumors are excluded
B (65%–80%)	Tumor localized, usually incomplete resection
	Stage 2A; macroscopic residual tumor; <10%
	Stage 2B; ipsilateral lymph nodes positive
	Stage 3; infiltration beyond median
	Patients with amplification positive tumors are excluded
C (20%–30%)	Tumor metastatic
	Risk groups A and B in case amplification is positive
D (75%–80%)	Stage 4s

Clinical Significance of *N-myc* Amplification

An important prognostic variable for patients with neuroblastoma is the clinical stage. Patients with disease stages I and II have a good prognosis with 75%–90% 2-year disease-free survival, while patients with stages III and IV have a poor prognosis with 10%–30% 2-year survival. Surveys of several hundred neuroblastomas revealed that a strong correlation exists between *N-myc* amplification and stages III and IV (Bartram and Berthold 1987; Brodeur et al. 1984; Nakagawara et al. 1988; Seeger et al. 1985). A number of patients have been identified with stages I or II carrying amplification. In all instances these tumors which on the basis of conventional diagnostic possibilities were of good prognosis, progressed later and turned out to be fatal. A peculiar stage IVs characterized by frequently spontaneous regression rarely shows amplification (7%); three cases with *N-myc* amplification have been published (Carlsen et al. 1986; Cohn et al. 1987; Tonini et al. 1987), and all tumors underwent progression. These observation clearly show that *N-myc* amplification is a reliable prognostic parameter for a poor prognosis in patients with low stage or IVs tumors.

Current therapeutic strategies for the treatment of neuroblastoma depend on the prognosis for survival which is evaluated on the basis of tumor stage, on the degree to which the tumor can be removed surgically, and on the basis of genomic analyses of the tumor cells. The pilot study of the German Neuroblastoma Study Group advises treatment of patients according to protocols that are specific for each of four risk groups (Table 1). Risk group A included patients with a localized tumor that can be surgically removed to at least 90% (prognosis 90%–100% for survival of patients). Risk group B includes patients with a localized tumor that extends beyond the area of the organ of origin and usually cannot be removed completely (prognosis 65%–80%). Risk group C includes patients who carry a metastatic tumor or a localized tumor that cannot be removed after four cycles of chemotherapy (prognosis 20%–30%). Risk group D includes only patients with a stage IVs tumor that frequently shows spontaneous regression (prognosis 75%–80%). Patients that on the basis of conventional parameters would be included in risk groups A and B are transferred to risk group C if there is *N-myc* amplification. Patients included in risk group C receive the most intensive treatment. It remains to be seen whether or not the same is advisable for patients of risk group D.

Chromosome 1p Deletion

In addition to amplification, a larger proportion of neuroblastomas carry non-random deletion at chromosome 1p. Deletions of chromosome 1p were first described in 1973 (Biedler et al. 1973). Even though the breakpoints of the deletion were found to vary, the portion of the chromosome distal to band p32 seemed to be most consistently deleted (Brodeur et al. 1981). In all cases, the deletions appear to involve only one chromosome. From cytogenetic analyses the portion deleted appears to be lost from the genome, which means that the cells are monosomic for this genetic material (Brodeur et al. 1981). At this point, the nature of the genetic material deleted and its significance to tumorigenesis can only be the subject of speculation. There is a good possibility that the deletion involves genetic information essential for the normal differentiation of certain neutral cells. Loss of this gene could result in abnormal differentiation and could be a factor contributing to tumorigenesis. In a similar way, lack of genetic information identified by cytogenetic analysis in specific regions of other chromosomes seems to contribute to other types of tumors, in particular Wilms' tumor, retinoblastoma, lung cancer, and certain forms of colon cancer (for a review, see Hansen and Cavanee 1987). The general idea is that presence of this genetic information suppresses tumorigenesis, and its lack allows tumors to develop. Genes behaving as suppressors of tumorigenesis have been termed "tumor suppressor genes," but their functions and the mechanisms by which they contribute to tumorigenesis are largely obscure. In pursuit of defining the role that loss of genetic information from 1p36 might have in neuroblastoma, the frequency and the architecture of the deletion were analyzed. The approach chosen depended on first generating a panel of DNA probes closely positioned to each other by generating a micro-clone library specific for the distal part of chromosome 1p (Martinsson et al. 1989). The dense distribution of probes should be advantageous for this study in different respects. Firstly, small deletions should be detectable with a higher probability. Secondly, it should provide the ability to detect allelic loss even in cases where adjacent loci were not informative due to homozygosity. Thirdly, it should be possible to define the borders of deleted regions within narrow limits and to determine a small region commonly deleted in different tumors.

Applying this strategy, it was possible to discover allelic deletions in a high proportion of tumors (at least 90%) analyzed. These studies revealed that

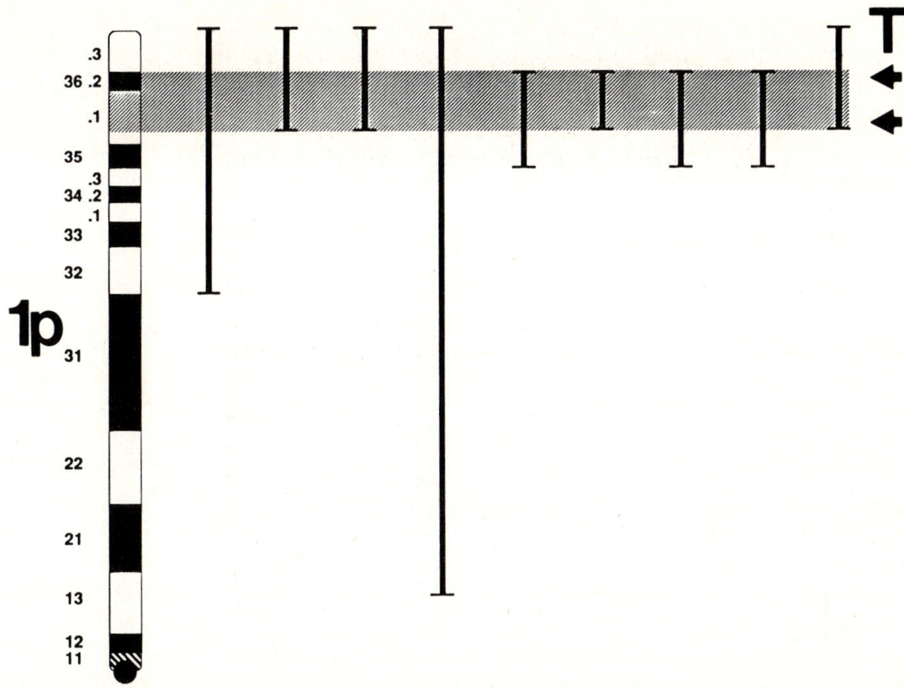

Fig. 2. Deletion of chromosome 1p in neuroblastomas. Although the size of the deletion differs among various neuroblastomas, the smallest overlapping deletion at 1p36.1–2 can be identified. This region is also the size of recurrent translocation breakpoints in neuroblastomas (*arrows*)

distal 1p material indeed was lost from the genome of the tumor cells (Weith et al. 1989). In another study of chromosomal deletions in neuroblastomas (Fong et al. 1989), loss of heterozygosity was also detected in 1p36, though the frequency described was lower (28%) than indicated by cytogenetic analyses. The higher overall frequency of loss of genetic material from the 1p region among stages III and IV tumors as compared with the frequency found by Fong et al. (28% vs. 90%) is probably due to the fact that probes generated by microcloning are from within the consensus deletion and are located closer to the putative tumor suppressor gene related to neuroblastoma. The number of tumors displaying allelic loss with these probes exceeded that showing cytogenetically detectable rearrangements. One may suspect that small deletions are likely to remain undetectable upon microscopic investigation.

Several tumors carried interstitial 1p deletion (Weith et al. 1989) that allowed the delineation of the smallest region of overlap at subbands 1p36.1–2 (Fig. 2). A rough estimate can be made as to the size of this deleted DNA segment. The entire 1p36 band comprises about 0.7% of the total haploid chromosome length. Predicting an even distribution of the DNA along the chromosomes, 1p36 would contain about 20 Mbp (megabase pairs) of DNA

(0.7% of the total 3×10^9 bp as the haploid DNA content). 1p36.1–1p36.2 represents roughly half of the 1p36 band. Hence, the genomic region included in the common deletion would span about 10 Mbp of DNA. Future studies should result in establishing a long-range restriction map of this region with pulsed field gel electrophoresis. This long-range map will provide information on the presence and location of CpG-rich islands, which often signify the 5′-regions of genes (Bird 1987) and therefore will be a tool for the identification of coding DNA sequences in this region.

Conclusions

Research into the molecular biology of human cancers is presently pursued under chiefly three perspectives. First is the aim to identify the types of genetic alteration within the framework of the cancer cell and to find out if particular genetic alterations occur at random or define specific forms of cancer. Second, it appears important to find out if tumor-specific genetic alterations can be employed as diagnostic tools to determine the prognosis and to aid in the design of existing therapeutical regimens. Third, the functions of cellular oncogenes and tumor suppressor genes have to be defined to identify their role in normal and malignant growth and to find avenues for causal therapies. Understanding the mechanisms of oncogene function might enable us to design antagonists against abnormal oncogene activity.

Cytogenetic studies of human and animal cancer cells have brought to light the presence of chromosomal abnormalities diagnostic for the presence of amplified DNA and have provided an entrance point for molecular studies of various human cancers. Evidence is emerging now that between 20% and 30% of certain solid tumors carry amplified cellular oncogenes. Amplification does not affect cellular oncogenes at random. There appears to be a preference for members of the *myc* gene family (*myc*, *N-myc*, or *L-myc*) and the *EGF*-receptor family (*EGFR* or *ERB*B2) to become amplified. The basis for the preferential amplification of genes encoding either nuclear phosphoproteins or cell surface receptors is unknown. Amplification of cellular oncogenes has been found associated with particularly malignant versions of certain human cancers and for this reason is of predictive value for evaluating the course the disease might take. This is especially true for neuroblastoma and breast cancer. The amplification of *N-myc* in neuroblastomas is an independent parameter for identifying patients that require an intensive therapeutic regimen.

Although the amplification of cellular oncogenes is associated with more aggressively growing forms of cancer, it is unclear at which stage of tumorigenesis amplification comes into play. Is amplification an early or a late event during tumorigenesis? There are indications that amplification is present from early on in certain tumors, such as neuroblastomas, and therefore, may be an early event. But for other tumors the situation is less clear, and it remains to be determined whether amplification is an element in initiation or in progression.

Structural analyses have revealed that most of the amplified DNA encompassing the gene *N-myc* in neuroblastomas is arranged in a surprisingly regular fashion. This regular arrangement, which is stable over many cell generations, is quite in contrast to the usually heterogeneous and unstable arrangement of amplified DNA in cells resistant to cytotoxic drugs. It is unclear at this moment whether or not the different arrangements of amplified DNA-encompassing oncogenes or drug-resistance genes reflect different mechanisms of DNA amplification. But it is also unclear whether or not other cellular oncogenes like *ERB*B2 in breast cancer cells are arranged as regularly as the *N-myc* gene.

There are principally three reasons why we should attribute etiological significance to gene amplification in cancer cells. First, amplification increases the copy number of cellular genes whose ability to alter the growth pattern has been demonstrated in other settings; second, amplification of cellular oncogenes is often a recurrent genetic abnormality in cancer cells that have a particularly aggressive growth behavior, as if amplification was the cause and malignant growth the consequence; and, third, amplified DNA persists during countless rounds of cell divisions as if providing a selective advantage to the host cell within a particular tissue architecture. Altogether, genetic damage by DNA amplification encompassing cellular oncogenes appears to occupy an important place in the development of at least many forms of human cancers.

Summary

Increased dosage of cellular oncogenes resulting from amplification of DNA is a frequent genetic abnormality of tumor cells. Certain types of human tumors carry a specific amplified cellular oncogene at frequencies of up to 50%–60%. Human neuroblastoma has been prototypic for a contribution of amplification to tumorigenesis, and evidence is emerging that amplification may be an early event involved in a malignant form of this cancer. It is unclear at which stage amplification plays a role in other cancers. Amplification of cellular oncogenes is a good predictor for clinical outcome in some human malignancies and is a paradigm for the application of oncogene research in a clinical context. In particular, the amplification of the gene *N-myc*, which was the first gene identified nonrandomly in a human cancer, is a reliable genetic alteration indicating a poor prognosis independent of other clinical parameters.

References

Alitalo K, Winqvist R, Lin CC, de la Chapelle A, Schwab M, Bishop JM (1984) Aberrant expression of an amplified c-*myb* oncogene in two cell lines from a colon carcinoma. Proc Natl Acad Sci USA 81:4534

Amler LC, Schwab M (1989) Amplified *N-myc* in human neuroblastoma cells is often arranged as clustered tandem repeats of differently recombined DNA. Mol Cell Biol 9:4903–4913

Barker P (1982) Double minutes in human tumor cells. Cancer Genet Cytogenet 5:81

Bartram CR, Berthold F (1987) Amplification and expression of the *N-myc* gene in neuroblastoma. Eur J Pediatr 146:162–165

Bernard O, Reid H, Bartlett PF (1989) Role of the c-*myc* and *N-myc* protooncogenes in the immortalization of neural precursors. J Neurosci Res 24:9

Biedler JL, Spengler BA (1976) Metaphase chromosome anomaly: association with drug resistance and cell-specific products. Science 191:185

Biedler JL, Helson L, Spengler BS (1973) Morphology and growth, tumorigenicity, and cytogenetics of human neuroblastoma cells in continuous culture. Cancer Res 33:2643–2652

Bird A (1987) CpG islands as gene markers in the vertebrate nucleus. Trends Genet 3:342–347

Brodeur GM, Green AA, Hayes FA, Williams KJ, Williams DL, Tsiatis AA (1981) Cytogenetic features of human neuroblastomas and cell lines. Cancer Res 41:4678–4686

Brodeur G, Seeger RC, Schwab M, Varmus HE, Bishop JM (1984) Amplification of *N-myc* in untreated human neuroblastomas correlates with advanced disease stage. Science 224:1121–1124

Carlsen NLT, Christensen IJ, Schroeder H, Bro PV, Hesselberg K, Jensen KB, Nielsen KH (1986) Prognostic value of different staging systems in neuroblastomas and completeness of tumour exision. Arch Dis Child 61:832–842

Cohn SL, Herst CV, Maurer HS, Rosen ST (1987) *N-myc* amplification in an infant with stage IV-s neuroblastoma. J Clin Oncol 5:1441–1444

Collins S, Groudine M (1982) Amplification of endogenous *myc*-related DNA sequences in a human myeloid leukaemia cell line. Nature 298:670

Cowell JK (1982) Double minutes and homogeneously staining chromosomal regions: gene amplification in mammalian cells. Annu Rev Genet 16:21

Cox D, Yuncken C, Spriggs A (1965) Minute chromatin bodies in malignant tumours of childhood. Lancet 2:55

Dalla-Favera R, Wong-Staal F, Gallo RC (1982) *onc* Gene amplification in promyelocytic leukaemia cell line HL-60 and primary cells of the same patient. Nature 299:63

Dildrop R, Ma A, Zimmermann K, Hsu E, Tesfaye A, de Pinoh R, Alt F (1989) IgH enhancer-mediated deregulation of *N-myc* gene expression in transgenic mice: generation of lymphoid neoplasias that lack c-*myc* expression. EMBO J 8:1121

Fong CT, Dracopoli NC, White P, Merrill PT, Griffith RC, Housman DE, Brodeur GM (1989) Loss of heterozygosity for the short arm of chromosome 1 in human neuroblastomas; correlation with *N-myc* amplification. Proc Natl Acad Sci USA 86:3753–3757

Gudkov AV, Kopnin BP (1987) Gene amplification and multidrug resistance. Sov Sci Rev [D] 7:95

Hansen MF, Cavanee WK (1987) Genetics of cancer predisposition. Cancer Res 47:5518–5527

Ibson JM, Rabbits PH (1988) Sequence of a germ-line *N-myc* gene and amplification as a mechanism of activation. Oncogene 2:399

Kohl N, Kanda K, Schreck PR, Bruns G, Latt S, Gilbert F, Alt F (1983) Transposition and amplification of oncogene related sequence in human neuroblastomas. Cell 35:359

Levan G, Levan A (1982) Transitions of double minutes into homogeneously staining regions and C-bandless chromosomes in the SEWA tumor. In: Schimke RT (ed) Gene amplification. Cold Spring Harbor Press, Cold Spring Harbor, p 91

Martinsson T, Weith A, Cziepluch C, Schwab M (1989) Chromosome 1 deletions in human neuroblastomas: generation and fine mapping of microclones from the distal 1p region. Genes Chromosomes Cancer 1:67–78

Mukhergee AB, Krawczum MS (1983) Double minutes and other chromosomal aberrations in two malignant cell lines of the German cockroach, *Blatella germanica*. Cancer Genet Cytogenet 10:11

Nakagawara A, Ikeda K, Tsuda T, Higashi K (1988) Biological chracteristics of *NMYC* amplified neuroblastoma in patients over one year of age. In: Evans A, d'Angio G, Knudson AG, Seeger RC (eds) Advances in neuroblastoma research. Liss, New York, pp 31–39

Rosenbaum H, Webb E, Adams JM, Cory S, Harris AW (1989) *N-myc* transgene promotes B lymphoid proliferation elicits lymphomas and reveals cross-regulation with c-*myc*. EMBO J 8:749

Schimke RT (1984) Gene amplification in cultured animal cells. Cell 37:705

Schwab M (1985) Amplification of *N-myc* in human neuroblastomas. Trends Genet 1:271

Schwab M (1986) Amplification of proto-oncogenes and tumor progression. In: Kahn P, Graf T (eds) Oncogenes and growth control. Springer, Berlin Heidelberg New York, pp 332

Schwab M (1990) Oncogene amplification during tumor development and progression. Crit Rev Oncog 2:35–51

Schwab M, Bishop JM (1988) Sustained expression of the human protooncogene *MYCN* rescues rat embryo cells from senescence. Proc Natl Acad Sci USA 85:9585

Schwab M, Alitalo K, Klempnauer KH, Varmus HE, Bishop JM, Gilbert F, Brodeur G, Goldstein M, Trent J (1983) Amplified DNA with limited homology to *myc* cellular oncogene is shared by human neuroblastoma cell lines and a neuroblastoma tumor. Nature 305:245

Schwab M, Varmus HE, Bishop JM, Grzeschik KH, Sakaguchi A, Brodeur G, Trent J (1984) Chromosome localization in normal human cells and neuroblastomas of a gene related to c-*myc*. Nature 308:288–291

Schwab M, Ramsay G, Alitalo K, Varmus H, Bishop JM, Martinsson T, Levan G, Levan A (1985a) Amplification and enhanced expression of the c-*myc* oncogene in mouse SEWA tumor cells. Nature 315:345

Schwab M, Varmus HE, Bishop JM (1985b) The human *N-myc* gene contributes to tumorigenic conversion of mammalian cells in culture. Nature 316:160

Schweigerer L, Breit S, Wenzel A, Tsunamoto K, Ludwig R, Schwab M (1990) Augmented *MYCN* expression advances the malignant phenotype of human tumor cells. Cancer Res 50:4411–4416

Seeger RC, Brodeur GM, Sather H, Dalton A, Siegel WE, Wong KY, Hammond D (1985) Association of multiple copies of the *N-myc* oncogene with rapid progression of neuroblastomas. N Engl J Med 313:111–116

Small M, Hay N, Schwab M, Bishop JM (1987) Neoplastic transformation by the human gene *N-myc*. Mol Cell Biol 7:1638

Tonini GP, Verdona G, de Bernardi B, Sansone R, Massimo L, Cornaglia-Ferraris P (1987) *N-myc* oncogene amplification in a patient with IV-s neuroblastoma. Am J Pediatr Hematol Oncol 9:8–10

Van Lohuizen M, Breuer M, Berns A (1989) *N-myc* is frequently activately by proviral insertion in MuLV-induced T cell lymphomas. EMBO J 8:133

Weith A, Martinsson T, Cziepluch C, Brüderlein S, Amler LC, Berthold F, Schwab M (1989) Neuroblastoma consensus deletion maps to chromosome 1p36.1–2. Genes Chromosomes Cancer 1:159–166

Beckwith-Wiedemann Syndrome, Tumorigenesis and Imprinting

C. Junien

The Unusual Genetics of Beckwith-Wiedemann Syndrome

The Beckwith-Wiedemann syndrome (BWS) occurs with an incidence of 1 in 13 700 live births and is characterized by numerous growth abnormalities, including exomphalos, macroglossia, visceromegaly and gigantism. These features show variable expression and can be found in association with multiple abnormalities including neonatal hypoglycemia, ear lobe creases and pits, and hemihypertrophy. The clinical findings in BWS patients are highly variable, tending to become less distinctive with age. The syndrome may therefore be underdiagnosed in adults. An increased incidence (7.5%) of different types of childhood tumors is observed, including the following tumors: Wilms' tumor (59%), adrenocortical carcinoma (15%) and a few instances of hepatoblastoma, rhabdomyosarcoma and neuroblastoma (Wiedemann 1983). Hemihypertrophy, nephrogenic rest, Wilms' tumor and BWS commonly occur together.

Although 85% of cases of BWS are sporadic, BWS can also occur in association with a duplication of region 11p15.5 and in familial forms. The mode of transmission is apparently autosomal dominant with a threefold excess of female transmitters. This can be explained by reduced fecundity and higher penetrance when the defect is transmitted via the maternal line (Moutou et al. 1991). Interestingly, eight cases of monozygotic twins with BWS have been reported and all were discordant for the syndrome. The involvement of region 11p15 is based on three types of observations: (1) more than a dozen reported cases presented with constitutional duplications of region 11p15 resulting either from de novo rearrangements or from malsegregation of balanced paternal translocations; (2) linkage analysis using 11p15 markers revealed that the locus for the familial form also mapped to this region (Turleau and de Grouchy 1985; Koufos et al. 1989); (3) in three out of eight sporadic cases uniparental paternal disomy was observed (Henry et al. 1991).

Altogether, these findings suggest that genomic imprinting may explain the sex-dependence. This hypothesis is also strongly supported by the parental bias in losses of alleles observed in the different types of associated tumors, i.e. nephroblastoma, rhabdomyosarcoma, and adrenocortical carcinoma.

Tumorigenesis

Nephroblastoma

Nephroblastoma or Wilms' tumor (WT) of the kidney is an embryonal tumor which affects approximately 1 in 10 000 children. Although sporadic forms are the most frequent (95%), the occurrence of bilateral tumors in 8% of the cases suggests the presence of a predisposing germline event in an even greater number, probably due to new mutations. The scarcity of familial cases (2%) did not facilitate linkage analysis. The first hint of the location of a gene predisposing to WT came from the observation of children (1%) with the complex syndrome WAGR associated with a deletion of band 11p13.

Genetic Predisposition

Two regions on the short arm of chromosome 11 are involved in malformation syndromes associated with a predisposition to WT. First, the deletion of region 11p13 is associated with a predisposition to WT (W), aniridia (A), genitourinary (GU) abnormalities, and mental retardation (R) – the so-called WAGR syndrome (Francke et al. 1979). Second, as already discussed, region 11p15, contains a gene involved in BWS and in associated childhood tumors and in progression of several adult malignancies.

When markers for regions 11p13 and 11p15 were used to investigate the location of the gene involved in familial predisposition, both regions were excluded. This suggests that a third as yet unmapped locus, WT3, is involved in predisposition to WT (Huff et al. 1988; Grundy et al. 1988).

Predisposition to WT is associated with several other malformation syndromes, including Drash syndrome (Pelletier et al. 1991), hemihypertrophy (Mannens et al. 1988, Grundy et al. 1991) and genitourinary abnormalities (Junien 1986) (Table 1).

Chromosomal Rearrangements in Tumors

Cytogenetics

Cytogenetic analyses on WT have revealed that chromosomes other than 11 play an important role in tumorigenesis. Structural abnormalities of both arms of 1, 7, 16, and 17, as well as quantitative abnormalities including trisomy 12, 6, 8 and 18 (Wang-Wuu et al. 1990), are characteristic features of WT.

Losses of Alleles

By analogy with retinoblastoma (Cavenee et al. 1983), losses of alleles for markers mapping to the same 11p region as the genes for predisposition to WT were described (Koufos et al. 1984). However, due to the presence of two

Table 1. WT: different loci are involved in predisposition and progression

	Syndrome	Mode	Map localization
WT1	WAGR	Deletion	11p13
	DRASH	Mutation	
WT2	BWS	Duplication families disomy	11p15
?	Hemihypertrophy	disomy	11p15
WT3	Familial WT	Families	? (Not linked to 11p)

different loci and to limited informativeness of the markers it was not always possible to determine whether the loss of alleles corresponded to the loss of the second allele at the same locus. Some sporadic cases of WT have a loss of alleles limited to region 11p13, while other tumors show a loss of heterozygosity for markers within 11p15 but not 11p13 (Mannens et al. 1988). In three WAGR patients with a constitutional del11p13, the allele loss was limited to region 11p15 (Henry et al. 1989). This may suggest that, as with hereditary and non-hereditary forms of colon carcinoma, a cascade of multiple genetic events is involved in WT. Furthermore, in del11p13 patients the somatic loss of the unique WT1 allele may not be necessary for the tumor to develop. Unlike retinoblastoma, there are only five cases described to date with a homozygously deleted WT1 gene.

The loss of heterozygozity for region 11p15 is an event common to several childhood and adult tumors. This region may thus contain one or several genes involved in rhabdomyosarcomas (Scrable et al. 1987, 1989), testicular tumors (Lothe et al. 1989), renal cell carcinoma (Zbar et al. 1987), bladder cancer (Fearon et al. 1985) and breast cancer (Ali et al. 1987).

Genomic Imprinting and Tumorigenesis

Whenever identifiable, the 11p alleles lost in WT (26/27) and in rhabdomyo-sarcoma (6/6) were of maternal origin, and, although not fully demonstrated, the vast majority concerned region 11p15, not 11p13. This preferential retention of paternal alleles could have different explanations: first, hypermutability of paternal gametes; second, differential genomic imprinting. A preferential paternal origin for deletion of band 11p13 appearing as new mutations is the only observation arguing in favor of the first explanation, if the WT1 locus was the one affected by allele loss. More likely, and in favor of the second explanation, is the unusual parental allele involvement in the different etiologic forms of BWS: first, in cytogenetic forms of BWS the duplicated segment of 11p15 sequences was of paternal origin (11/12 cases), due to malsegregation of a paternal balanced translocation; second, in families with BWS there was a threefold excess of female carriers due not only to reduced fecundity in affected males but also to a higher probability of being affected when born to a

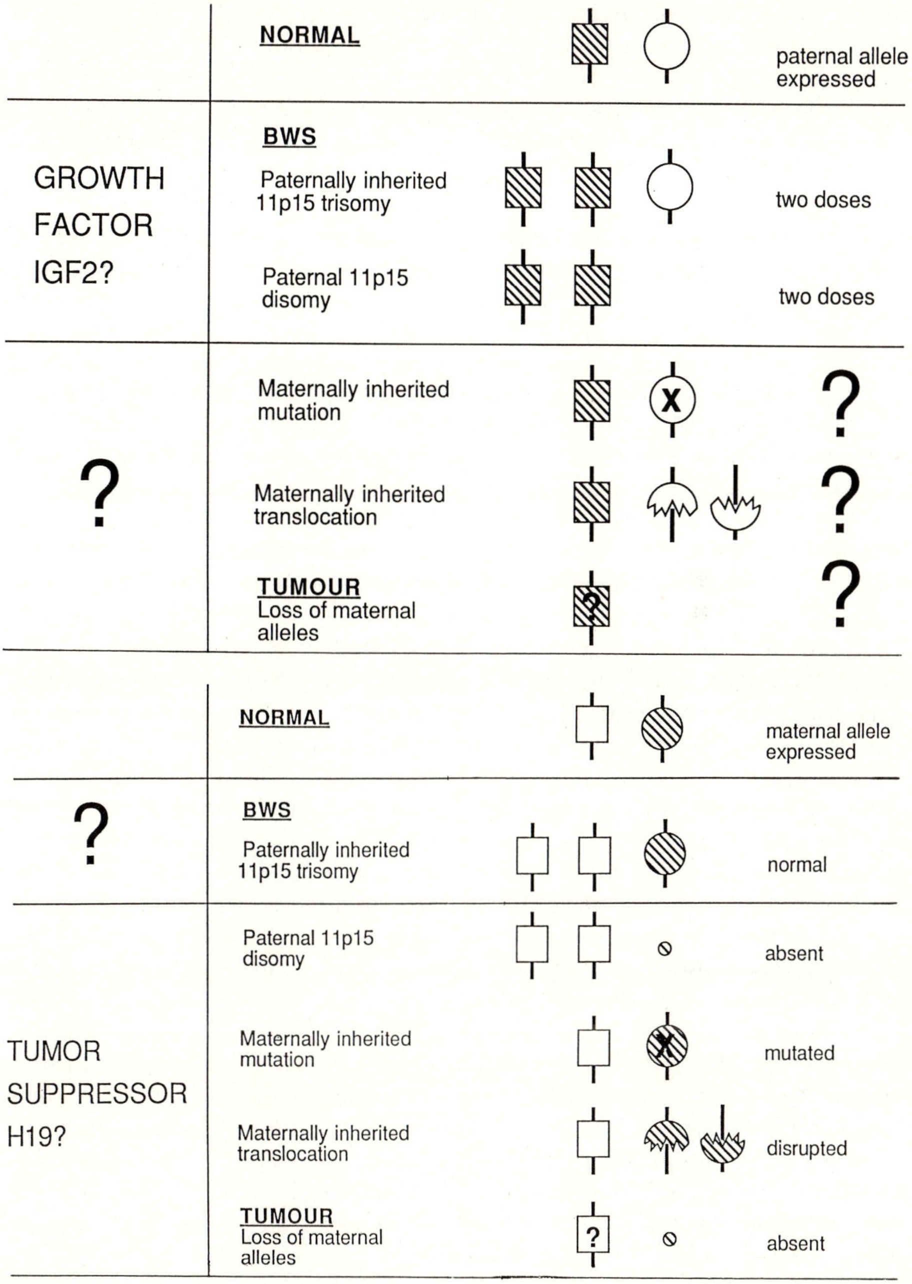

GROWTH FACTOR IGF2?
?
NORMAL
paternal allele expressed
BWS
Paternally inherited 11p15 trisomy
two doses
Paternal 11p15 disomy
two doses
Maternally inherited mutation
?
Maternally inherited translocation
?
TUMOUR
Loss of maternal alleles
?
NORMAL
maternal allele expressed
?
BWS
Paternally inherited 11p15 trisomy
normal
Paternal 11p15 disomy
absent
TUMOR SUPPRESSOR H19?
Maternally inherited mutation
mutated
Maternally inherited translocation
disrupted
TUMOUR
Loss of maternal alleles
absent

Figure 1

carrier woman (sex-dependent transmission) (Moutou et al. 1991); third, in sporadic cases of BWS uniparental paternal disomy limited to 11p15 markers was described in three of eight cases (Henry et al. 1991). Altogether, these observations suggest that the BWS locus undergoes genomic imprinting (Fig. 1).

However, the different observations are apparently contradictory under a single locus hypothesis. First, it can be proposed that the BWS/WT gene is a tumor suppressor gene expressed from the maternal allele (H19?). This explanation is in agreement with all observations except with the paternal duplication: it is difficult to admit that the duplication of a silent (paternal) allele could lead to an overgrowth syndrome. Second, it can be hypothesized that the BWS gene is a growth factor, expressed from the paternal allele (IGF2?). This hypothesis is incompatible with maternal transmission in familial cases and with the loss of the maternal allele in tumors, which would imply that the alteration or the loss of an inactive allele could be responsible for the observed phenotypes. Alternatively, other explanations could account for these findings: first, harmonious growth could be dependent on the strict balance of maternal and paternal alleles, implying that both alleles have to be active, at least during some stages of development or in specific cell types; second, BWS could be a so-called contiguous gene syndrome involving several interacting genes or genes with different patterns of imprinting.

Imprinting for two mouse genes, Igf2 and H19, has recently been demonstrated (DeChiara et al. 1991; Bartolomei et al. 1991). For H19, the expression is limited to the maternal allele, while for Igf2, only the paternal allele is expressed in a large majority of tissues examined. Interestingly, a duplication of the mouse region that carries these two closely linked genes leads to fetal overgrowth, a finding similar to that in BWS (Ferguson-Smith et al. 1991).

The isolation of the 11p15 WT/BWS locus will be necessary to test this concept and understand the nature of the underlying mechanisms. If a locus involved in tumorigenesis undergoes genomic imprinting, this would infer that the loss of the second allele is not necessary. This could be supported by the following observations: in WT, Poisson statistical analysis of the frequency of bilateral tumors predicts that 38% of all cases are hereditary (Knudson 1971); however, familial cases are estimated to represent approximately 2% of observed WT, while 8% of the victims develop bilateral tumors; Knudson's findings thus imply that the vast majority of bilateral cases as well as a portion of unilateral cases represent de novo germline mutations at either of the three loci for predisposition; alternatively, this may also suggest that imprinting of the 11p15 locus would require only one additional event, the loss of the maternal allele, for the tumor to develop. Imprinting would be the equivalent of the germline mutation in hereditary cases.

References

Ali IU, Lidereau R, Theillet C et al. (1987) Reduction to the homozygosity of genes on chromosome 11 in human breast neoplasia. Science 238:187

Bartolomei MS, Zemel S, Tilghman S (1991) Parental imprinting of the mouse H19 gene. Nature 351:153–155

Cavenee WK, Dryja P, Phillips et al. (1983) Expression of recessive alleles by chromosomal mechanisms in retinoblastoma. Nature 305:779–784

DeChiara TM, Robertson EJ, Efstratiadias A (1991) Parental imprinting of the mouse insulin-like growth factor II gene. Cell 64:849–859

Fearon ER, Feinberg AP, Hamilton SH et al. (1985) Loss of genes on the short arm of chromosome 11 in bladder cancer. Nature 381:377–380

Ferguson-Smith AC, Cattanach BM, Barton SC et al. (1991) Embryological and molecular investigations of parental imprinting on mouse chromosome 7. Nature 351:667–670

Francke U, Holmes LB, Atkins L et al. (1979) Aniridia-Wilms' tumor association: evidence for specific deletion of 11p13. Cytogenet Cell Genet 24:185–192

Grundy P, Koufos A, Morgan K et al. (1988) Familial predisposition to Wilms' tumor does not map to the short arm of chromosome 11. Nature 336:374–376

Grundy P, Telzerw P, Peterson MC, Haber D, Herman B, Li F, Garber L (1991) Chromosome 11 uniparental isodisomy predisposition to embryonal neoplasms. Lancet 338: 1079–1080

Henry I, Grandjouan S, Couillin P et al. (1989) Tumor-specific loss of 11p15.5 alleles in del11p13 Wilms' tumor and in familial adrenocortical carcinoma. Proc Natl Acad Sci USA 86:3247–3251

Henry I, Bonaïti-Pellié C, Chehensse V et al. (1991) Uniparental paternal disomy in sporadic Beckwith-Wiedemann syndrome with Wilms' tumor suggests genomic imprinting. Nature 351:665–667

Huff V, Compton DA, Chao LY et al. (1988) Lack of linkage of familial Wilms' tumor to chromosomol band 11p13. Nature 336:377–378

Junien C (1986) Les antioncogènes. Médecine/Science 2:238–254

Knudson AG (1971) Mutation and cancer: statistical study of retinoblastoma. Proc Natl Acad Sci USA 4:820–823

Koufos A, Hansen MF, Lampkin BC et al. (1984) Loss of alleles at loci on human chromosome 11 during genesis of Wilms' tumor. Nature 309:170–172

Koufos A, Grundy P, Morgan K et al. (1989) Familial Wiedemann-Beckwith syndrome and a second Wilms' tumor locus both map to 11p15.5. Am J Hum Genet 44:711–719

Lothe RA, Fossa SD, Stenwig AE (1989) Loss of 3p or 11p alleles is associated with testicular cancer tumors. Genomics 5:134–138

Mannens M, Slater RM, Heyting C et al. (1988) Molecular nature of genetic changes resulting in loss of heterozygosity of chromosome 11 in Wilms' tumor. Hum Genet 81:41–48

Moutou C, Junien C, Henry I et al. (1992) A demonstration of the mechanisms responsible for the excess of transmitting females. J Med Genet (in press)

Pelletier J, Bruening W, Kashtan CE, Mauer SM, Manivel JC, Striegel JE, Houghton DC, Junien C, Habib R, Fouser L, Fine RN, Silverman BL, Haber DA, Housman D (1991) Germline mutations in the Wilms' tumor suppressor gene are associated with abnormal urogenital development in Denys-Drash syndrome. Cell 67:437–447

Scrable HJ, Witte DP, Lampkin BC et al. (1987) Chromosomal localization of the human rhabdomyosarcoma locus by mitotic recombination mapping. Nature 329:645–647

Scrable HJ, Cavenee W, Ghavimi F et al. (1989) A model for embryonal rhabdomyosarcoma tumorigenesis that involves genome imprinting. Proc Natl Acad Sci USA 86:7480–7484

Turleau C, de Grouchy J (1985) Beckwith-Wiedemann syndrome: clinical comparison between patients with and without 11p15 trisomy. Ann Genet 28:93–96

Wang-Wuu S, Soukup S, Bove K et al. (1990) Chromosome analysis of 31 Wilms' tumor. Cancer Res 50:2786–2793

Wiedemann HR (1983) Tumors and hemihypertrophy associated with Wiedemann-Beckwith syndrome. Eur J Pediatr 414–129

Zbar B, Brauch H, Talmadge C et al. (1987) Loss of alleles of loci on the short arm of chromosome 3 in renal cell carcinoma. Nature 327:721–724

Remarks on the Detection of Chromosomal Aberrations by Nonisotopic In Situ Hybridization

P. Lichter

Recent advancements in nonisotopic in situ hybridization protocols facilitate the highly specific delineation of targeted DNA sequences. Individual chromosomes, chromosomal subregions, or small DNA segments can be visualized by using appropriate nucleic acid probes or probe sets. Specific painting of whole chromosomes is achieved by using library DNA from sorted human chromosomes as a pool. In order to stain chromosomal subregions, pools of cloned DNA can be used. New approaches to the generation of subregional probe sets include DNA derived from microdissected chromosome regions and species-specific DNA sequences amplified from interspecies hybrid cell DNA. The specific amplification is achieved with the polymerase chain reaction (PCR), using primers that recognize species-specific sub-sequences of interspersed repetitive DNA (IRS-PCR). The efficiency of labeling chromosomal target sites with single, cloned DNA fragments increases with the size of the target region. Cosmid probes generally allow visualization of more than 90% of the chromosomal sequences. Details of the methodology are described in Lichter et al. (1991).

The high specificity and efficiency in delineating DNA sequences permits the diagnosis of structural chromosome aberrations at the one-cell level. Even small structural aberrations which can be very difficult to assess can be easily detected using appropriate DNA fragments as hybridization probes. The potential of this approach is increased by simultaneous hybridization and multicolor detection of several probes in the same preparation. The analysis of chromosomal aberrations can be performed not only on metaphase chromosomes, but also in interphase nuclei (for review, see Lichter et al. 1991 and Lichter and Ward 1990). The principles of such an analysis are shown schematically in Fig. 1. A DNA probe which specifically labels one chromosomal target site allows the immediate confirmation of a disomic status of the respective chromosomal region by counting two signals in metaphase and interphase cells, respectively (Fig. 1a). Accordingly, a trisomy can be detected by three visible signals. Figure 1b illustrates the case for a disomic (white signal) and a trisomic (black signal) chromosome.

The detection of small (even submicroscopic) deleted regions is a challenging task for cytogeneticists, and one which is of particular importance in cases where the deletion of a tumor suppressor gene is thought to play a role in tumor development. Using a suitable probe, a deletion can be detected if only one signal is present, i.e., only one homolog of the respective chromosomal

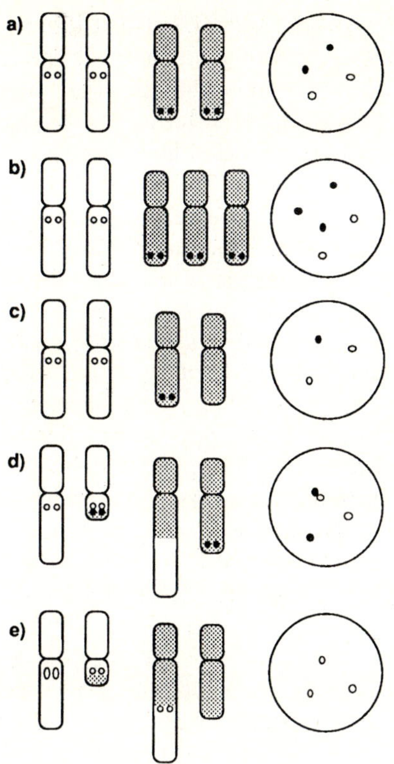

Fig. 1a–e. Schematic illustration of the detection of chromosomal aberrations by in situ hybridization using specific DNA probes. Two chromosomes of interest from a single metaphase plate are depicted in the left half of the scheme for each panel, whereas the right half displays the signals in an interphase nucleus of the corresponding karyotype. a A normal karyotype with two probes confirming disomies for the respective chromosomes. b A trisomy of one chromosome visible by three signals in metaphase and interphase versus two signals of a chromosome with normal copy number. c An internal deletion within one chromosome homolog visible by only one signal (from a probe specifically delineating the undeleted region of the normal homolog) versus two signals with a probe from a control chromosome. d A translocation visible by the specific joining of two regions from different chromosomes. e A translocation visible by the splitting of a signal from a large probe set depicting the region that spans the translocation break point (resulting in three instead of two signals)

region can be seen in metaphase or interphase nuclei (see Fig. 1c). The detection of specific translocations can be achieved by a dual color experiment using the two differentially labeled sequences from different chromosomes which are joined by the translocation event. Two closely juxtaposed signals (of different colors) can be seen, and this juxtaposition serves to distinguish the translocation from the normal status even in interphase nuclei (compare Fig. 1d and 1a). Furthermore, a specific translocation can be detected by using a probe set of sufficient complexity to cover the whole area of possible breakpoints. Hybridization to translocated chromosomes then reveals three signals instead of two (compare Fig. 1e and 1a).

The detection of specific chromosomal aberrations in human tumor cells and other cases of clinical cytogenetics as well as the practical value of various types of probe sets for detecting different kinds of aberrations are discussed in Lichter and Ward (1990) and Lichter et al. (1991). This approach will greatly benefit from the advent of large sets of cloned and mapped human DNA sequences, which will be established in the course of the human genome project.

As a result of their potential in the analysis of chromosome aberrations in interphase nuclei, these techniques are becoming increasingly important in tumor diagnostics. From many kinds of tumors, metaphase spreads are hard (if at all possible) to prepare. Furthermore, when metaphases without chromosomal changes are obtained, it is often unclear whether these are derived from tumor cells or from nontumor cells stimulated during the culturing of the cells. This problem can be overcome in many cases by adopting the interphase cytogenetics approach using uncultured cells. At present, interphase cytogenetics is being introduced into the area of early tumor diagnostics. Cell types thought to be early stages of various types of carcinomas are analyzed with large batteries of probe sets in order to detect chromosome aberrations specific for the corresponding tumor type or for the cell type considered as an early stage. This kind of analysis might be of use in developing diagnostic approaches for the early detection of tumor development.

References

Lichter P, Ward DC (1990) Is non-isotopic in situ hybridization finally coming of age? Nature 345:93–95
Lichter P, Boyle AL, Cremer T, Ward DC (1991) Analysis of genes and chromosomes by non-isotopic in situ hybridization. Genet Anal Techn Appl 8:24–35

Antibodies to the Human Papillomavirus 16 and 18 E7 Proteins: A Possible Diagnostic Marker for Cervical Cancer*

M. Müller, I. Jochmus, C. Bleul, K.V. Shah, R.K. Viscidi,
and L. Gissmann

Introduction

Human papillomavirus (HPV) types 16 and 18 belong to a heterogeneous group of epitheliotropic viruses which induce benign proliferations of the skin or mucosa (for review, see de Villiers 1989). During the past few years it became evident that they are associated with malignant tumors of the anogenital tract, particularly of the uterine cervix (for review, see zur Hausen 1989). Besides the demonstration of the transforming activity of the early viral genes E6 and E7 *in vitro*, the strongest evidence for a causative role of HPV 16 and HPV 18 in tumor development arose from the frequent detection of their genomes in tumor biopsies as well as in cell lines derived therefrom. After the tumorigenic properties of HPV 16 and 18 had become apparent, it was assumed that detection of the virus in healthy individuals could be of diagnostic value for determining the risk of developing cancer of the uterine cervix. Subsequent studies, however, demonstrated that the viruses quite frequently persist in clinically normal cervical epithelium, and it is not yet clear how frequently a latent infection may lead to a clinically overt lesion and finally to a malignant tumor.

Development of Serologic Methods

Searching for more informative diagnostic markers, we decided to develop serological tests for the detection of antibodies to HPV proteins in human sera. The immune response to PV infections so far is only poorly characterized because the viral proteins are not readily available to be used as antigens in serological assays. The reason for this shortage is the inability to amplify PV in experimental systems. Since the genomic clones of all known HPV types are available, expression of individual genes can be achieved in appropriate bacterial vectors. In a first attempt, fusion proteins were developed and used as antigens in Western blot experiments. For this purpose, the open reading frames (ORF) E4 and E7 of HPV 16 were ligated to pBR 322-derived expression vectors carrying 13 N-terminal amino acids of the lambda CII protein or

*This work was supported by the Deutsche Forschungsgemeinschaft (Gi 128/2-2) and by U.S. Public Health Service grant PO5 AI16959.

the 100 N-terminal amino acids of the bacteriophage MS2 polymerase, respectively. Both sequences had been cloned downstream to the inducible PL promoter of the bacteriophage lambda (Jochmus-Kudielka and Gissmann 1990). Fusion proteins were partially purified from the bacteria, separated through SDS-polyacrylamide gels, and blotted onto nitrocellulose strips. Human sera were diluted 1:20 and incubated with the antigen. Binding of human IgG was monitored by reaction with a peroxidase-linked human-specific antibody and staining with diaminobenzidine. All sera were tested at least three times. False-positive samples were identified by including the MS2 and CII portion of the fusion proteins into each test. In addition, only those samples which reacted with both the CII and MS2 fusion proteins were scored positive in order to exclude the reaction with a contaminating bacterial protein of identical size to one or the other fusion proteins. In addition, by this strategy, binding of antibodies to an epitope generated at the junction of the two peptides could be identified (Jochmus-Kudielka et al. 1989). In fact, about 7% of the sera reacted with the CII or MS2 E4 protein exclusively, whereas in case of E7 only 2% of the samples gave an inconsistent result when tested with both fusions (Jochmus-Kudielka 1991).

As an alternative approach to detect HPV antibodies in human sera, an enzyme-linked immunosorbent assay (ELISA) was developed. In comparison with the Western blotting procedure, this assay was assumed to have some advantages such as practicability if many samples have to be handled and the possibility of providing quantitative data. Because of possible false-positive results due to reactivity of human sera with prokaryotic peptides as discussed before, we did not use the bacterial fusion proteins as antigens in microtiter wells but synthetic peptides of immunoreactive regions identified within the individual HPV proteins.

For the detection of seroreactive regions two approaches were employed (Müller et al. 1990; Bleul et al. 1991):

1. Testing of overlapping dekapeptides synthesized on polyethylene pins (pep-scan; Geysen et al. 1984) with human sera as well as with rabbit hyperimmune sera and mouse monoclonal antibodies, the latter two obtained after immunization with HPV fusion proteins. By this approach, reacting regions of about 20 amino acids represented by five to six neighboring peptides within the HPV 16 E4 and HPV 18 E6 and E7 proteins could be identified. In some instances, isolated peptides reacted with the antisera, but their reactivity could not be confirmed when the respective peptide was synthesized and used for ELISA in microtiter wells. This indicates that unspecific binding of immunoglobulins to this pin-bound peptide had occurred. It further demonstrates that the pep-scan method is only a prescreening, and the results have to be confirmed by an independent technique.

2. Immune screening of bacteriophage fd expression libraries constructed with random HPV DNA fragments. Sheared fragments of cloned HPV DNA were ligated into the gene III of the double-stranded replicative intermediate DNA of bacteriophage fd which carries a tetracycline resistance marker (Smith 1985). The DNA is transfected into *E. coli* cells, and tet-resistant bacteriophage

particle-producing colonies were obtained. These particles were used to infect a susceptible *E. coli* strain, and the plaques were screened for HPV peptide expression with rabbit hyperimmune sera as mentioned above. Positive recombinants were isolated and repeatedly retested. The specific insert was characterized by direct sequencing of the insertion site within the gene III of the single-stranded fd DNA. As shown in Fig. 1, different recombinants with overlapping sequences were obtained. This figure also demonstrates the specificity of the immune screening method since only regions of specific ORFs (in this case of the HPV 16 E1 and E2 ORFs) were identified with the hyperimmune serum, although fragments of the whole HPV 16 genome including the plasmid vector were used for preparing the libraries. In total, seroreactive regions of the HPV 16 E1, E2, E4, E6, E7, and L1 and HPV 18 E1, E6, and E7 proteins were identified by this approach (Müller et al. 1990; Bleul et al. 1991).

Presence of Antibodies to HPV Proteins in Human Sera

Antibodies to the HPV 16 and HPV 18 E7 proteins were determined. The E6 and E7 proteins are involved in transformation (Münger et al. 1989) and are constantly expressed in tumor cells (Schwarz et al. 1985; Yee et al. 1985). Therefore, it was speculated that antibodies against these proteins may be prevalent in cancer patients.

In a first series of experiments, sera obtained from 131 cervical cancer patients were tested by Western blot in comparison with sera from an equal number of age-matched controls (Jochmus-Kudielka 1991). There was a 15-fold higher prevalence of HPV 16 E7-specific antibodies in cervical cancer patients (19.9% positive) than in nontumor controls (1.3% positive). Despite this statistically highly significant difference, only about one-fifth of the tumor sera reacted with the E7 fusion protein. As in this series the HPV type within the patients' tumors could not be determined and only 40%–70% of cervical cancer biopsies are associated with HPV 16 (for review, see Ikenberg 1991), it was anticipated that in sera from HPV-16-positive tumor patients the prevalence is at least twofold higher.

This assumption was indeed confirmed when sera from 116 cervical cancer patients and 178 age-matched controls were tested (Müller et al. 1991). Some 39 of the 116 tumor biopsies contained HPV 16 DNA as demonstrated by Southern blot hybridization (Guerrero, personal communication), 77 were positive for another HPV type (e.g., HPV 18, 31) or were devoid of any detectable HPV DNA. Using the HPV 16 E7 peptides E701 (PTLHEYMLDLQPETTDLYCYEQLNDSSEEE) and E702 (NDSSEEEDEIDGPAGQAEPDRAHYN) in an ELISA (Müller et al. 1990), 51.3% of the sera from HPV 16 DNA-positive but only 18.2% of sera from HPV 16 DNA-negative tumor patients and 8.9% of controls were shown to be reactive. These data suggest that the antibodies to the HPV 16 E7 peptides are reacting in a type-specific manner. A similar conclusion was drawn when

sequence	position
region E1-1090	
NGWFYVEAVVEKKTGDAISDDENENDSDTGEDLVDFIVNDNDYLT	aa 16-60
NENDSDTGEDLVDFIVND	aa 38-55
MADPAGTNGEEGTGCNGWFYVEAVVEKKTGDAISDDENENDSDTGEDLVDFIVNDNDYLT	aa 1-60
EDLVDFIVNDNDYLT	aa 46-60
EDLVDFIVNDNDYLTQAETETAHALFTAQEAKQH	aa 46-79
NENDSDTGEDLVDFIVNDNDYLTQAETETAHALFTAQEAKQHRDAVQVLKRKYL	aa 38-91
region E1-1059	
GSPLSDIS	aa 92-99

sequence	position
region E2-1066	
DKILTHYENDS	aa 13-23
DKILTHYENDSTDLRDHI	aa 13-30
region E2-1170	
DLRDHIDYWKH	aa 25-35
region E2-1074	
AIYYKAREMGFKHINHQVVPTLA	aa 41-63
AIYYKAREMGFKHINHQVVPTLAVSKNKAL	aa 41-70
YYKAREMGFKHINHQVVPTLAVSKN	aa 43-67
INHQVVPTLAVSKNKALQAI	aa 55-73
INHQVVPTLAVSKNKAL	aa 55-70
TLAVSKNKALQAIELQLTLETIYNSQYSNEKWTLQDV	aa 61-76
region E2-1112	
QLTLETIYNSQYSNEKWTLQDVSLE	aa 76-100
TLETIYNSQYSNEK	aa 78-91
region E2-1158	
TSVFSSNEVSSPEII	aa 197-211
VFSSNEVSSPEIIRQHLANHPASTHTKAVALGTEET	aa 199-234
region E2-1102	
EIIRQHLANHPASTHTKAVALGTEETQTTIQRPRSEP	aa 209-245
TEETQTTIQRPRSEPDTGN	aa 231-249

Fig. 1. Seroreactive regions on the human papillomavirus (HPV) 16 E1 and E2 proteins. A phage expression library containing randomly generated, subgenomic fragments of HPV 16 DNA was screened using HPV 16 E1 and E2-specific polyclonal antisera. Seroreactive recombinants were identified and analyzed by sequencing of the inserted HPV-DNA fragments. Usually, of every type of recombinant several isolates were identified. The amino acids derived from the nucleotide sequence and their positions on the E1 or E2 ORF are indicated. On the HPV 16 E1 proteins, two antibody reactive regions (E1-1090 and E1-1059) could be identified which were represented by six (overlapping) and one different phage clone, respectively. Six seroreactive regions (E2-1066, -1170, -1174, -1112, -1158, -1102) represented by different numbers of individual recombinants were identified on the HPV 16 E2 protein.

cervical cancer sera were tested for the presence of antibodies directed against an HPV 18 E7 seroreactive region. Four of 8 sera from patients with proven HPV 18 DNA within the tumor biopsy reacted in the HPV 18 E7-specific ELISA in contrast to 0/13 sera from HPV-16-positive patients and 0/3 sera from patients whose tumors either harbored another HPV type or were devoid of any detectable HPV genomes (Bleul et al. 1991). In fact, none of 395 sera tested both with the HPV 16 E701 and with the HPV 18 E7 peptide was found to react with both epitopes. Since both peptides were derived from regions within the HPV 16 or HPV 18 E7 protein which share considerable sequence homology (Fig. 2), it was concluded that there should be no cross-reactivity with antibodies directed against the E7 proteins of even more distantly related HPV types.

```
HPV 18 E701p:   SD-SEEENDEIDGVNHQHLPARRAEPQR-H
                 * **** *****       **   *** * *
HPV 16 E702p:   NDSSEEE-DEIDG------PAGQAEPDRAHYN
```

Fig. 2. Comparison of the amino acid sequences of peptides derived from seroreactive regions of HPV 16 and HPV 18 E7 (Müller et al. 1990; Bleul et al. 1991)

As shown in the previous section antibodies to the HPV 16 or HPV 18 E7 protein clearly correlate with cervical cancer and may represent a marker for virus persistence. It is an interesting question, however, why only about one-half of cancer sera reacts with the HPV 16 or HPV 18 E7 peptide. The following explanations can be considered:

1. There are subtypes of HPV 16 and HPV 18 which differ in their E7 epitope from the prototype whose sequences were used for the respective synthetic peptides. This hypothesis will be tested by sequencing of individual isolates obtained from seronegative patients.
2. There are additional, possibly conformational epitopes which have escaped detection as in our studies only linear epitopes were tested. In fact, additional cervical cancer sera were shown to be positive when an E7 protein produced by in vitro translation was used for immunoprecipitation (Müller et al. 1991).
3. In a certain number of cases, the antibody response is impaired since PV interfere with MHC class II expressing cells within the infected epithelium. This hypothesis is testable, and the appropriate experiments are in progress in our laboratory.

4. The anti-E7 response correlates with the size of the tumor and grade of invasion and hence is a marker for tumor progression. Analysis of sera from cervical cancer patients with tumors in different stages will verify this possibility.

From the data obtained in our studies as well as by others (Krchnak et al. 1990; Mann et al. 1990), it is evident that antibodies to HPV 16 or HPV 18 correlate with cancer of the uterine cervix. It remains to be elucidated, however, whether testing human sera for these antibodies can be used as a screening test for cervical tumors.

Summary

The early protein E7 of the human papillomavirus (HPV) types 16 and 18 which are associated with cervical cancer proved to be responsible for malignant transformation of epithelial cells. Using bacterial fusion proteins in Western blot experiments and synthetic peptides in ELISAs cervical cancer patients were shown to contain E7-specific antibodies at a higher prevalence and with elevated titers than healthy controls.

Acknowledgement. We thank Dr. Harald zur Hausen for his support and for helpful discussions.

References

Bleul C, Müller M, Frank R, Gausepohl H, Koldovsky U, Mgaya HN, Luande J, Pawlita M, ter Meulen J, Viscidi R, Gissmann L (1991) Human papillomavirus type 18 E6 and E7 antibodies in human sera: increased anti-E7 prevalence in cervical cancer patients. J Clin Microbiol 29 (in press)

De Villiers E-M (1989) Heterogeneity of the human papillomavirus group. J Virol 63:4898–4903

Geysen HM, Meloen RH, Barteling SJ (1984) Use of peptide synthesis to probe viral antigens for epitopes to a resolution of a single amino acid. Proc Natl Acad Sci USA 81:3998–4002

Ikenberg H (1991) Human papillomavirus DNA in invasive genital papillomas. In: Gros G, Jablonska S, Pfister H, Stegner H-E (eds) Genital papillomavirus infections. Springer, Berlin Heidelberg New York, pp 87–112

Jochmus-Kudielka I (1991) Untersuchung der humoralen Immunantwort gegen frühe Proteine der menschlichen Papillomviren (HPV) Typ 1, 11, 16 und 18. PhD thesis, University of Munich

Jochmus-Kudielka I, Gissmann L (1990) Expression of human papillomavirus type 16 proteins in *Escherichia coli* and their use as antigens in serological tests. In: Alitalo KK, Hutala ML, Knowles J, Vaheri A (eds) Recombinant systems in protein expression. Elsevier, Amsterdam, pp 87–93

Jochmus-Kudielka I, Schneider A, Braun R, Kimmig R, Koldovsky U, Schneweis K-E, Seedorf K, Gissmann L (1989) Antibodies against human papillomavirus type 16 early proteins in human sera: anti E7 reactivity correlates with cervical cancer. JNCI 81:1698–1704

Krchnak V, Vagner J, Suchnkova A, Krzmar M, Ritterova L, Vonka V (1990) Synthetic peptides derived from E7 region of human papillomavirus type 16 used as antigens in ELISA. J Gen Virol 71:2719–2724

Mann VM, Loo de Lao S, Brenes M, Brinton LA, Rawls JA, Green M, Reeves WC, Rawls WE (1990) Occurrence of IgA and IgG antibodies to select (sic) peptides representing human papillomavirus type 16 among cervical cancer cases and controls. Cancer Res 50:7815–7819

Müller M, Gausepohl H, de Martynoff G, Frank R, Brasseur R, Gissmann L (1990) Identification of seroreactive regions of the human papillomavirus type 16 proteins E4, E6, E7 and L1. J Gen Virol 71:2709–2717

Müller M, Viscidi RP, Sun Y, Guerrero E, Hill PM, Shah F, Bosch FX, Muñoz N, Gissmann L, Shah KV (1991) Antibodies to HPV-16 E6 and E7 proteins as markers for HPV-16-associated invasive cervical cancer. Virology (in press)

Münger K, Phelps WC, Bubb V, Howley PM, Schlegel R (1989) The E6 and E7 genes of the human papillomavirus type 16 together are necessary and sufficient for transformation of primary human keratinocytes. J Virol 63:4417–4421

Schwarz E, Freese UK, Gissmann L, Mayer W, Roggenbuck B, Stremlau A, zur Hausen H (1985) Structure and transcription of human papillomavirus sequences in cervical carcinoma cells. Nature 314:111–114

Smith GP (1985) Filamentous fusion phage: novel expression vectors that display cloned antigens on the virion surface. Science 228:1315–1317

Yee C, Krishnan-Hewlett I, Baker CC, Schlegel R, Howley PM (1985) Presence and expression of human papillomavirus sequences in human cervical carcinoma cell lines. Am J Pathol 119:361–366

Zur Hausen H (1989) Papillomaviruses as carcinomaviruses. In: Klein G (ed) Advances in viral oncology, vol 8. Raven, New York, pp 1–26

Summary of Discussion: Session 6

H. Brauch

Cytogenetics

Chromosomal aberrations are characteristic of neoplastic cells, both benign and malignant. Classic and modern cytogenetic techniques for detection of these aberrations in cancer diagnosis were discussed.

An overview of karyotypic changes in various types of tumors was given in the contribution by Nils Mandahl. Hematologic disorders often have simple characteristic karyotypic changes. Cytogenetic analysis has become important in the diagnosis and prognosis of leukemias. Solid tumors present a difficulty because they often display an abundance of karyotypic changes like translocations, monosomies, trisomies, inversions, and isosomies. In solid tumors with complex karyotypes the cytogeneticist is faced with the task of distinguishing "random" from "nonrandom" aberrations. The terms "random" and "nonrandom" in cytogenetics and the bias obtained from metaphases prepared from cell cultures were discussed.

There is no quantitative definition of the terms "random" and "nonrandom." They refer to the subjective expression of the observations of individual cytogeneticists. A cytogenetic aberration is considered to be a frequent event if found in 40% or more of the metaphases studied. A cytogenetic aberration is considered to be a nonrandom event if 10% of the metaphases evaluated contain this particular aberration and the other metaphases are pure. Cytogenetic changes found in fewer than 10% of the metaphases are considered to be random events.

Metaphases obtained directly from primary tissue are usually not satisfactory. To obtain metaphases that can be interpreted unambiguously, cells should be in a single cell suspension and viable. For this reason, metaphases should be prepared from cultured cells. However, restrictions apply in interpreting the results because cultured cells may not represent the composition of the original primary tumor. Cultured cells may only be a subpopulation which was able to adapt to the culture conditions and to respond to growth selection. Coincidentally, these could be the cells with gross cytogenetic changes. These changes may not reflect any specific and critical event involved in tumorigenesis. Some bias may occur even if there is no growth selection. Because of cell cycles in culture, the cells may undergo additional cytogenetic changes and therefore reflect a situation similar to an advanced tumor stage. Cytogenetic aberrations found in these cells would not reflect primary changes.

An update on in situ hybridization techniques and their applicability in the early detection of cancer was given in the contribution by Peter Lichter. In situ hybridization techniques are widely used to visualize specific DNA sequences in preparations of chromosomes, single cells, or tissue sections. Nonisotopic hybridization techniques provide fast, sensitive, and simultaneous analyses of chromosomal domains using either conventional microscopy or digital imaging microscopy. The benefit of these techniques is their applicability to the detection of genomic features on metaphase chromosomes and on interphase nuclei. Since nonisotopic, in situ hybridization allows one to paint and delineate chromosomes in any stage of the cell cycle, this is the method of choice to identify directly chromosomal aberrations in the more numerous examples of interphase nuclei instead of mitotic cells of solid tumors. This method overcomes the limitation of metaphase cytogenetics in solid tumors and allows the detection of duplications, deletions, and translocations in clinical specimens.

The probes used for hybridization in this novel technique are cosmids, composite chromosome probe sets, or more complex probe sets such as a pool of clones from an individual chromosome library of sorted human chromosomes. The efficiency of the probe to detect its chromosomal target sequence increases with the size of the probe. Since the number of repetitive sequences increases with the size of the probe, competitive DNA is required in order to suppress nonspecific hybridization of these repetitive elements.

There were discussions concerning the specificity of the method and its applicability in the detection of amplified sequences and detection of chromosomal aberrations on tissue sections. Deletions can be resolved and identified in 85%–90% of the interphase nuclei studied. The presence of both alleles in the remaining 10%–15% of interphase nuclei can be explained by a technical failure of the probe to hybridize completely and/or by the presence of a small percentage of tetraploid cells resulting in additional signals. High specificity can also be obtained in the detection of numerical chromosome changes using chromosome specific probes like clones of the alphoid DNA repeat family. Alphoid DNA repeats are amplified in a polymerase chain reaction (PCR), and the reaction mixture is used for nonisotopic labeling and hybridization to interphase nuclei. Since multiple copies at different target sites are present, such probes are qualified to decorate or paint chromosomes. To detect amplification the nonisotopic, in situ, hybridization signals need to be evaluated by quantitative fluorescence microscopy. It would be desirable to have better internal standards available.

The applicability of the method for testing and evaluating tissue sections for chromosomal aberrations depends on the capability of the probe to penetrate. This works better for the amplified alphoid probes than for single copy probes. Improvement in the detection of structural chromosomal abnormalities in tissue sections is expected from the use of yeast artificial chromosomes in nonisotopic, in situ hybridization.

Molecular Genetics

Genetic alterations found in human neoplasms can explain different mechanisms involved in tumorigenesis. Such mechanisms may include (1) amplification of cellular oncogenes, (2) inactivation of the two homologues of a tumor suppressor gene, (3) genomic imprinting and preferential inactivation of one parental allele, (4) integration and activation of viral DNA sequences in the human genome.

Amplification of DNA sequences has been observed in tumorigenesis and accounts for an increase of gene dosage of cellular oncogenes. Amplification of the MYCN gene in the childhood tumor neuroblastoma, its correlation with staging of the disease, and its prognostic value were presented by Manfred Schwab. In neuroblastoma, amplification is the selective multiplication of a DNA sequence containing the MYCN gene on extrachromosomal genetic elements and in homogeneously staining regions on chromosomal regions other than the MYCN locus on chromosome 2. This amplification correlates with a more aggressively advancing disease and may have prognostic value for survival.

Along a different line of evidence neuroblastoma is associated with a characteristic deletion on the short arm of chromosome 1. Specific chromosomal deletions in several types of tumors have led to the discovery of tumor suppressor genes. Tumor suppressor genes are involved in normal development and/or differentiation. According to Knudson's two-hit theory of tumorigenesis, two homologues of a tumor suppressor gene must be inactivated. This theory explained the underlying mechanism of tumorigenesis in retinoblastoma, neurofibromatosis type 2, multiple endocrine neoplasia, and von Hippel–Lindau disease. The existence of hereditary forms of these diseases allowed determination of genetic linkage of a disease to a genetic locus and determination of the parental origin of two homologous alleles. By including the parents of a patient in the genotype analysis, identification of the allele that was carrying the germline defect and the allele that was lost in the tumor became possible. Inactivation of a tumor suppressor gene by a recessive mechanism was shown in tumors in which the wild type allele was deleted and the allele with the germline defect retained. Families with a genetic predisposition for a neoplastic disease are therefor a prerequisite to identify a putative tumor suppressor gene. The involvement of a tumor suppressor gene in neuroblastoma is unknown. Evidence for a genetic predisposition is rare. Difficulties in determining the incidence and penetrance of an inherited susceptibility to neuroblastoma derive from undiagnosed tumors that have undergone regression or spontaneous maturation to benign ganglioneuroma, as well as from early deaths or long-term treatment that preclude reproduction and multigenerational pedigrees. Since large pedigrees are missing, linkage of neuroblastoma to a 1p locus cannot be tested. Preferential loss of a certain parental allele in neuroblastoma is also unknown.

The significance of MYCN amplification and chromosome 1p deletion as prognostic parameters in neuroblastoma is stressed by the natural occurrence of spontaneous regression in a small proportion of cases with stage IVs. There is no 1p deletion, and MYCN amplification is a rare event in stage IVs cases. Based on 4 stage IVs patients, who died after initial regression but had amplification of MYCN, the unfavorable prognosis in tumors with MYCN amplification is confirmed.

Knudson's two-hit theory is based on the assumption that there is no difference in function between maternally and paternally derived alleles. If this theory applies to other neoplasms, it implies that the deletions found in sporadic tumors should be random. Both alleles, paternal and maternal, should be affected with the same statistical frequency. The observation of a non-random maternal loss of 11p alleles in patients with sporadic Wilms' tumor made clear that the prediction of random loss was not fulfilled for this neoplasm. It became necessary to extend and refine the two-hit theory of carcinogenesis, taking into consideration the phenomenon of genomic imprinting. The preferential inactivation of the maternal allele suggested that the two homologues of a gene may differ in their functional activity due to differential expression of the maternal and paternal genome. This is known as genomic imprinting. Hypermutability of the gametes may be responsible for this parental bias.

Claudine Junien introduced the principle of genomic imprinting as a mechanism involved in the tumorigenesis of Beckwith–Wiedemann syndrome (BWS). BWS predisposes to Wilms' tumor and other neoplasms. A combined approach of gene dosage and restriction fragment length polymorphism (RFLP) analysis allowed determination of the parental origin of a constitutional rearrangement in patients with BWS. This rearrangement resulted from a mitotic recombination event which included the region 11p15.5 leading to duplication of the paternal allele and absence of the maternal allele. If the maternal allele is the active one, its absence results in an impaired function implicated in the tumorigenesis of BWS. If the paternal allele is the active one, its duplication may account for a dose-dependent activation of a transforming gene responsible for the genetic predisposition to BWS. Additional evidence that the presence of only one of the parental alleles predisposes to BWS comes from the experimental evidence that constitutional homozygosity at the 11p15 locus is more common among sporadic BWS patients compared with the normal population. This constitutional homozygosity may reflect uniparental hemizygosity, which may aid the preclinical diagnosis of patients at risk.

Human papillomavirus infection is considered to cause cancer. Lutz Gissmann presented the correlation between the presence of certain types of human papillomaviruses (HPV 16, 18, 31, 33) and the incidence of cervical uterine carcinoma. The causal role of the physical presence, integration into the host genome, expression of viral genes, and presence of viral proteins involved in cellular transformation was discussed.

HPV DNA persists regularly in primary and metastatic tumor biopsies of patients with uterine cervix carcinoma and in established cervical cancer cell lines. In benign genital lesions, the viral genome persists episomally. In the majority of cancers, the virus genome is integrated into the host genome under conservation of the E6 and E7 open reading frames, resulting in translation of two biologically active products in vitro. The viral proteins E6 and E7 are specific for each HPV type. Their presence is considered to be circumstantial evidence for a developing cervical cancer. E6 and E7 proteins are considered to be responsible for the induction of transformation and maintenance of the transformed stage. E6 can bind to p53, and E7 can bind to the Rb protein, suggesting a direct interaction of viral protein with host protein. It is unclear whether or not p53 and Rb protein are involved in a selective regulation of HPV gene expression.

Despite the fact that HPV infection is considered the prime risk factor for the development of cervical cancer, its significance is hampered by the long latency period of about 30 years between HPV infection and the development of cervical cancer and the low tumor/infection ratio. The prevalence of HPV infection throughout the population is higher than the number of women developing cervical carcinoma. Recent PCR studies showed that about 45% of sexually active, nondiseased women were carriers of HPV virus. The majority of infected women will not develop cervical cancer during their lifetime. This underlines that HPV infection per se is not sufficient for carcinoma induction and suggests that co-factors must be involved in HPV-linked carcinogenesis. Such a multistep mechanism of HPV infection and activation may include endogenous and exogenous co-factors. Endogenous ones may include hormones, factors involved in immune response mechanisms, and cellular components controlling HPV expression. The consequence of dysregulation may result in failure of the host cell to respond to HPV infection. Exogenous factors may include carcinogenic substances introduced by bacterial or protozoal infection, as well as cigarette smoking, and uptake of mutagenic food metabolites. Additional virus infection, e.g., cytomegalovirus and viruses from the herpes group, could result in an activation of HPV gene expression. Little is known about the mechanisms of action of such putative co-factors.

The answer to the fundamental question of whether or not HPV viruses are needed at all for the development of cervical carcinoma is expected to come from further epidemiological studies. Vaccination against viral proteins should protect women from HPV infection and should bring down the frequency of this cancer. Production of HPV-type specific antisera requires enough virus particles for immunization. Difficulties arise from the fact that HPV viruses cannot be propagated in culture. For antisera production significant amounts of virus particles are needed. The virus particles need to be purified from the respective lesions and heterotransplanted into athymic mice in order to produce significant amounts of virus particles from the infected tissue for immunization. Availability of suitable antisera would enable the surveillance of viral proteins in infected individuals and improve the diagnosis of translated viral genes. If HPV viruses play a causal role in the development of cervical carcinoma, the ultimate outcome of successful vaccination would be the prevention of cervical cancer.

SESSION 7

Epidemiology

Chairman: J. Wahrendorf

Epidemiological Aspects of Early Detection Programs

A.B. MILLER

Introduction

It is generally assumed that early detection of cancer results in an improvement of prognosis. This, and simpler therapy, are the major benefits expected from screening programs. However, these benefits are not always realized. For some cancers, this is because the natural history of the disease, or the sensitivity of the screening test used for early disease, is such that application of presently available tests may not result in the reduction of deaths from cancer. For other cancers, it seems that organizational issues are impeding the achievement of the expected effect in several populations. In this paper, some general principles that affect the evaluation of screening are presented, and then the possibilities that screening may result in an important reduction in cancer mortality are discussed for a number of cancer sites.

Evaluation of Screening

Screening involves the application of tests or other procedures to asymptomatic persons in the hope of detecting disease sufficiently early in its natural history so that treatment will result in cure or at least reduced morbidity. However, unless the tests are completely free of risk there is a possibility of harm as well as benefit (Miller 1988). This is because of a risk from the diagnostic procedures following screening as well as a risk from the test itself.

The application of screening results in the person screened being classed as positive or negative to the test. If positive, diagnostic tests are required to identify those with the disease. Those with positive tests found not to have the disease (false-positive) will have had the inconvenience, costs, and risks of the diagnostic tests unnecessarily. Those negative to the test will be reassured, but for those who have the disease (false-negative) the reassurance will be false, and there is a risk that they will ignore symptoms when their disease presents subsequently. To identify the false-negatives requires close follow-up. The sensitivity of the test can be determined as the proportion of those who have the disease who test positive. The corresponding measure of validity is specificity, the proportion of those free of the disease who test negative. Thus, the higher the proportion of those free of disease who test positive (false-positive), the lower the specificity of the test. A process measure used to assess screening tests is the predictive value positive, the proportion of those who test positive who have the disease.

For screening to be applicable as public health policy the disease has to be an important health problem, and it has to be demonstrated that treatment of disease found by the application of screening tests results in a reduction of deaths from cancer. This is not equivalent to prolongation of survival for cases detected on screening compared with the survival experienced by cases detected in the absence of screening. This is because of four biases: lead time, length bias, selection bias, and overdiagnosis bias. Lead time is the prolongation of the observation time by the detection of cases earlier in their natural history. Length bias is the propensity of screening to detect preferentially the slower growing cancers, as fast growing cancers tend to present for diagnosis with intrusive symptoms and are diagnosed before screening starts or in the interval between screens. Selection bias is the effect of recruiting volunteers into screening programs who are more health conscious and therefore have a better survival. Overdiagnosis bias is the tendency for screening to identify borderline abnormalities which are labelled cancer though they may lack true biologic potential for malignancy.

Although less satisfactory designs have been used to evaluate the effectiveness of screening in populations, in practice effectiveness can only be unequivocally established by controlled trials, when mortality (deaths from the disease in the population) is used as the endpoint in the screened and control groups, as mortality is not affected by the biases. However, other endpoints and other evaluation designs can be used under special circumstances. Thus, reduction in the incidence of a cancer can be expected if the screening test detects a precursor, such as in screening for cancer of the cervix. Further, when mortality is the appropriate endpoint, reduction in the cumulative prevalence of advanced cancer can be expected to precede the mortality reduction. In terms of application of screening in the population, the full effect cannot be anticipated unless those at high risk for the disease are screened, and this implies high population compliance with screening.

Case control studies, time trend analyses, and quasi-experimental studies have been used to evaluate screening. The major difficulty with these designs is selection bias, and it may be very difficult to control for this, as risk factor information may either not be available or insufficient for its control (Miller et al. 1990).

Screening for Specific Cancer Sites

Oral Cancer

There is indirect evidence that inspection of the mouth could be used to promote early detection of oral cancer (Prorok et al. 1984). This has been evaluated in Sri Lanka, where it has been confirmed that primary health care workers can detect the disease (Warnakulasuriya et al. 1984). In many countries, dentists are urged to inspect the mouth for oral cancer. Unfortunately, this approach is unlikely to have a major impact on control of the disease because those at high risk of oral cancer do not usually attend dentists.

Colorectal Cancer

A number of controlled trials of colorectal cancer screening have been conducted or are in progress. The earliest evaluated rigid sigmoidoscopy as part of a multiphasic health screen. Although a reduction in mortality from colorectal cancer was seen in the study group, this is probably due to chance and not due to the effect of sigmoidoscopy (Selby et al. 1988). All the other trials are evaluating the effect of the fecal occult blood test (FOBT). Of these, two in the USA have been running long enough for results on mortality to be expected. One of these, in New York, is evaluating the effect of the addition of the FOBT to routine sigmoidoscopic screening. It was not randomized, and the results are difficult to interpret. Although the mortality results for these who had not attended the screening center before have been presented in a review (Winawer et al. 1991) suggesting a borderline significant result in favor of screening, these results were only for a segment of the population, and the overall results suggest no mortality reduction from screening (Miller 1991). The other, in Minnesota, used the FOBT alone, annually in one group, biennially in another. A decision has been taken to resume screening in that trial (stopped by design a few years ago), so mortality results cannot be expected for some years. In the meantime, it is clear from the Minnesota trial that a major difficulty with screening using the FOBT is lack of specificity, especially if the test is rehydrated, and that this results in major increase in use of health services and raised costs (Chamberlain et al. 1986; Miller et al. 1990).

In the absence of firm evidence that it will result in reduced mortality from the disease, screening for colorectal cancer or its precursors cannot be recommended as part of a cancer control program. There is no evidence that a different policy should be applied to those judged to be at increased risk, though some special high-risk groups, such as family members with familial polyposis, or those with a previous diagnosis of colorectal adenoma or carcinoma, should be placed on clinical surveillance programs.

Lung Cancer

There is good evidence that screening for lung cancer using either sputum cytology over and above 6-monthly chest X-radiographs or 4-monthly chest X-radiographs and sputum cytology in comparison with recommended annual chest X-radiographs and sputum cytology does not reduce mortality from the disease (Prorok et al. 1984). This evidence was derived from three randomized trials in asymptomatic smoking males over the age of 45 years conducted in the USA. Two of these evaluated sputum cytology screening, and the other the combination of chest X-radiograph and sputum cytology screening. Chest X-radiograph screening alone had previously been evaluated in other studies with no evidence of mortality reduction, while a case control study in the former East Germany found no evidence of benefit from 2-yearly mass miniature radiography screening (Ebeling and Nischan 1987). Screening for lung cancer cannot therefore be recommended as public health policy.

Breast Cancer

There is good evidence that screening for breast cancer can reduce mortality from the disease in women over the age of 50 years (Day et al. 1986). The data in support of this have come from two randomized trials (Shapiro et al. 1988; Tabar et al. 1989), three case control studies (Collette et al. 1984; Verbeek et al. 1985; Palli et al. 1986), and one quasi-experimental study (UK Trial of Early Detection of Breast Cancer Group 1988). In addition, three trials have shown some indication of effectiveness in women aged 50 years or more. In the Malmö trial, the relative risk among women aged 55–69 years on entry was 0.79 (95% confidence interval 0.51–1.24), data compatible with a protective effect of screening 5–10 years after initiation of screening (Andersson et al. 1988). A similar effect was seen in the Stockholm trial (Rutqvist et al. 1990) but only for women aged 55–59 years on entry in the Edinburgh trial (Roberts et al. 1990).

The HIP trial, the Utrecht study, and the UK quasi-experimental study used the combination of mammography and physical examination. The other studies were based on mammography alone, though in the Two-County Swedish trial the screening process incorporated a visual examination of the breasts, and the women received a pamphlet advising them to practice breast self-examination (BSE) and explaining the technique. Mammography was single view in the Two-County Swedish trial (mediolateral oblique) and in Nijmegen (lateral); in the UK study, the mammographic technique was a single mediolateral oblique view of each breast, although in Edinburgh in the first round a cephalocaudal view was also taken; in the other studies, mammography was double view. Screening was given annually only in the HIP study. In Utrecht, the intervals were 18 months, 2 years, and then 4 years; in Nijmegen and Malmö screening was biennial; in Florence, every 2.5 years; in the Two-County Trial in Sweden, every 21 months in women aged 40–49 years, every 33 months in older women. In the UK study, physical examination was given annually and mammography every 2 years.

Indirect evidence on the optimal frequency of rescreening is obtained from the studies that used a long interval between screens by determining the proportion of the expected incidence of breast cancer (measured in the control group or from other data) that presents in the interval between screens. Data from both the Two-County Swedish (Day et al. 1988) and Nijmegen (Day and Chamberlain 1988) studies indicate that screening every 2 years is satisfactory in women over the age of 50 years, but that annual screening would be required if programs were to be introduced for younger women.

All the studies except those in Malmö and Edinburgh had a similar order of effectiveness in women aged 50 years or more, approximately a 40% reduction in breast cancer mortality at 5–7 years after initiating screening. Clearly, this order of effectiveness can be achieved by mammography alone; whether physical examination (and BSE) provides most of the benefit from the combination with mammography, or can substitute for mammography, is under investigation in the Canadian National Breast Screening Study (NBSS) (Miller et al. 1981). Early results suggest that in women aged 50–59 years on entry, there is little or no benefit from the addition of mammography to physical examination, at least in the first 7 years after initiation of screening (Miller et al. 1991b).

The largest breast screening project was the US Breast Cancer Detection Demonstration Project (BCDDP). This involved over 280 000 women in the 1970s aged 35 years or more who were screened with mammography and physical examination. This project was uncontrolled, and for many years the only data available were on case detection (Baker 1982) or on survival (Seidman et al. 1987). Estimates of mortality have been made, however, and compared with that expected from the general population (Morrison et al. 1988). The difference in observed mortality from breast cancer from that expected is not large, and no difference was seen in the first five years for women under the age of 50 years. For women over that age who attended for routine screening, however, the difference between observed and expected breast cancer mortality was approximately 40%. These results are difficult to interpret, as lower breast cancer mortality compared with the general population might be expected in women who volunteer for screening who are often health conscious.

Only the HIP study has so far produced any evidence that screening is effective in women aged 40–49 years, and only on long-term follow-up (Shapiro et al. 1988). In the Malmö study, there was a suggestion of an increase in breast cancer mortality in the first 5 years following screening in women aged 45–54 years (Andersson et al. 1988). In the Swedish Two-County trial (Tabar et al. 1985), the Nijmegen study (Verbeek et al. 1985), and the Stockholm trial (Rutqvist et al. 1990), there was also a suggestion of an early excess of breast cancer mortality in women under the age of 50 years. The NBSS in Canada also supports no indication of early benefit (Miller et al. 1991b). Even if an assumption is made that benefit will eventually be seen more than 10 years after initiation of screening, screening women in this age group is unlikely to be cost-effective (Eddy et al. 1988). Although none of the projects using more modern mammography has yet reached the period of follow-up in which in the HIP study's apparent benefit in younger women began to be seen, they have at least lasted long enough to confirm that even if benefit in younger women is eventually seen, it will be delayed compared with women over the age of 50 years. The reason for this age difference in time to effect is still unclear. One possible reason could be the relatively poorer sensitivity of the screen, or a biological difference in the response to therapy of advanced disease detected by screening in younger women.

When mammography is used for screening, the importance of high quality and the necessity for the skills to be available in the community to localise and diagnose impalpable lesions cannot be too strongly emphasised. Ensuring high quality requires constant attention to the details of positioning and compression, film type and screen, darkrooms, development of film, as well as kilovoltage, phototiming, and dosage, to ensure films of adequate contrast and definition. In the NBSS, these aspects were supervised by a reference physicist. We also had a reference radiologist who assessed the performance of the radiologists reading the films. In spite of such care, there is clear evidence that mammography quality increased as the NBSS proceeded (Baines et al. 1990).

The UICC project on screening for cancer drew the following conclusions on the state of the art of breast cancer screening (Miller et al. 1990):

Screening for breast cancer by mammography every 1 to 3 years can reduce breast cancer mortality substantially in women age 50–70. In women under age 50 there is little evidence for a benefit, at least in the first 10 years after screening is initiated. The cost-effectiveness of screening every 2–3 years by mammography for women age 50–70 compares well with many other medical procedures.

The time taken for a reduction in breast cancer mortality to appear will depend on the initial quality of the screening modalities used. The level of effect in the target population will be strongly dependent on the degree of compliance and on the quality of the mammography. The effect on mortality will be reduced if the screening sensitivity is inadequate.

Physical examination, for women over 50, has lower sensitivity than mammography, and in some studies was inferior to mammography in specificity and predictive value. In programmes with high quality mammography physical examination may not be a cost-effective adjunct to mammography as a screening procedure.

The introduction of mass screening into a population should be planned in a way such that the initial and long-term outcome measures can be evaluated.

Non-randomized studies of the effectiveness of breast screening in which screened women are compared with women who refused screening will give an incorrect estimate of the effect of screening in the population if the non-compliers are at substantially different underlying risk from the rest of the population. The results of studies in which this source of bias is not specifically examined need to be treated with extra caution. Study designs which specify women who attended, who refused and who had no opportunity to be screened may reduce this problem.

There has been some controversy over whether or not screening for breast cancer should be recommended in women under the age of 50 years. Policy recommendations should reflect findings from well-conducted studies, not anecdotal evidence or opinion. Although breast cancer in women aged 40–49 years is a very important cause of death, the participants in a national workshop in Canada did not recommend screening in this age group but left it to the provinces to decide (Workshop Group 1989). As already reported, the UICC project noted little evidence of a benefit in this age group, at least in the first 10 years after screening is initiated (Miller et al. 1990), and the US preventive Services Task Force did not recommend mammography screening in this age group, though other US groups do (Miller 1990). It should also be noted that although mammography is often advocated for women under the age of 50 years at high risk, such as those with a strong family history, there is no evidence as yet that it will be beneficial in such women.

Mammography is a more sensitive screening test than physical examination, with 85% of the cancers found by mammography when both tests are used compared with about 50% for physical examination alone. However, evaluation of physical examination in relation to the false-negative results that present over the next 6 months suggests that the sensitivity for progressive breast cancer is of the order of 80% (Baines et al. 1989).

There is little evidence for the effectiveness of BSE in reducing breast cancer mortality. A case control study of advanced breast cancer in Seattle suggests that benefit may be restricted to compliers with adequate BSE practice (Newcomb et al. 1991), but a cohort study in Finland suggests benefit in women age 40–69 years (Gastrin et al., in preparation). Other studies are ongoing. Only BSE has the potential to improve the outlook for interval cancers, while its teaching probably reduces false reassurance.

Providing programs are successful in recruiting a high proportion of the eligible women aged 50–69 years and maintain adequate quality control so that the results obtained in the research studies are replicated in the general population, it can be estimated that a 25% reduction in breast cancer mortality would result.

Cancer of the Cervix

A number of reviews (Hakama et al. 1985; Task Force 1976, 1982) have concluded that screening for cancer of the cervix is effective in reducing the incidence and mortality from the disease, but that for maximal effectiveness, attention needs to be paid to the organizational aspects of screening. It is the organized programs that have shown the greatest effect while using fewer resources than the unorganized programs.

Essential elements of an organized program include:

– The individual women in the target population are identifiable
– Measures are available to guarantee high coverage and attendance, such as a personal letter of invitation
– Adequate field facilities for taking the smears and adequate laboratory facilities to examine them
– An organized quality control program on taking of the smears and on interpreting them
– Adequate facilities for diagnosis and for appropriate treatment of confirmed neoplastic lesions
– A carefully designed and agreed referral system for management of any abnormalities found and for providing information about normal screening tests
– Evaluation and monitoring of the total program is organized (Hakama et al. 1985)

Many programs for screening for cancer of the cervix lack the first two elements. It is a paradox that we accept without question that dentists can recall women for routine examinations, but we do not expect this of family physicians or gynecologists. A case control study in Toronto found that among women who had visited a physician in the last 5 years, the proportion of patients with cancer of the cervix who had had a cytology smear was significantly lower than in the neighborhood controls free of the disease; this difference was greater in the poor and the elderly (Clarke and Anderson 1979). This observation suggests that not all physicians are aware of the importance of screening.

An element of the organization of cervical cancer screening programs that has caused great controversy has been the optimal frequency of rescreening and the appropriate ages to initiate and stop screening. The results of an IARC study based on the records of a number of screening programmes in Europe and Canada show that one, or preferably two negative smears, are followed for at least 5 years by low risk (IARC Working Group on Cervical Cancer Screening 1986). The findings were used to estimate the optimal frequency of rescreening. Starting screening at age 25 and stopping at age 64 years with 3-year intervals gives 90% of the maximal protection and only requires 13 tests a lifetime. Screening starting at age 20 years with annual screens gives only just over 90% protection yet requires 45 tests a lifetime. Thus, the marginal yield in a population from annual compared with 3-yearly screening is minimal. The problem with recommending annual tests is that resources will be wasted which could be used to target those who are at high risk. The concern over women at high risk is not whether or not they should have annual screening but whether or not they are screened at all. The elderly indigent woman who has never been screened, or was screened many years before, is at particularly high risk. Organized programs are more likely to bring such women into screening than opportunistic screening.

A recent analysis of British Columbia screening data has provided no evidence that women born in 1944–1948 had a more rapid progression of dysplasia or carcinoma in situ than women who belonged to older birth cohorts (Miller et al. 1991c). There seems therefore to be little justification for annual screening at any age. However, there is an urgent need in many countries to ensure that the unscreened or poorly screened are screened regularly, and this seems unlikely to be accomplished unless the organizational principles summarized above are followed.

Recently, a Canadian workshop proposed revised recommendations on screening for cancer of the cervix (Miller et al. 1991a). These include:

- Governments should encourage and support the development of organized cervical cytology screening programmes designed to reduce the morbidity and mortality from carcinoma of the cervix.
- All women who have had sexual intercourse who are aged 18 years and over should be encouraged to enter a cervical cytology screening program.
- Such women should generally be advised to be rescreened every 3 years to the age of 69 years.
- Women over the age of 69 years who have never had biopsy-confirmed

severe dysplasia or carcinoma in situ (CIN III) and who have had at least two satisfactory normal smears and no positive smears in the past 9 years can be dropped from a screening program for squamous cell cancer of the cervix.

The workshop group emphasized that the recommended screening frequencies should only be established as formal policy when high quality laboratory services for the reading of cytology smears with quality control systems established and information systems to monitor the frequencies and to issue reminders to attend at the recommended intervals are in place. Recommendations were made over the establishment of information systems, over laboratories, concerning recruitment of women into screening, and other aspects.

It seems likely that screening women aged 20–69 years should reduce the incidence of the disease by at least 60%. This is lower than the theoretical maximum of 90% from the simulations conducted by the IARC Working Group on Cervical Cancer Screening (1986), because it is probably unrealistic to expect much more than a population compliance of 80% (rather than the assumption made in the simulation of 100%) and in recognition of the fact that part of the reduction in incidence of cancer of the cervix in some countries in the past 20 years has come from screening. It is relevant, for example, that if the Canadian incidence rate is compared with that from Finland (the country with the most effective screening program for cancer of the cervix in the world), the proportion of the disease preventable by screening in Canada is 48%, and it is likely that Finland has not yet seen the final plateauing of its incidence from the disease.

Ovarian Cancer

In many countries, ovarian cancer is now the most important gynecological cause of cancer mortality. Screening is thus being considered for this disease. Two screening tests are under evaluation, ultrasound and a monoclonal antibody (Ca 125). However, both seem to be relatively nonspecific, though research is underway in a number of centers on their use (Miller et al. 1990). At present, therefore, screening for ovarian cancer cannot be recommended as public health policy.

Prostate Cancer

There is interest in the possibility of screening for prostate cancer using the digital rectal examination and/or ultrasound, as well as other potential screening tests such as that for a prostate specific antigen. There are, however, insufficient data available as to whether these are valid screening tests, though pilot studies are in progress in some countries. It is clear, however, that there are many obstacles in the way of an effective screening program for a disease that is a relatively unimportant cause of premature mortality. Not only has an acceptable and valid screening test to be available, but there must also be an acceptable and effective treatment for the preclinical lesions found as a result of screening. This problem is particularly acute for prostate cancer because of the increasing frequency of latent prostatic carcinoma with increasing age and the not inappreciable morbidity and mortality of the radical procedures usually used to treat it (Miller et al. 1990). Nevertheless, prostate cancer is an important disease in elderly men, and when these problems are solved, it will be appropriate to evaluate the effectiveness of screening programs for prostate cancer by well-designed, randomized trials.

Malignant Melanoma

Screening for malignant melanoma has been advocated in the form of total skin examinations by a professional, especially of those who are believed to be at high risk through operation of the risk factors such as fair skin and a tendency to burn after sun exposure. Such screening is at an early stage of development. In Australia and New Zealand as well as in the UK, public education programs have been mounted to enhance individual awareness of the problem of melanoma and to encourage self-referral for suspicious lesions. Substantial increases in the patient load at skin diagnostic clinics have been documented, with a large number of early cancers found. However, no evaluation studies have been completed to determine the impact of screening on mortality (Miller et al. 1990). Until such data are available, screening for malignant melanoma is not recommended as public health policy.

Bladder Cancer

Although urine cytology has been used for surveillance of some occupational groups at increased risk of bladder cancer, there is insufficient evidence available on its efficacy to justify recommending screening for bladder cancer as public health policy (Prorok et al. 1984).

Endometrial Cancer

Programs for screening for endometrial cancer have been considered, but there has been little enthusiasm for their use, largely because of the low mortality from the disease. There is no evidence that routine pelvic examinations are effective in reducing mortality. The cervical cytology smear is insensitive for endometrial cancer, and although other procedures have been proposed, none have been properly evaluated (Hakama et al. 1985). Screening for endometrial cancer cannot therefore be recommended as public health policy.

Stomach Cancer

Screening for stomach cancer is a major cancer control measure used in Japan, where the incidence and mortality from the disease are high. The screening test used is a standard 6-view, barium meal X-radiograph of the stomach with image intensification, usually administered through mass mobile units. The evidence that this program is effective in reducing mortality from the disease is slim (Hirayama et al. 1985), though a case control study produced suggestive evidence of efficacy (Oshima 1988).

In many countries, incidence and mortality from stomach cancer are much lower than in Japan and falling. In view of this and the uncertainty over whether screening even in Japan is effective, screening for stomach cancer in such countries cannot be recommended as part of a cancer control program (Miller et al. 1990).

Summary

There has to be much care taken over evaluation of the effectiveness of screening and in applying screening as public health policy. Currently, only screening for cancer of the cervix for women aged 25–60 years and for cancer of the breast for women aged 50–69 years can be regarded as established. Even for these sites, the reduction in cancer mortality that can be expected overall is only of the order of 6% in women. For all other cancer sites, screening must be considered to be experimental. Only when screening for these sites has been fully evaluated will we know whether it could make a more important contribution to reduction in cancer mortality.

References

Andersson I, Aspegren K, Janzon L et al. (1988) Mammographic screening and mortality from breast cancer: the Malmo mammographic screening trial. Br Med J 297:943–948
Baines CJ, Miller AB, Bassett AA (1989) Physical examination. Its role as a single screening modality in the Canadian National Breast Screening Study. Cancer 63:1816–1822
Baines CJ, Miller AB, Kopans DB et al. (1990) Canadian National Breast Screening Study: assessment of technical quality by external review. AJR 155:743–747
Baker L (1982) Breast Cancer Detection Demonstration Project: five-year summary report. CA 32:194–225
Chamberlain J, Day NE, Hakama M, Miller AB, Prorok PC (1986) UICC workshop of the project on evaluation of screening programmes for gastrointestinal cancer. Int J Cancer 37:329–334
Clarke EA, Anderson TW (1979) Does screening by "Pap" smears help prevent cervical cancer? Lancet 2:1–4
Collette HJA, Day NE, Rombach JJ, de Waard F (1984) Evaluation of screening for breast cancer in a non-randomized study (the Dom project) by means of a case-control study. Lancet 1:1224–1226
Day NE, Chamberlain J (1988) Screening for breast cancer: workshop report. Eur J Cancer Clin Oncol 24:55–59
Day NE, Baines CJ, Chamberlain J, Hakama M, Miller AB, Prorok P (1986) UICC project on screening for cancer: report of the workshop on screening for breast cancer. Int J Cancer 38:303–308
Day NE, Walter SD, Tabar L et al. (1988) The sensitivity and lead time of breast cancer screening: a comparison of the results of different studies. In: Day NE, Miller AB (eds) Screening for breast cancer. Huber, Toronto, pp 105–109

Ebeling K, Nischan P (1987) Screening for lung cancer – results from a case-control study. Int J Cancer 40:141–144

Eddy DM, Hasselblad V, McGivney W, Hendee W (1988) The value of mammography screening in women under age 50 years. JAMA 259:1512–1519

Hakama M, Chamberlain J, Day NE et al. (1985) Evaluation of screening programmes for gynaecological cancer. Br J Cancer 52:669–673

Hirayama T, Hisamichi S, Fujimoto I et al. (1985) Screening for gastric cancer. In: Miller AB (ed) Screening for cancer. Academic, Orlando, pp 367–376

IARC Working Group on Cervical Cancer Screening (1986) Summary chapter. IARC Sci Publ 76:133–142

Miller AB (1988) The ethics, the risks and the benefits of screening. Biomed, Pharmacother 42:439–442

Miller AB (1990) Breast cancer screening. Who should be included? J Gen Intern Med 5:S19–S22

Miller AB (1991) Colorectal cancer screening. JNCI 83:1111–1112

Miller AB, Howe GR, Wall C (1981) The National Study of Breast Cancer Screening. Clin Invest Med 4:227–258

Miller AB, Chamberlain J, Day NE, Hakama M, Prorok PC (1990) Report on a workshop of the UICC project on evaluation of screening for cancer. Int J Cancer 46:761–769

Miller AB, Anderson G, Brisson J et al. (1991a) Report of a national workshop on screening for cancer of the cervix. Can Med Assoc J 145:1301–1325

Miller AB, Baines CJ, To T, Wall C (1991b) The Canadian National Breast Screening Study. In: Miller AB et al. (eds) Cancer screening. Cambridge University Press, Cambridge, pp 45–55

Miller AB, Knight J, Narod S (1991c) The natural history of cancer of the cervix, and the implications for screening policy. In: Miller AB et al. (eds) Cancer screening. Cambridge University Press, Cambridge, pp 142–152

Morrison AS, Brisson J, Khalid N (1988) Breast cancer incidence and mortality in the Breast Cancer Detection Demonstration Project. JNCI 80:1540–1547

Newcomb PA, Weiss NS, Storer BE et al. (1991) Breast self-examination in relation to occurrence of advanced breast cancer. JNCI 83:260–265

Oshima A (1988) Screening for stomach cancer: the Japanese program. In: Chamberlain J, Miller AB (eds) Screening for gastrointestinal cancer. Huber, Toronto, pp 65–70

Palli D, del Turco MR, Buiatti E et al. (1986) A case-control study of the efficacy of a non-randomized breast cancer screening program in Florence (Italy). Int J Cancer 38:501–504

Prorok PC, Chamberlain J, Day NE, Hakama M, Miller AB (1984) UICC workshop on the evaluation of screening programmes for cancer. Int J Cancer 34:1–4

Roberts MM, Alexander FE, Anderson TJ et al. (1990) Edinburgh trial of screening for breast cancer: mortality at seven years. Lancet 335:241–246

Rutqvist LE, Miller AB, Andersson I et al. (1990) Reduced breast cancer mortality with mammography screening – an assessment of currently available data. Int J Cancer [Suppl] 5:76–84

Seidman H, Gelb SK, Silverberg E et al. (1987) Survival experience in the Breast Cancer Detection Demonstration Project. CA 37:258–290

Selby JV, Friedman GD, Collen MF (1988) Sigmiodoscopy and mortality from colorectal cancer: the Kaiser Permanente Multiphasic Evaluation Study. J Clin Epidemiol 41:427–434

Shapiro S, Venet W, Strax P, Venet L (1988) Current results of the breast cancer screening randomized trial: the Health Insurance Plan (HIP) of greater New York study. In: Day NE, Miller AB (eds) Screening for breast cancer. Huber, Toronto, pp 3–15

Tabar L, Fagerberg CJG, Gad A et al. (1985) Reduction in mortality from breast cancer after mass screening with mammography. Lancet 1:829–832

Tabar L, Fagerberg G, Duffy SW, Day NE (1989) Recent results from the Swedish two-county trial of mammographic screening for breast cancer. J Epidemiol Community Health 43:107–114

Task Force (1976) Cervical Cancer Screening Programs. Can Med Assoc J 114:1003–1033

Task Force (1982) Cervical Cancer Screening Programs 1982. Health Services and Promotion Branch, Health and Welfare, Ottawa

Warnakulasuriya KAAS, Ekanayake ANI, Sivayoham S et al. (1984) Utilisation of primary health care workers for early detection of oral cancer and precancer cases in Sri Lanka. Bull WHO 62:243–250

Winawer SJ, Schottenfeld D, Flehinger BJ (1991) Colorectal cancer screening. JNCI 83:243–253

Workshop Group (1989) Reducing deaths from breast cancer in Canada. Can Med Assoc J 141:199–201

UK Trial of Early Detection of Breast Cancer Group (1988) First results on mortality reduction in the UK trial of early detection of breast cancer. Lancet 2:412–416

Verbeek ALM, Hendriks JHCL, Holland R et al. (1985) Mammographic screening and breast cancer mortality: age-specific effects in Nijmegen project, 1975–82. Lancet 1:865–886

Summary of Discussion: Session 7

J. Chang-Claude

There were three main points brought up for discussion. With regard to whether screening would be beneficial for women between 40 and 49 years of age at high risk of breast cancer, A.B. Miller indicated that the Canadian data show no evidence of a difference in benefit between high and low risk women. There is a need to balance the lack of benefit and the anxiety caused by screening, and therefore it is not appropriate to disregard the psychological burden of patients being screened. A detailed surveillance of genetic factors should be conducted so that this additional information may be taken into account. Breast cancer may be a malignant disease in which the progression of smaller cancers can occur with variable time lengths. The experience of Canada is to conduct chemotherapy immediately after surgical procedures, and no interval after surgery is recommended.

With regard to the costs involved for management when there is a sizeable false-positive rate, A.B. Miller admitted that there are more false-positives seen in America than in Scandinavia. A detailed cost-benefit analysis is therefore of importance. However, additional biopsies do not affect benefit. The problem is how to show benefit especially for those younger than 50 years of age.

It was reported that the results of HIP showed a benefit for those over 50 years of age after 5–9 years and for those under 50 years of age, a benefit after 10 years. Therefore, in the Canadian trial the observation period may not have been long enough. There may have been undertreatment among young women, since the diagnosis of negative nodal involvement could have included instances of missed lymph nodes. A.B. Miller admitted that the lymph nodes may not have been adequately examined in patients with small cancers. If a benefit were to show for women between 40 and 49 years, this would be first observed in the Swedish trial. Tabar thought that if one waited long enough, this benefit would show. However, screening for breast cancer in women under 50 years as a public health policy has declined in importance as a result of the available evidence. If screening should be conducted among those under 50 years of age, the government will surely be able to show no substantial benefit relative to cost.

Summary of Round Table Discussion on Efficiency of Screening Programs for the Early Detection of Cancer?

G. DHOM and A. LUZ

Participants: K. Ebeling, D. von Fournier, H. Isele, E. Peters, E. Rauterberg, I. Vogt-Moykopf, and J. Wahrendorf

Participants in the round table discussed questions which remain open regarding the efficiency of the strategies of screening for early cancer in the FRG. Two basic viewpoints were represented, that of the general management of public health and that of the improvement of medical management of certain specific neoplastic diseases. The evaluation was based on the use of several criteria at different levels of the analysis.

General Criteria of Efficiency

The participants agreed with the statement of the epidemiologist J. Wahrendorf that recommendations for cancer screening must rely on statistically significant data. The most relevant criterion for efficiency is a decrease in mortality from certain specific neoplasias. The minimum criterion is an increase of cases detected at an early stage of malignancy. The latter includes the aspect of medical treatment of individual patients, since it helps to avoid debilitating treatment procedures. A direct proof of this effect can be derived from data in studies directed by the Humboldt University in Berlin, as K. Ebeling reported. Decisions concerning the application of screening procedures must be based on the criterion of significant efficiency. This should also be the case when counselling individual patients requesting cancer screening. P.E. Peters, a radiologist, remarked that in the case of diagnostic strategies which are not yet well established (ultrasonography, computed tomography, magnetic resonance imaging) screening may contain the danger that patients with false-positive results become subject to further – sometimes distressing – medical procedures.

Evaluation of the efficiency of cancer screening includes evaluation of cost/efficiency. E. Rauterberg from the Federal Ministry of Health commented on this point. She underlined the difficulty in expressing the social aspect of efficiency in numbers. Increases in lifespan could, in most cases, even mean more cost for the public. There is the quite different aspect of improvement in quality of life, which is difficult to measure.

Epidemiology and Screening Strategy

J. Wahrendorf and G. Dhom (pathologist and consultant from the Saarland Cancer Registry) both regretted that neither of the two registries which existed in the FRG at the time when the public cancer screening program was started in 1971 (Saarland and Hamburg) were included in the national cancer screening program. At that time, cancer epidemiology was not well established and not even well recognized. Due to the cancer registry laws existing in Saarland, Hamburg, and Nordrhein-Westfalen, it is difficult to perform longitudinal studies. Wahrendorf reported on one such study in Saarland. The aim was to investigate the effect of screening (haemoccult test) on cancer mortality. Due to the data protection law, personal data from the individual cases in the Saarland cancer registry were not available for this study. In place of these data, Drs. Wahrendorf and Dhom established a much more time-consuming and costly evaluation program. Patients' data are collected by tracing backwards from the pathology database. This should allow the evaluation of the different age cohorts in a cross-sectional study. Both authors appreciate the optimal cooperation of the practicing physicians in this study, but they also stress the necessity of organizing longitudinal evaluation when a new cancer screening program is established in the FRG.

D. von Fournier mentioned that tracing of individual cases whilst protecting the individuality of persons is ensured in the German mammography study which he directs.

K. Ebeling and P.E. Peters stressed that the lowest state of the art in diagnostic techniques – especially in radiology – limits the real efficiency of a screening program. E. Rauterberg explained that details of the diagnostic strategies in the German cancer screening program are the responsibility of the "Bundesausschuß der Ärzte und Krankenkassen" and do not come under the auspices of the Ministry of Health. Cancers at present included in screening are cancer of the uterus, breast cancer, prostate cancer, colorectal cancer, and malignant melanoma.

Compliance

H. Isele, representing physicians in general practice, and E. Rauterberg regretted the relatively low percentage of the German population participating in the cancer screening program offered by the public health service. In 1989, the mean proportion of participants was 34% in women and 13% in men. The age dependence of this percentage differed between the sexes: 40% of 35–39-year-old women participated in cancer screening with a continuous decrease beyond the age of 50 years. In men, the percentage of participants increased from the age of 45 to the age of 60 years, at which time 15% participate. In general, the compliance of women seems to be increasing. H. Isele pointed to the relatively low absolute number of cancers detected by the screening program as a consequence of low compliance (5244 cases out of 7.3 million women and 2452 cases out of 1.3 million men).

H. Isele recommended the development of education programs on cancer prevention which should be included into health education in schools. E. Rauterberg proposed education programs for the general population more directly designed to encourage participation in the screening for specific neoplastic diseases. A study organized by the "Zentralinstitut für die Kassenärztliche Versorgung" is intended to investigate details of the motivation of people participating in the cancer screening program. Some minor problems with regard to the data protection law have inhibited the start of the study, but these problems should be solved in the near future.

Screening for Specific Neoplastic Diseases

Cervical Cancer

This is the most successful example of cancer screening. About two-thirds of cervical cancer cases could probably be prevented by this strategy, and in many positive cases the early stage at detection of the disease allows preservation of the uterus (D. von Fournier). G. Dhom reported the data from the Saarland cancer registry where the incidence has decreased by about 60%. The lack of further decrease might be due to the low participation of older women in the screening program. Mortality from cervical cancer decreased by about one-half from 1970 to 1983. The incidence was originally higher in urban and industrial populations as compared with rural areas and is now very similar in both areas.

The occurrence of cervical cancer within a short space of time after the last screening has sometimes been explained as cancer development in a single act (G. Dhom). K. Ebeling and D. von Fournier stressed that in most cases retrospective studies revealed failure of the cytologic diagnosis in the previous screening. This failure was related to both the sampling technique and the microscopic screening. The latter is complicated by the factor of fatigue (there are only about 6 positive cases per 1000 first round cases tested and 2 positive cases per 100 second round cases tested!). In addition, there is the problem of cancer developing beneath the intact epithelium or within the cervical glands, with a low chance of shedding cells into the vaginal lumen. Detection of these cases might be especially low when there are long screening intervals.

Mammary Cancer

D. von Fournier (who is a member of the German mammography study which is organized by Dr. Robra, Department of Epidemiology, Hannover Medical School, is financed by the Ministry of Research and Technology, and has centers in Esslingen, Hamburg, Heidelberg, and Cologne) reported that there are already promising results with respect to the detection of breast cancer by mammography. Particularly near Heidelberg (with a high degree of compliance) more than 60% of the positive cases could be treated surgically with preservation of the breast.

D. von Fournier pointed to results in the literature. A 20%–30% decrease in mortality was reported in studies performed in Sweden and The Netherlands.

Mammography is even able to detect nonpalpable cancers. In the USA more than 20% of the cases detected belong to the group of carcinoma in situ, which can probably be cured. The quality of mammography in hospitals away from the mammography centers will be supported by including several of them into the framework of the German mammography study. (This includes training courses once a year and control of selected X-radiographs by a central reference center.) H. Isele mentioned the problem of low compliance due to the painful breast compression during mammography. According to the experience of D. von Fournier, this problem might be solved by the new generation of mammography equipment which automatically limits the pressure to minimal values. In addition, the date of the investigation should be related to the cyclic changes in the breast, i.e., investigation is best about 1 week after menstruation.

The cost for a routine mammography (4 photographs) is DM 63, while an additional photograph in an oblique direction costs DM 34–41.

E. Rauterberg told participants that after a final positive evaluation of the German mammography study (after the end of 1991), mammography is likely to become part of the cancer screening program in 1992/1993.

Colorectal Cancer

G. Dhom pointed out that the digital rectal examination is not as successful in detecting early cancer as described in older textbooks. H. Isele assumed from personal experience that the efficiency of the screening program must be low, since no case of colon cancer had been diagnosed in his practice by the methods applied. He thought that repeated application (2–3 times) of the "haemoccult test" (he quoted a local study) and immunological techniques for blood assay might be more successful in detecting early colon cancer than the single test applied up to now. He claimed that the gynecologist often omitted the digital rectal examination in female genital cancer screening, as patients had told him. In addition, he stressed the danger of false-positive findings in patients undergoing aspirin treatment, which often seemed to be overlooked.

J. Wahrendorf explained that the haemoccult test was introduced in 1977 (with the idea of improving the screening) after the original screening started in 1971 with only digital examination. At present, there is no proof of the efficiency of the method. Wahrendorf and Dhom have started a case control study in the Saarland cancer registry which is still under way.

Prostate Cancer

The practising physician H. Isele has only detected one case, with a small cancer of the prostate gland, during the entire period of the screening program.

G. Dhom (quoting literature data and the report by A.B. Miller during this meeting) underlined the lack of benefit of screening for early prostate cancer. This is also the experience of the Humboldt University as K. Ebeling demonstrated. One out of three men aged 45 years or more, and every second man aged 70 years, may have latent prostate cancer. On the one hand, it is known that a high percentage of these cancers will never become life-threatening (as a Swedish urologist described it, these cancers are like accompanying dogs). On the other hand, experience shows that cancer of the prostate holds the second place in the order of frequency of cancer deaths in males. The problem is that prostate cancer cannot at present be classified correctly according to its biological behaviour, and only about 60% of palpable nodular changes are histological cancer. In addition, there is a considerable danger of overtreatment. (But there is no scientific basis for the claims of Hackethal in newspapers and magazines that surgical treatment might stimulate the progression of small cancers.)

Testicular Cancer

H. Isele has detected four cases of testicular cancer in his general practice. Three of these patients were 18–23 years old. Only one case complained of physical symptoms. H. Isele would like to recommend an earlier age for the start of screening for testicular cancer. Based on the data of the Saarland cancer registry E. Rauterberg calculated that there are about 1900 new cases of testicular cancer per year (as related to the population of the former West Germany). An earlier start to testicular cancer screening is under consideration. With regard to the screening methods, P.E. Peters recommended a controlled study using ultrasonography in addition to physical examination. The results gained with this method are promising, but there is as yet no exact proof of its usefulness. G. Dhom proposed a pilot study with ultrasonography during the investigation of the health status of young men prior to military service. According to the experience of P.E. Peters, magnetic resonance imaging might be of additional help in individual cases. It was possible to detect testicular cancers of 3–4 mm diameter in the contralateral testis of cases with cancer at one site by this method (see also the report by P.E. Peters during this meeting).

Malignant Melanoma

E. Rauterberg stressed the frequency of malignant melanoma. There are about 6000 new cases (equal numbers of men and women) per year (again related to the population of the former West Germany). H. Isele experienced an increase in requests by patients for skin cancer screening in general practice, clearly as a consequence of information to the public.

Lung Cancer

At present, there seems to be no efficient strategy for early detection of lung cancer. Considering the frequency of this lesion, this is clearly a challenging problem and induced a very lively discussion.

I. Vogt-Moykopf mentioned the former X-radiography screening for pulmonary tuberculosis, which has been cancelled. About 15–20 peripheral lung cancers were detected per 10000 X-radiographs. This type of lung cancer has a fair chance of being cured. However, I. Vogt-Moykopf conceded that according to epidemiological experience X-radiography and sputum cytology were not successful in detecting early lung cancer by mass screening of the general population. As K. Ebeling stressed, even the stricter X-radiography screening and registration performed in the former East Germany did not lead to a decrease in lung cancer mortality. There was not even a demonstrable decrease in debilitating surgery. P.E. Peters quoted a study by the Mayo Clinic with X-radiography and cytology examination every 4 months which found no improvement in the early diagnosis of lung cancer.

Nevertheless, I. Vogt-Moykopf discussed in detail whether there might be any chance – at least for the sick patient – to improve life expectancy. He pointed out that there could still be some gap in the diagnostic strategy for lung cancer. According to his experience, the delay in the diagnosis by the symptomatic patient himself and by his physician might together be about 12 months. This does not seem to have changed in recent years. The technique of diagnostic X-radiography is probably not performed with the same efficiency by all practitioners (especially in the detecting of indirect signs of bronchial cancer) and demands a better training of physicians in radiology of the chest. The former X-radiography screening was also done with less well experienced physicians. I. Vogt-Moykopf assumed that it would be useful to study persons at high risk, i.e., heavy smokers. He proposed X-radiography study twice a year for these persons and, in the case of negative results but symptomatic patients, further detailed diagnostic procedures. This might at least lead to a diagnosis at an earlier stage and could also decrease the costs of the disease. A fair chance – as mentioned above – might be given for successful treatment of the 20% of cancers located in the peripheral part of the lung. The increase of 5-year survival from 5% to 11%, observed by I. Vogt-Moykopf during the past few years, might offer some hope. There was no general acceptance of the proposal for limited screening made by I. Vogt-Moykopf, again because of experience with the studies performed up to now. In addition, D. von Fournier raised the ethical question of giving public financial support to people who decided to undertake an enjoyment well-known to be dangerous.

K. Ebeling claimed that the challenge of the sick patient should result in recommendations to the public to stop smoking. Possibly, people could also be made more sensitive to the early symptoms of lung cancer.

According to the experience of I. Vogt-Moykopf, medical diagnostics could be more sensitive for the early signs of lung cancer.

Future Screening

E. Rauterberg explained that – despite some skepticism with regard to particular neoplasms – there seemed to be no strong reason for reducing the present screening program. E. Rauterberg underlined that the Ministry of Health does not itself decide which neoplasms are selected for screening. However, studies analyzing the efficiency of screening programs are supported by the Ministry of Health in cooperation with the Ministry of Employment and the Ministry of Research and Technology. New plans are under consideration with regard to the starting age for screening for genital cancer in women (20 years), for breast cancer in women (30 years), for colon cancer and skin cancer (45 years). The screening intervals (in every case annual? for mammography, probably about 2 years) are the subject of discussion. There is some consideration of the possibility of more direct integration of screening programs into the general cancer treatment program.

With regard to other neoplasms which should be screened, the division of the Ministry of Health which is responsible (and which was also responsible when still a part of the Ministry of Employment) has initiated a study by the Institute for Health Research in Kiel. This study is considering cancer of the upper alimentary and respiratory tract, stomach cancer, lung cancer, and cancer of the lower urinary tract as possible topics for future screening programs. As mentioned above, this study is also considering an earlier start for the screening of testicular cancer.

Subject Index

Printing: Druckerei Zechner, Speyer
Binding: Buchbinderei Schäffer, Grünstadt